WILLIAM HARVEY LIBRARY

This book is due for return on or before the last date shown below
28 DAY LOAN

2016

WITHDRAWN

Oxford Specialist Handbooks

General Oxford Specialist Handbooks

A Resuscitation Room Guide
Addiction Medicine
Day Case Surgery
Perioperative Medicine, 2e
Postoperative Complications, 2e
Renal Transplantation

Oxford Specialist Handbooks in Anaesthesia

Anaesthesia for Medical and Surgical Emergencies
Cardiac Anaesthesia
Neuroanaethesia
Obstetric Anaesthesia
Ophthalmic Anaesthesia
Paediatric Anaesthesia
Regional Anaesthesia, Stimulation and Ultrasound Techniques
Thoracic Anaesthesia

Oxford Specialist Handbooks in Cardiology

Adult Congenital Heart Disease
Cardiac Catheterization and Coronary Intervention
Cardiac Electrophysiology and Catheter Ablation
Cardiovascular Computed Tomography
Cardiovascular Magnetic Resonance
Echocardiography, 2e
Fetal Cardiology
Heart Failure
Hypertension
Inherited Cardiac Disease
Nuclear Cardiology
Pacemakers and ICDs
Pulmonary Hypertension
Valvular Heart Disease

Oxford Specialist Handbooks in Critical Care

Advanced Respiratory Critical Care

Oxford Specialist Handbooks in End of Life Care

End of Life Care in Cardiology
End of Life Care in Dementia
End of Life Care in Nephrology
End of Life Care in Respiratory Disease
End of Life in the Intensive Care Unit

Oxford Specialist Handbooks in Neurology

Epilepsy
Parkinson's Disease and Other Movement Disorders
Stroke Medicine

Oxford Specialist Handbooks in Paediatrics

Paediatric Dermatology
Paediatric Endocrinology and Diabetes
Paediatric Gastroenterology, Hepatology, and Nutrition
Paediatric Haematology and Oncology
Paediatric Intensive Care
Paediatric Nephrology, 2e
Paediatric Neurology, 2e
Paediatric Radiology
Paediatric Respiratory Medicine
Paediatric Rheumatology

Oxford Specialist Handbooks in Pain Medicine

Spinal Interventions in Pain Management

Oxford Specialist Handbooks in Psychiatry

Child and Adolescent Psychiatry
Forensic Psychiatry
Old Age Psychiatry

Oxford Specialist Handbooks in Radiology

Interventional Radiology
Musculoskeletal Imaging
Pulmonary Imaging
Thoracic Imaging

Oxford Specialist Handbooks in Surgery

Cardiothoracic Surgery
Colorectal Surgery
Hand Surgery
Hepatopancreatobiliary Surgery
Neurosurgery
Operative Surgery, 2e
Oral Maxillofacial Surgery
Otolaryngology and Head and Neck Surgery
Paediatric Surgery
Plastic and Reconstructive Surgery
Surgical Oncology
Urological Surgery
Vascular Surgery

Oxford Specialist Handbooks in Cardiology

Echocardiography

Second edition

Edited by

Paul Leeson

Consultant Cardiologist and BHF Senior Fellow
John Radcliffe Hospital
and University of Oxford, UK

Daniel Augustine

Specialist Trainee in Cardiology &
Cardiovascular Research Fellow
John Radcliffe Hospital
and University of Oxford, UK

Andrew R.J. Mitchell

Consultant Cardiologist
General Hospital, St Helier,
Jersey, Channel Islands, UK

Harald Becher

Professor of Medicine
Mazankowski Alberta Heart Institute,
University of Alberta, Edmonton, Canada

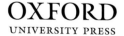

OXFORD
UNIVERSITY PRESS

OXFORD
UNIVERSITY PRESS

Great Clarendon Street, Oxford OX2 6DP,
United Kingdom

Oxford University Press is a department of the University of Oxford.
It furthers the University's objective of excellence in research, scholarship,
and education by publishing worldwide. Oxford is a registered trade mark of
Oxford University Press in the UK and in certain other countries

British Library Cataloguing in Publication Data

Data available

Library of Congress Cataloging in Publication Data

Data available

ISBN 978–0–19–959179–4

Printed in Great Britain by

Ashford Colour Press Ltd, Gosport, Hants

Preface to the second edition

Over the last five years echocardiography as a specialty has evolved dramatically. When the first edition of this book was published, people were still exploring the potential for clinical uses of 3D echocardiography, new echocardiography-guided transcatheter interventions were being evaluated, and routine use of echocardiography in the intensive care and emergency departments was being considered. All of these developments are now sufficiently established in day-to-day clinical practice to warrant inclusion in this essential handbook-guide on how to perform echocardiography.

Importantly, all the basics still form the bulk of the new handbook, so that even the complete novice can pick up the text and start to learn how to acquire good quality images and interpret what they see. These sections have now been enhanced with colour images and video loops as well as having been reviewed to ensure the information is consistent with numerous new guidelines released by international echocardiography societies.

We are delighted with the success and widespread appeal of this handbook. When we wrote the first edition, however, we did not expect to have to update so much, so soon. This is a reflection of how rapidly echocardiography as a specialty develops and has allowed us to produce an even better echocardiography handbook. We hope you enjoy it.

PL
DA
ARJM
HB
2012

Preface to the first edition

Why another book on echocardiography? There are numerous textbooks, some with excellent descriptions, accompanied by images of normal and abnormal findings.

This handbook originates from the demands of our trainees and sonographers for a new approach based on practical guidelines that describe how to apply current imaging technology to address the common, key issues in adult echocardiography. The book follows the natural workflow of echocardiography, detailing what to record, and how to analyse and report studies. These demands have also been heard by the professional organizations like the British and American Society of Echocardiography and the European Association of Echocardiography who have started to provide guidelines for specific questions. Therefore this handbook combines the standard acquisition protocols, analysis and reporting for adult transthoracic and transoesophageal echocardiography, starting from a minimal recording dataset, with all the current guidelines relevant to clinical practice.

The book was designed as a comprehensive compendium of focused approaches for specific clinical questions. We hope it will be used both as a means to learn how to perform echocardiography and as a trusted, easily accessible reference for those who are already proficient.

PL
AM
HB

Contents

Acknowledgements

We would like to express our sincere thanks to the many individuals who read the text during its preparation and gave advice on its development.

Contributors

We would like to express our sincere thanks to the contributors to the original edition and the following people for their expert contributions and advice that were used as the basis for the following sections in the new edition (in alphabetical order):

Harald Becher
Professor of Cardiology,
Mazankowski Alberta Heart
Institute,
University of Alberta, Edmonton,
Canada
*Chapters 4 and 7: 3D left
ventricular and right ventricular
function*
*Chapter 9: Contrast
echocardiography*

Will Bradlow
Specialist Trainee in Cardiology,
John Radcliffe Hospital, Oxford,
UK
*Chapters 4 and 7: 2D right
ventricular function*

John Chambers
Consultant Cardiologist,
Cardiothoracic Centre, Guy's and
St. Thomas' Hospital, London, UK
Chapter 3: Aortic stenosis

Jonathan Choy
Cardiologist & University of
Alberta Echo Lab Director,
University of Alberta, Edmonton,
Canada
*Chapter 4: 3D left ventricular
function*

Claire Colebourn
Consultant Intensivist, Programme
Lead Oxford Critical Care Echo
Fellowship, John Radcliffe Hospital,
Oxford, UK
Chapter 11: Acute echocardiography

Jonathan Goldman
Consultant Cardiologist, VA
Hospital, San Francisco, CA, USA
Chapter 4: Left atrial measures

Lucy Hudsmith
Consultant Cardiologist in Adult
Congenital Heart Disease,
The Queen Elizabeth Hospital,
Birmingham, UK
*Chapters 3, 4, 6, and 7: Tricuspid
valve, Pulmonary valve, and
Congenital heart disease*

Xu Yu Jin
Consultant in Surgical Echo-Cardi-
ology, John Radcliffe Hospital,
Oxford, UK
*Chapter 5: Intraoperative
transoesophageal echocardiography*

Theodoros Karamitsos
Honorary Consultant Cardiologist
and University
Research Lecturer,
John Radcliffe Hospital and
University of Oxford, UK
*Chapter 10: Stress
echocardiography*

Justin Mandeville
Senior Critical Care Echo Fellow,
John Radcliffe Hospital,
Oxford, UK
Chapter 11: Acute echocardiography

Thomas Marwick
Director, Center for
Cardiovascular Imaging, Heart and
Vascular Institute, Cleveland
Clinic, Cleveland, OH, USA
Chapter 4: Left ventricular function

Andrew R.J. Mitchell
Consultant Cardiologist,
General Hospital, St. Helier,
Jersey, Channel Islands, UK
*Chapter 8: Intracardiac
echocardiography*

Saul Myerson
Consultant Cardiologist, John
Radcliffe Hospital, Honorary
Senior Clinical Lecturer, University
of Oxford, UK
*Chapters 3 and 6: Aortic
regurgitation*

Jim Newton
Consultant Cardiologist, John
Radcliffe Hospital, Oxford, UK
*Chapters 3 and 6: 3D TOE
prosthetic valvular assessment and
Transcatheter aortic valve
implantation*

Steffen Petersen
Honorary Consultant Cardiologist,
Centre Lead for Advanced
Cardiovascular Imaging, Barts and
The London NIHR Biomedical
Research Unit, The London Chest
Hospital, London, UK
Chapter 4: Cardiomyopathies

Susanna Price
Consultant Cardiologist and
Intensivist, Royal Brompton &
Harefield NHS Foundation Trust,
London, UK
Chapter 6: MitraClip®

Oliver Rider
Clinical Lecturer Cardiovascular
Medicine, John Radcliffe Hospital,
Oxford, UK
Chapter 1: Ultrasound

Michael Stewart
Consultant Cardiologist,
Cardiothoracic Unit, The James
Cook University Hospital,
Middlesborough, UK
Chapters 4 and 7: Aorta

Jon Timperley
Consultant Cardiologist,
Northampton General Hospital,
Northampton, UK
*Chapters 3 and 6: Mitral stenosis
and mitral regurgitation*

James Willis
Research Cardiac Physiologist,
Royal United Hospital, Bath, and
University of Bath, UK
DVD

This new edition was compiled and revised by Paul Leeson and Daniel
Augustine. The text was illustrated by Paul Leeson and Daniel Augustine.
Paul Leeson, Daniel Augustine, Andrew Mitchell, and Harald Becher edited
the final version.

Symbols and abbreviations

📖	cross-reference
~	approximately
2D	two-dimensional
3D	three-dimensional
A	A-wave velocity
A4C	apical 4-chamber
Ao	aorta
AR	aortic regurgitation
AS	aortic stenosis
ASD	atrial septal defect
AV	aortic valve
BSA	body surface area
CFM	colour flow mapping
CHD	congenital heart disease
CMR	cardiovascular magnetic resonance
CO	cardiac output
CRT	cardiac resynchronization therapy
CSA	cross-sectional area
CT	computed tomography
CW	continuous wave (Doppler)
d	diastole
DET	deceleration time
E	E-wave velocity
ECG	electrocardiogram
ed	end-diastole
EF	ejection fraction
EROA	effective regurgitant orifice area
HFNEF	heart failure with a normal ejection fraction
Hz	hertz
ICE	intracardiac echocardiography
IVC	inferior vena cava
IVRT	isovolumetric relaxation time
JVP	jugular venous pressure
LA	left atrium
LLPV	left lower pulmonary vein
LUPV	left upper pulmonary vein

LV	left ventricle
LVID	left ventricular internal diameter
LVOT	left ventricular outflow tract
LVPW	left ventricular posterior wall
LVS	left ventricular septum
MHz	megahertz
MPR	multiplanar reformatting
MR	mitral regurgitation
MS	mitral stenosis
MV	mitral valve
MVA	mitral valve area
PA	pulmonary artery
PDA	patent ductus arteriosus
PFO	patent foramen ovale
PISA	proximal isovelocity surface area
PLAX	parasternal long axis view
PR	pulmonary regurgitation
PRF	pulse repetition frequency
PS	pulmonary stenosis
PSAX	parasternal short axis view
PV	pulmonary valve
PW	pulse wave (Doppler)
RA	right atrium
RLPV	right lower pulmonary vein
RUPV	right upper pulmonary vein
RV	right ventricle
RVOT	right ventricular outflow tract
s	systole
SAX	short axis
SV	stroke volume
SVC	superior vena cava
TAVI	transcatheter aortic valve implantation
TGC	time-gain compensation
TOE	transoesophageal echocardiography
TR	tricuspid regurgitation
TTE	transthoracic echocardiography
TV	tricuspid valve
V	volt/s
VSD	ventricular septal defect
vti	velocity time integral

References

Reference Textbooks (alphabetical order)

Feigenbaum H (2004). *Echocardiography* 6th edition. Philadelphia, PA: Lippincott, Williams & Wilkins.

Galiuto L, Badano L, Fox K, Sicari R, Zamorano J (2011). *The EAE Textbook of Echocardiography*. Oxford: Oxford University Press.

Otto CM (2004). *Textbook of Clinical Echocardiography*, 3rd edition. WB Saunders and Co Ltd.

Perrino AC, Reeves ST (2007). *A Practical Approach to Transesophageal Echocardiography* 2nd edition. Philadelphia, PA: Lippincott, Williams & Wilkins.

Rimmington H, Chambers J (2007). *Echocardiography: Guidelines for Reporting—A Practical Handbook*, 2nd edition. New York: Informa Healthcare.

Sidebotham D, Merry A, Legget M, Bashein G (2003). *Practical Perioperative Transoesophageal Echocardiography*. Philadelphia, PA: Butterworth-Heinemann Ltd.

Zamorano J, Bax J, Rademakers F, Knuuti F (2009). *The ESC Textbook of Cadiovascular Imaging*. Boston, MA: Springer.

Websites

- American Heart Association ℘ http://www.americanheart.org
- American Society of Echocardiography ℘ http://www.asecho.org
- British Cardiovascular Society ℘ http://www.bcs.com
- British Heart Foundation ℘ http://www.bhf.org.uk
- British Society of Echocardiography ℘ http://www.bsecho.org
- European Association of Echocardiography ℘ http://www.escardio.org/bodies/associations/EAE
- European Society of Cardiology ℘ http://www.escardio.org

Papers and guidelines

Lancellotti P, Tribouilloy C, Hagendorff A, et al. European Association of Echocardiography recommendations for the assessment of valvular regurgitation. Part 1: aortic and pulmonary regurgitation (native valve disease). *European Journal of Echocardiography* 2010; **11**:223–44.

Rudski L, Lai W, Afilalo J, et al. Guidelines for the echocardiographic assessment of the right heart in adults: a report from the American Society of Echocardiography endorsed by the European Association of Echocardiography. *J Am Soc Echocardiogr* 2010; **23**:685–713.

Aune E, Baekkevar M, Rodevand O, *et al.* Reference values for left ventricular volumes with real time 3 dimensional echocardiography. *Scandinavian Cardiovascular Journal* 2010; **44**:24–30.

Horton K, Meece R, Hill J. Assessment of the right ventricle by echocardiography: a primer for cardiac sonographers. *J Am Soc Echocardiogr* 2009; **7**:776–92.

Saito K, Okura H, Watanabe N, *et al.* Comprehensive evaluation of left ventricular strain using speckle tracking echocardiography in normal adults: comparison of three dimensional and two dimensional approaches. *J Am Soc Echocardiogr* 2009; **22**(9):1025–30.

Recommendations for evaluation of the severity of native valvular regurgitation with two-dimensional and Doppler echocardiography. A report from the American Society of Echocardiography's Nomenclature and Standards Committee and The Task Force on Valvular Regurgitation, developed in conjunction with the American College of Cardiology Echocardiography Committee, The Cardiac Imaging Committee Council on Clinical Cardiology, the American Heart Association, and the European Society of Cardiology Working Group on Echocardiography. *J Am Soc Echocardiogr* 2003; **16**:777–802.

Recommendations for chamber quantification: a report of the American Society of Echocardiography Guidelines and Standards Committee and the Chamber Quantification Writing Group, developed in conjunction with the European Association of Echocardiography. *J Am Soc Echocardiogr* 2005; **18**:1440–63.

Waggoner AD, Ehler D, Adams D, *et al.* Guidelines for the cardiac sonographer in the performance of contrast echocardiography: recommendations of the American Society of Echocardiography. *J Am Soc Echocardiogr* 2001; **14**:417–20.

Masani N, Chambers J, Hancock J, *et al. BSE Echocardiogram Report: Recommendations for Standard Adult Transthoracic Echocardiography.* From the British Society of Echocardiography Education Committee.

Becher H, Chambers J, Fox K, *et al.* British Society of Echocardiography Policy Committee. BSE procedure guidelines for the clinical application of stress echocardiography, recommendations for performance and interpretation of stress echocardiography: a report of the British Society of Echocardiography Policy Committee. *Heart* 2004; **90**(Suppl 6):vi23–30.

Chapter 1

Ultrasound

Introduction

Echocardiography is a non-invasive method for imaging the living heart.
- It is based on detection of echoes produced by a beam of ultrasound pulses transmitted into the heart. A working knowledge of the principles and basic concepts of ultrasound imaging is fundamental to understanding clinical applications and is necessary for accreditation examinations.
- Understanding the limitations both of fundamental physics and current technology can ensure image acquisition is performed in a way that drastically reduces image distortion and artefacts. This will reduce the chance of misdiagnoses.
- An understanding of the concepts behind how images are generated helps the operator to optimize, interpret, and analyse images.
- This chapter is aimed at a basic review of the fundamental principles of echocardiography that will help the clinician get the most out of, and understand the limitations of the technique.

Sound waves and ultrasound

Sound waves are often simplified to a description in terms of sinusoidal waves which are characterized by the properties (Fig. 1.1):
- The frequency (f, number of cycles per second).
- The wavelength (λ, the distance between two identical points on adjacent cycles).
- The velocity (v, the direction *and* speed of travel).

The relationship between these properties is described by the formula:

$$V = f\lambda$$

- In soft body tissues pressure waves travel at about 1500m/s (compared with 300m/s in air).
- Thus, in soft body tissues, at a frequency of 1000Hz (= Hertz, or cycles per second), the wavelength is 1.5m. Common-sense dictates that this wavelength is too great to image the heart, which is only about 15cm across and which contains structures less than 1mm thick. To achieve a wavelength of 1mm, the frequency has to be 1,500,000 Hz, or 1.5 MHz.
- The human ear responds only to frequencies from about 30 Hz to 15,000 Hz, and since the word *sound* implies a sensation generated in the brain, the term, *ultrasound* is used to describe the much higher frequencies used in echocardiography.

Compression waves

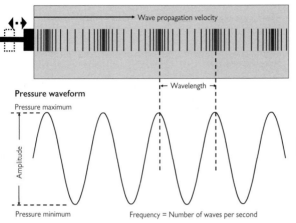

Fig. 1.1 Features of a wave.

Velocity of ultrasound in various tissues

- Bone: 2–4000m/s
- Blood: 1570 m/s
- Heart: 1540 m/s
- Water: 1520 m/s
- Fat: 1450 m/s
- Air: 300 m/s.

Calculating wavelength from frequency and velocity

Example: For a 3.5MHz echocardiography transducer:

$$V = f\lambda,$$

$$1540 = 3,500,000 \times \lambda$$

$$\lambda = 0.44mm$$

Transthoracic transducers

- The transducer (or 'probe') held on the patient's chest transmits high-frequency ultrasound waves into the thorax and detects echoes returning from the heart and great vessels (Figs. 1.2 and 1.3).
- The transducer contains a layer of piezoelectric crystals which have several properties:
  - They are able to generate and receive ultrasound waves.
  - When a current is applied the crystal expands and compresses which generates the ultrasound wave.
  - When an ultrasound wave strikes the piezoelectric crystal an electric current is generated.
- The transducer emits and then switches into receiving mode. The repetition of this cycle allows the scanner to build an ultrasound image.
- The velocity of these high-frequency sound waves generated by the transducer depends on the physical properties of the tissues through which it is travelling.
- Transducers for echocardiography typically generate frequencies in the range 1.5–7MHz.
- Denser tissues allow faster propagation. Thus, in softer body tissues like the heart, the waves travel slower (1540m/s) than in harder tissues like bone (2000–4000m/s).

Stand-alone probe

The stand-alone continuous wave (CW) Doppler probe comprises a single transmit element and a single receive element. The probe is considered to provide more accurate estimation of transaortic velocities (Fig. 1.4).

3D matrix array transducers

- Matrix array transducers (Figs. 1.2 and 1.3) are used to generate 3D pyramidal volumes in live real time (approximately 30° × 60° in size) or full volume datasets which are not in real time (approximately 100° × 104° in size).
- The transducer uses 3000–4000 elements arrayed in a 2D phase.

Differences between cardiac and vascular transducers?

- Vascular ultrasound uses linear array transducers as it is designed to image linear structures—blood vessels. The elements are aligned along an axis enabling the beam to be moved, focused, and deflected along a plane.
- As the objects of interest are closer to the probe, higher frequencies can be used for vascular imaging.
- 3D imaging using a matrix array probe is possible. Vascular 3D imaging tends to be based on scanning the artery and creating a 3D reconstruction from a series of 2D images.
- Cardiac transducers tend to have a curved array of elements to image a volume.

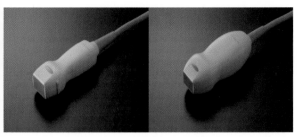

Fig. 1.2 Left: Toshiba 30BT phased array sector 2D probe. Right: Toshiba 25SX matrix sector 3D probe. Images courtesy of Toshiba medical systems, Europe.

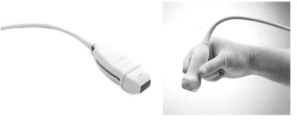

Fig. 1.3 Left: Phillips 3D X3-1 Probe. Right: Phillips X5-1 probe (2D/3D). Images courtesy of Phillips Healthcare UK.

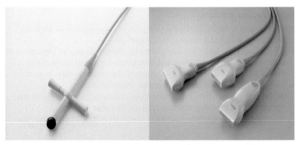

Fig. 1.4 Left: Toshiba PC20M stand alone probe. Right: Toshiba Vascular Probes. Images courtesy of Toshiba Medical Systems, Europe.

Transoesophageal transducers

- The probe (Fig. 1.5) is similar in construction to a gastroscope, but in place of the fibre-optic bundle used for light imaging, a miniature ultrasound transducer is mounted at its tip.
- The plane of the transducer array can be rotated by the operator to provide image planes that correspond to the orthogonal axes of the heart despite the fact that these are not naturally aligned with the axis of the oesophagus.
- Precautions have to be taken to prevent accidental harm to the patient through heating and the potential for it to apply 150V electrical impulses to the back of the heart requires it to be checked regularly to ensure integrity of the electrical insulation.

2D imaging from a transducer positioned in the oesophagus has advantages:
- There is no attenuation from the chest wall.
- It can operate at higher frequencies (up to 7.5MHz), improving image quality.

3D transoesophageal imaging is increasingly being used, e.g. analysis of valvular structure and to guide interventional procedures:
- The most recent 3D transoesophageal echocardiography (TOE) probes utilize fully sampled matrix array transducers to allow real-time 3D imaging.
- A 2–7MHz transducer incorporates 2500 elements that allow acquisition of a pyramidal 3D data set.

Other transducers

Intracardiac probes

- Intracardiac echocardiography (ICE) allows visualization of cardiac structures within the heart (see Chapter 8).
- ICE probes (Fig. 1.6) have been used for almost 30 years. They provide improved resolution imaging but due to the high frequency of the transducers (20–40MHz), penetration of the earlier probes was poor.
- The latest ICE probes have improved characteristics:
  - Linear phased array and lower multifrequency range (5–10MHz).
  - Capability of both pulsed and colour Doppler imaging.
  - Improved manipulation with the use of multidirectional steerable devices.
  - A steering lock to maintain catheter angulation.

Intravascular ultrasound probes

- High frequency intravascular transducers (30–40MHz) allow imaging from within the coronary arteries.
- The probe positioned in the lumen of the artery emits ultrasound waves which penetrate into the vascular wall. Reflections are created at interfaces between tissue components of different acoustic properties (e.g. plaque, calcification and thrombus).
- High-resolution cross-sectional images are produced allowing measurement of luminal diameter and characterization of the vessel wall.

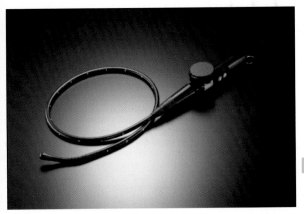

Fig. 1.5 Toshiba TEE 512 transoesophageal probe. Image courtesy of Toshiba Medical Systems, Europe.

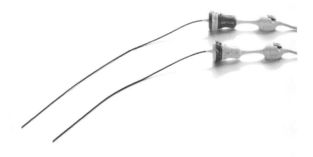

Fig. 1.6 AcuNav intracardiac echocardiography catheters. Image courtesy of Biosense Webster, Inc.

Echocardiography modes (Figs. 1.7, 1.8)

- Modern echocardiography machines use arrays of crystals which send out several ultrasound waves across the sector of view.
- Each line of reflected ultrasound waves is then collated to produce an image of the heart.
- Returning echoes strike the piezoelectric crystals, first from structures closest to the transducer, followed in succession by those from more distant interfaces.
- The minute electrical signals generated are amplified and processed to form a visual display showing the relative distances of reflecting structures from the transducer, with the signal intensities providing some information about the nature of the interfaces.
- Repeating this sweep of ultrasound waves across the sector multiple times per second allows a moving image to be produced. Hence the spatial resolution of the image is determined by the distance between scan lines and number of scan lines per sector; the temporal resolution is determined by the number of sweeps across the sector per second (frame rate).

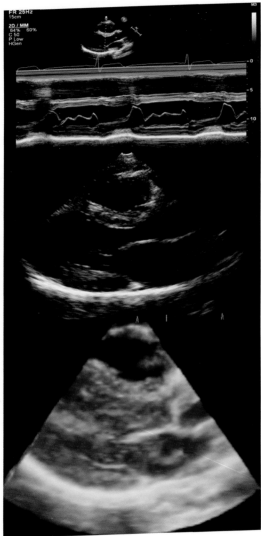

Fig. 1.7 Example of M-mode through mitral valve. M-mode images show structures intersected by a stationary ultrasound beam.

A (amplitude)-mode echocardiography

- The oldest type of ultrasound generation was created using A-mode echocardiography. Here, the amplitude of the reflected ultrasound wave is plotted against the distance from which the reflection originates (not in clinical use).

B (brightness)-mode echocardiography

- In B-mode imaging the amplitude of the reflected ultrasound wave is recorded by the brightness (intensity) of a dot (not in clinical use).

M (motion)-mode echocardiography

- The reflection of the ultrasound signals are recorded and displayed as monochromic dots over time (Fig. 1.8).
- The direction of the ultrasound beam is fixed, and interrogates structures along a single axis over time, allowing a very high temporal resolution when compared to 2D techniques (1000 lines/second compared to 25 lines/second for a 2D image).

2D echocardiography

- Transducer technology allows the ultrasound beam to be scanned rapidly across the heart to produce 2D tomographic images.

3D echocardiography

- The latest transducers are able to instantly acquire the image contained in a pyramidal volume enabling the generation of a 3D data set.

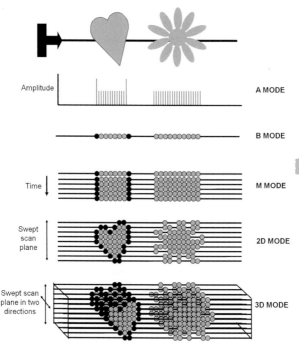

Fig. 1.8 Types of image: A (amplitude)-mode traces amplitude of a reflection against distance from probe (of historical interest as one of the first type of ultrasound image). B (brightness)-mode represents amplitude as intensity or brightness of a dot. M (motion)-mode traces change in brightness over time. 2D images are generated from sweeping across the field of interest.

Behaviour of ultrasound in tissue

- When ultrasound waves pass through tissue they undergo *reflection*, *refraction* or *scattering* (Fig. 1.9).

Reflection

- As ultrasound waves pass through the chest towards the heart they encounter several interfaces between different body tissues, e.g. pericardium and myocardium.
- Some of the incident energy is reflected at these interfaces as they act like a mirror, in the same way as light bounces back off a shiny surface.
- Reflected sound waves are termed 'echoes', and having undergone 'specular' (mirror-like) reflection they are termed 'specular echoes'.
- The reflected 'echoes' are transmitted back to the transducer and vibrate the piezoelectric crystals to form a signal from an electrical signal, from which a picture of the heart can be built.
- The minute electrical signals generated are amplified and processed to form a visual display showing the relative distances of reflecting structures from the transducer, with the signal intensities providing some information about the nature of the interfaces.

Refraction

- Refraction is the change in direction of a wave due to a change in its speed. This is most commonly observed when a wave passes from one medium to another at any angle other than 90° or 0°.
- Refraction of light is the most commonly observed phenomenon, (e.g. the apparent bending of the angle of a pencil sitting in a glass of water) but any form of wave, including ultrasound waves are subject to refraction.

Scattering

- Specular echoes used to form images of the heart arise from tissue interfaces.
- When ultrasound encounters much smaller structures, it interacts with them differently: instead of being *reflected* along a defined path they are scattered equally in all directions.

Reflection, scattering, and image quality

- Some tissues within the heart allow a lot of specular reflection (pericardium, epicardium, endocardium, and valves) and have high signal intensity on echocardiography, others produce a lot of scattering (i.e. myocardium).
- Blood produces very little reflection and as such has very low signal intensity on echocardiography. This allows the myocardium to be easily differentiated from the blood.

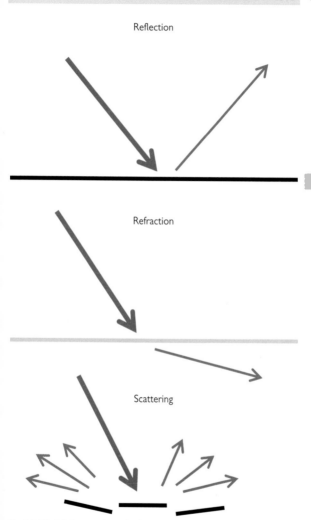

Fig. 1.9 (Top) Reflection: the angle of the transmitted ultrasound influences the reflection back from the boundary of a medium. (Middle) Refraction: the transmitted ultrasound wave is transmitted from one medium to another causing a change in direction. (Bottom) Scattering: echoes are generated from smaller objects and are less intense and less angle dependent.

Reflection, attenuation, and depth compensation

Ultrasound waves are quite severely attenuated (Fig. 1.10) as they pass through 'spongy' tissues such as fat and muscle. The degree of attenuation depends greatly on the ultrasound frequency.

- The proportion reflected at a tissue interface depends mainly on the difference in density of the tissues. Where there is a large difference—such as an interface with air or bone—most of the incident wave is reflected, creating an intense echo but leaving little to penetrate further to deeper structures. It is for this reason that the operator has to manipulate the transducer to avoid ribs and lungs, and that a contact gel is used to eliminate any air between the transducer and the chest wall.
- In contrast, there is relatively little difference in the densities of blood, muscle, and fat, so echoes from interfaces between them are very small—about 0.1% of the incident amplitude.
- Not only is this a very small signal to detect, but the amplification level required would be vastly greater than that needed for the same interface closer to the transducer. To overcome this problem, the machine provides depth compensation or time-gain compensation (TGC). This automatically increases the amplification during the time echoes from a particular pulse return, so that the last to arrive are amplified much more than the first.
- Most of this compensation is built into the machine, but the user can fine-tune it by means of a bank of slider controls that adjust the amplification at selected depths.
- The reflection and attenuation characteristics of various media can be used to help in their identification. In particular, an interface with air generates a very strong reflection at the proximal boundary, beyond which the air strongly attenuates the beam casting a dark shadow.

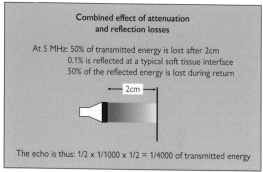

**Combined effect of attenuation
and reflection losses**

At 5 MHz: 50% of transmitted energy is lost after 2cm
0.1% is reflected at a typical soft tissue interface
50% of the reflected energy is lost during return

2cm

The echo is thus: 1/2 × 1/1000 × 1/2 = 1/4000 of transmitted energy

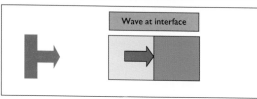

Wave at interface

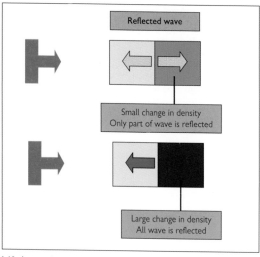

Reflected wave

Small change in density
Only part of wave is reflected

Large change in density
All wave is reflected

Fig. 1.10 Attenuation.

Reverberation artefacts

- Reverberation artefacts are produced by the presence of structures with transmission and attenuation characteristics very different from that of soft tissue (i.e. the heart).
- The reflected echoes bounce back and forth between the highly reflective object and the transducer (Fig. 1.11).
- In a reverberation artefact, the ultrasound wave is reflected back into the chest from the transducer–skin interface and are common sources of misinterpretation of images creating secondary 'ghost' images. Under normal circumstances this effect is not seen because soft-tissue reflections are so weak and secondary reflections are too small to register.
- However, if the object is a very strong reflector such as a calcified or prosthetic valve, then the secondary or higher-order reverberation echoes are strong enough to be detected.
- The clue to their recognition is that they are always exactly twice as far away from the transducer as a high-intensity echo, and if the primary structure moves a certain distance, the multiple reflection echo moves twice as far.

Clues to avoid and recognize reverberation artefacts

- Beware of objects that are only seen in one imaging plane.
- Beware of objects that do not respect anatomical boundaries, e.g. a valve lying over a chamber wall or a line lying outside the heart.
- Beware of objects that are twice as far from the transducer as intense reflectors.
- Use the minimum power necessary to obtain an image.
- Use adequate ultrasound gel.
- Rotating the patient or changing the angle probe to move the artefact if it is in the required field of view.

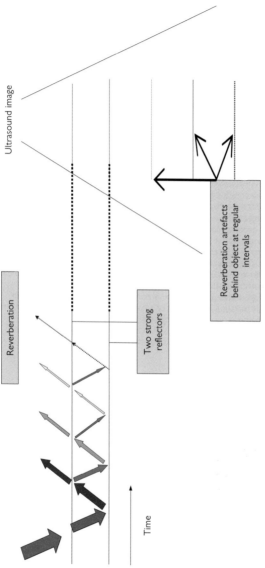

Fig. 1.11 Reverberation artefacts.

Transmit power

- The amplitude (ultrasound strength) of the transmitted ultrasound wave is controlled by the transmit power (or mechanical index).
- Commercially available echocardiography systems are usually set to a default transmit power to ensure there are no adverse effects on the tissue being imaged, e.g. for native imaging MI >1.0.
- The adjustment of the transmit power is particularly important during contrast opacification studies to reduce contrast bubble destruction.

Gain

- The brightness of an image depends on the amount of ultrasound signal received by the probe from the reflected echoes.
- The intensity of the reflected signal is dependent on the depth of the structure being imaged (increased distance reduces signal) and the inherent reflective properties of the object being imaged.
- Objects in the near field appear brighter than those in the far field. In order to compensate for this *depth compensation* or *time gain compensation* (TGC) is used, which enhances the intensity of signals returning later (and as such further away from transducer).
- TGC automatically increases the amplification during the time echoes from a particular pulse return, so that the last to arrive are amplified much more than the first.
- Most of this compensation is built into the machine, but the user can fine-tune it by means of a bank of slider controls that adjust the amplification at selected depths.
- Too high levels of gain result in noise making images appear like 'a snowstorm' and difficult to interpret (Fig. 1.12).

Grey scale and compress

- The intensity of an echo depends on the nature of the tissue interface. There are a wide range of echo intensities, with a calcified structure generating an echo many thousands of times more intense than a boundary between, say, blood and newly formed thrombus.
- The limited dynamic range of the display system can only represent a fraction of this range (the difference in light intensity between 'black' ink printed on 'white' paper is only a factor of 30 or so). As a consequence, ultrasound images show all intense echoes as 'white', all weak echoes as 'black', and almost no grey tones.
- The number of levels of grey (or the dynamic range) can be altered so that a range of grey levels in between black and white appear, but at the expense of boundary definition (Fig. 1.12).

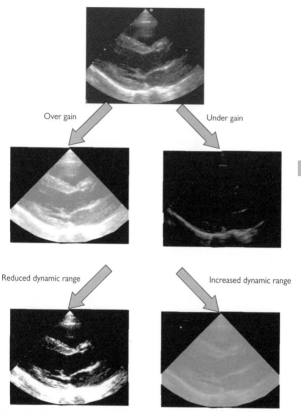

Fig. 1.12 Effects of changes in gain and dynamic range (grey scale) on image.
See 🎞 Video 1.1, 🎞 Video 1.2, 🎞 Video 1.3.

Image resolution

- *Temporal resolution* is the overall visualized image quality with respect to time, a compromise between the frame rate, angle width and depth. Shallower imaging depths and narrower sector widths will both increase temporal resolution.
- *Axial resolution* is the minimum separation needed so that two interfaces located in a direction parallel to the beam (i.e. above and below each other) can continue to be imaged as two separate sampling points rather than one. It can be optimized by employing a higher ultrasound frequency.
- *Lateral resolution* is the resolution side to side, across the 2D image: the minimum separation of two sampling points aligned perpendicular to the ultrasound beam so that they continue to be imaged as two separate interfaces rather than one. It is primarily determined by the distance from the transducer and, as the echo beam widens with increased depth the lateral resolution decreases.
- *Spatial resolution* is a measure of how close two reflectors can be to one another so that they can still be identified as different reflectors.

Focusing

- Lateral resolution is the chief factor limiting the quality of all ultrasound images and is worse than axial resolution by something like a factor of 10. To improve it, the ultrasound beam must be made narrower by focusing it.
- A plastic lens is fitted on the face of the transducer, in the same way that a glass lens focuses light, though less effectively. Transducers can be constructed with short-, medium-, or long-focus lenses.
- The pulsing sequence that steers the beam can be electronically modified to provide additional focusing. This adjustment can be made by the operator.

Transducer frequency and spatial resolution

- The frequencies of various probes differ depending on the application (see Table 1.1).
- The choice of transducer frequency is determined by the depth of imaging and the resolution required.
- Low frequency transducers have good penetration but because of the longer wavelength, poorer resolution.
- High frequency transducers have good resolution but poor penetration.
- Higher frequency transducers with better resolution can be used where less depth is required, e.g. when imaging children or TOE.
- Intravascular ultrasound requires very little penetration but very high resolution and therefore uses very high frequencies.

Table 1.1 Different ultrasound probes and their specific frequencies

Probe type	Transducer frequency
Transthoracic echocardiography	2–5Mhz
Transoesophageal echocardiography	5–7.5Mhz
Vascular probes	10Mhz
Intravascular probes	30–40Mhz

The effect of transducer frequency on image quality

- Axial resolution is dependent on the wave frequency (calculated as ~2 × λ).
- When using a 3.5Mhz probe the axial resolution is around 1mm. Using a high frequency cardiac probe (>3.5MHz) rather than a standard 2.5MHz probe will increase axial resolution, but will do so at the expense of tissue penetration, which is lower at lower wavelengths.

Second harmonic imaging

- The frequency of the ultrasound wave sent out is the fundamental frequency.
- The target tissue expands and compresses in response to the wave which in turn causes distortion of the sound wave. This distortion generates additional frequencies called harmonics.
- This change in wave shape can be shown mathematically to be due to the addition of a frequency twice that of the original transmitted frequency (called its 'second harmonic') (Fig. 1.13).
- Harmonic frequencies are larger than the fundamental frequency.
- Both harmonic and fundamental frequencies will return to the transducer but by filtering out the original fundamental frequency it is possible to receive the higher harmonic frequencies preferentially.

Advantages

- Harmonic imaging combines the penetration power of a transmitted low fundamental frequency with the improved axial image resolution of the harmonic frequency which is twice that of the fundamental frequency.
- The harmonic image is derived from deeper structures and thus reduces artefacts from proximal objects such as ribs.
- The harmonic image away from the central beam axis is relatively weak and thus not so susceptible to off-axis artefacts.

Disadvantages

- As the image is now formed from echoes of a single frequency, some 'texture' is lost and structures such as valve leaflets may appear artificially thick.
- If the quality of the fundamental frequency image is very good, such that second harmonic mode offers little benefit, it may be better not to use it, but in most patients the improvement in image quality greatly outweighs this minor disadvantage.

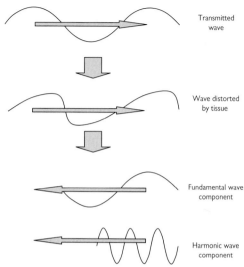

Transmitted
wave

Wave distorted
by tissue

Fundamental wave
component

Harmonic wave
component

Fig. 1.13 Harmonic imaging relies on analysing the harmonics of reflected waves to generate an image.

Doppler echocardiography

Doppler imaging allows the determination of the direction and speed of blood flow and is used for the detection and assessment of cardiac valvular insufficiency and stenosis as well as a large number of other abnormal flow patterns.

The Doppler effect (Fig. 1.14)

- First described in 1842, Doppler hypothesized that certain properties of light emitted from stars depend upon the relative motion of the observer and the wave source.
- Consider a ship setting sail from the shore with an incoming tide with a wave frequency of one wave per minute. As the ship is moving out to sea would it meet the waves with more frequency than one per minute? The converse is also true that if the same ship turned around to set sail to shore, it would meet less than one wave per minute.
- Although initially described for light, the Doppler effect applies to all waveforms including ultrasound. As blood is moving, the frequency of the backscattered echoes is modified by the Doppler effect, termed 'the Doppler shift'.
- The change in frequency of reflected echo waves will be either increased if blood is travelling towards the probe or decreased if travelling away from the probe, with the size of the Doppler shift determines the speed of the blood.

The Doppler equation describes the change in frequency that occurs:

$$\Delta_F = \frac{2f_o \; V \cos \theta}{C}$$

- Δ_F is the Doppler shift in frequency.
- f_o is the ultrasound frequency of the transducer.
- V is the velocity of the blood.
- θ is the angle between the flow and the ultrasound beam.
- C is the velocity of ultrasound in tissue (1540 m/s).

The returning ultrasound signal is demodulated to extract the Doppler shift and the velocity is then determined.

Doppler shifts are usually in the audible range (20Hz–20KHz) and heard during the Doppler examination, the higher the pitch of the sound the higher the Doppler shift and blood velocity.

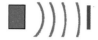

Transmitted wave

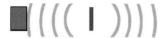

**Reflected wave
stationary object**

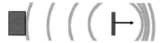

**Reflected wave—
object moving away from probe**

Received
wavelength
increases

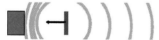

**Reflected wave—
object moving towards probe**

Received
wavelength
decreases

Fig. 1.14 The Doppler effect.

Continuous wave Doppler

- Continuous wave (CW) Doppler requires transmission of a continuous train of ultrasound waves, with simultaneous reception of the returning backscattered echoes (Fig. 1.15).
- The frequency of backscattered echoes from moving blood is different to that from the transmitted frequency. This difference is known as the Doppler shift or Doppler frequency.
- As blood in an artery does not flow at a constant rate, the ultrasound beam generates a large number of different Doppler frequencies, all of which are used by the machine to generate the spectral Doppler display.
- This all requires two piezoelectric crystals (one for transmission one for reception) rather than the one used in pulsed wave Doppler (Fig. 1.16).
- Different probes have different arrangements of crystals with stand alone 'pencil' probes having separate transmit and receive crystals and normal probes assigning crystal groups to either a transmit or receive.
- As transmission and reception of ultrasound is continuous it can't provide depth discrimination, and a particular Doppler shift may have arisen from anywhere along the beam axis.
- Although this would appear to be a problem, it usually is not the case in clinical practice, since identification of the source of a high-velocity jet is usually apparent from the 2D image and from the flow velocity profile.
- The density of the spectral trace is proportional to the amplitude of the signal at each Doppler frequency and thus a representation of the blood flow at that velocity.

Limitations of CW Doppler for measuring pressure gradients

- For successful application of CW Doppler the ultrasound beam needs to be aligned accurately with the direction of blood flow (within 15° of the flow, for which the cosine is 0.97 and error in the value of $[velocity]^2$ is <7%).
- A colour-flow image can be used to guide beam alignment and in the case of aortic stenosis the measurements should be checked by using two different views (e.g. apical and upper right parasternal).
- It is also necessary to align the beam with the centre of the jet passing through the restriction.
- The 'pencil probe', which is optimized for CW Doppler, is strongly recommended for recording high-velocity valve jets.

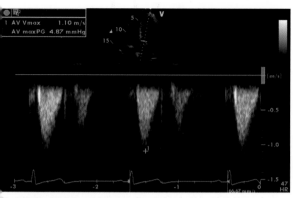

Fig. 1.15 Example of continuous wave Doppler.

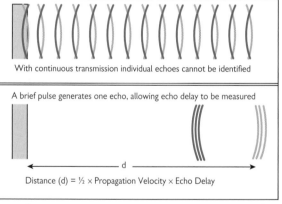

With continuous transmission individual echoes cannot be identified

A brief pulse generates one echo, allowing echo delay to be measured

Distance (d) = ½ × Propagation Velocity × Echo Delay

Fig. 1.16 Continuous wave and pulsed wave.

Pulsed wave Doppler

- This is a single piezoelectric crystal technique which uses alternating transmission and reception of ultrasound waves (Fig. 1.17).
- The depth of the region of interest ('sample volume') determines this interval between transmission and reception of the ultrasound waves.
- The cycle of alternating transmission and reception of pulses is termed the pulse repetition frequency (PRF).
- Information is gathered over a small sample, which can be moved to any region of interest.
- The main advantage of pulsed Doppler is the high spatial resolution that can be obtained (typically a 1–5mm sample size can be interrogated), and is useful for investigating velocities in specific areas, i.e. the left ventricular outflow tract.

Pulse repetition frequency

- With pulsed wave (PW) Doppler the time interval between sequential pulses must be sufficient so that the initial pulse has enough time to reach the target and return to the probe.
- If this interval between pulses is too short so that the second pulse is sent before the first is received back, then it is difficult to differentiate between reflected signals from the sample volume.
- The closer the region of interest to the probe, the higher the PRF.
- Lower PRFs are usually used to evaluate low velocities as the increased time between pulsed transmission–reception cycles allows better chance for the scanner to identify slower flow (e.g. venous).

Aliasing

- With pulsed Doppler, transmitted waves must be sampled at least twice in each cycle to allow determination of wavelength (this is an example of Nyquist's theorem).
- The maximum velocity (Doppler shift) that can be measured accurately is equal to half of the PRF (this value is the Nyquist limit).
- If pulsed Doppler waves travel to greater depths then the time interval to receive the reflected signal is increased and thus the PRF is lower. The Nyquist limit (aliasing level) is therefore lower at greater sampling depths.

Practical considerations of PW Doppler

- The practical effect of aliasing is that the 'tops' of the positive velocities that exceed the Nyquist limit are cut off and displayed as negative velocities (Fig. 1.18).
- Provided that the flow is predominantly towards or away from the transducer, and not bi-directional, the zero velocity baseline can be shifted to favour one direction at the expense of the other, and it is thus possible to increase the aliasing velocity by a factor of up to 2, but beyond this nothing can be done.
- When looking at the display of a pulsed wave trace if the flow being measured is laminar then the trace has a defined outline, if the flow is turbulent then flow fills in to form a more solid flow trace.

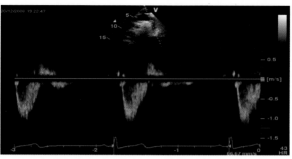

Fig. 1.17 Example of normal pulsed wave Doppler placed in aortic arch.

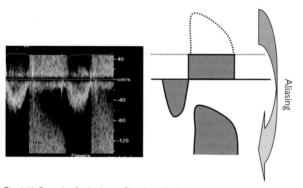

Fig. 1.18 Example of pulsed wave Doppler with aliasing.

High pulse repetition frequency PW Doppler

- This is the deliberate use of high PRFs to increase the aliasing velocity and thus increase the maximum velocity that can be measured with PW Doppler.
- Sequential pulses are transmitted without waiting for the original one to be received. This increases the PRF and allows a spectral trace which is not aliased.
- The trade off with using high PRFs to sample increased velocities is that some of the ultrasound waves will penetrate beyond the depth of interest and so signals from different sampling depths may be recorded.
- In practice this is overcome by judicious placement of the beam to ensure that the additional sample volumes do not arise from high-velocity areas that are not of interest.

Colour flow mapping

- The PW Doppler principle can be extended to display a pictorial representation of PW Doppler readings over a designated region of interest (determined on the 2D image).
- Pulses are rapidly emitted from the probe so that sequential pulses hit the same moving scatterer. Thus, a representation of how far the scatterer has moved either towards or away from the probe can be determined.
- Standard designation of colours occurs according to direction as Blue Away and Red Towards (BART) the probe (Fig. 1.19). On CW or PW Doppler, blood flowing towards the transducer would appear as a spectral trace above the time line, whereas blood flowing away from the transducer would appear as a spectral trace below the time line.

Limitations of colour flow mapping

Aliasing

- Simultaneous imaging and Doppler lower the effective PRF and aliasing in a colour flow image typically occurs at velocities above 0.5m/s.
- Aliasing manifests on a colour display as colour inversion: red turning to blue, and vice versa. For steady flow towards the transducer, a velocity of 0.4m/s is represented by pale red but as it increases to 0.6m/s it becomes pale blue (Fig. 1.20). At 1.0m/s (twice the aliasing velocity) the colour display again shows black, and with further increase in velocity red, then blue, and so on.

Turbulent flow (variance mapping)

- When flow is turbulent, there is a wide spectrum of local velocities: high and low, forward and reverse. This is indicated on a CW display as broadening of the spectral band, but cannot be indicated by colour Doppler, since it can only display flow velocity at one point and at one time by a single colour.
- A solution is provided by analysing the time-variance of local velocity, so that when the same pixel detects greatly different velocities in successive images, the display is modified, for example by showing those pixels in green.
- This is called variance mapping, but it places further strain on frame rates and aliasing velocity.

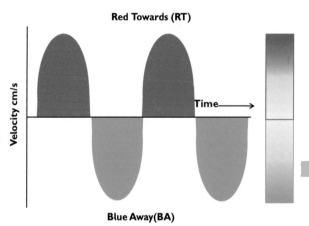

Fig. 1.19 Example of BART principle. On colour Doppler mapping flow away from the transducer is blue and a continuous or pulsed Doppler trace (blue spectra in figure) would appear as a spectral trace below the time line. Flow towards the transducer is red and a continuous or pulsed Doppler trace (red spectra in figure) would appear as a spectral trace above the time line.

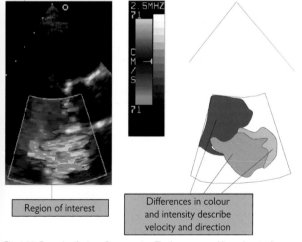

Fig. 1.20 Example of colour flow mapping. The homogenous blue colour in the left ventricle indicates blood flow away from the transducer. The flow becomes turbulent when the blood is pushed through the leaky mitral valve, which can be seen as a mosaic pattern of different velocities.

Tissue Doppler imaging

- Tissue Doppler imaging (TDI) allows the velocities of myocardial segments and other cardiac structures to be measured (Fig. 1.21).
- Whereas conventional Doppler techniques assess the velocity of blood flow by measuring high-frequency, low-amplitude signals from small, fast-moving blood cells, TDI uses the same Doppler principles to quantify the higher amplitude, lower-velocity signals of myocardial tissue motion (Figs. 1.21 and 1.22).
- TDI allows the measurement of myocardial motion relative to the adjacent myocardium rather than the transducer which is susceptible to tethering of adjacent tissue.
- High-velocity signals from blood are filtered out and amplification scales suitably adjusted so that Doppler signals from tissue motion can be recorded.

Practical considerations for tissue Doppler imaging

- The accuracy of TDI is angle dependent and only measures the vector of motion that is parallel to the direction of the ultrasound beam.
- High frame rates (100–150 frames per second) should be used in order to maximize the information gathered in the spectral trace.
- The sample volume should remain within the tissue of interest during the cardiac cycle.
- Respiratory motion can cause drifting of the strain curve as the sample volume moves out of the desired region of interest and therefore images should be acquired at end expiration.
- Tissues close to the body surface can cause false echoes from their reflections ('reverberation artefacts'). In PW TDI these can be seen as an increased intensity at zero velocity.
- The lowest readable gain setting should be used to acquire and analyse the spectral trace. Too much gain increases the width of the spectrum and increasing the gain intensity increases the peak TDI value.

Strain rate imaging by tissue Doppler

- Strain is a measure of the change in shape ('deformation') of a region of interest. The relative amount of this deformation over time is termed the strain rate.
- The peak systolic strain is the maximum deformation seen during systole.
- Peak systolic strain rate is the maximum rate of deformation during systole.
- Strain rate by tissue Doppler measures the velocity gradient between two points within a segment at a fixed distance apart.

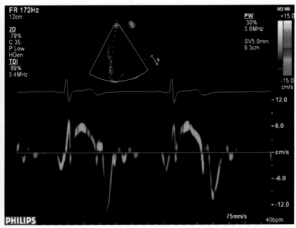

Fig. 1.21 Example of pulsed wave tissue Doppler imaging placed at basal left ventricular septum.

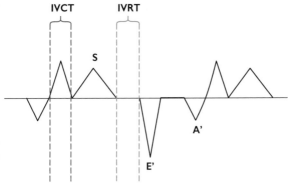

Fig. 1.22 Schematic of pulsed wave tissue Doppler trace showing the isovolumic contraction time (IVCT), the peak systolic myocardial velocity (S), the isovolumic relaxation time (IVRT), the early diastolic myocardial velocity (E') and the late diastolic myocardial velocity (A').

3D echocardiography

Introduction

- 3D image acquisition has the advantage of taking into account variation in ventricular shape in all directions rather than just the two of biplane measurements. It is dependent on capturing the whole left ventricle within the 3D-probe sector and requires images to have good endocardial border definition.
- 3D echocardiography is well suited for the evaluation of valvular disease and has the advantage of offering depth as an additional dimension over 2D echocardiography and the ability to view the valve from multiple different angles.
- 3D image acquisitions are either true 'live' images or near real-time (full volume) images. Live images offer instant feedback although are limited by a narrow display sector. Near real-time images occur when the electrocardiogram (ECG) recording is used to acquire individual subvolumes over sequential cardiac cycles (Fig. 1.23).

3D acquisition modes

Full volume 3D data sets

- This mode allows the generation of a 3D data set with the final image of the heart created by acquiring several subvolumes (usually 1–7 depending on the vendor) over the corresponding number of sequential cardiac cycles.
- A regular cardiac rhythm and adequate breath-holding capabilities of the patient are needed to reduce the incidence of artefact when the subvolumes are merged together.
- The greater the number of subvolumes used, the higher the frame rate and temporal resolution (Fig. 1.24).
- Once all of the subvolumes have been acquired a final image is formed. This image is therefore not 'live'.

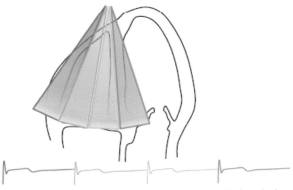

Fig. 1.23 Diagrammatic representation of subvolume acquisition. The first subvolume (red) is taken during the first cardiac cycle (red), the second subvolume (orange) is taken during the second cardiac cycle (orange) and so on. All subvolumes are merged together to create the final dataset.

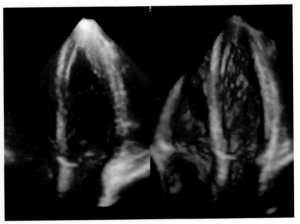

Fig. 1.24 2-beat 3D left ventricle (LV) full volume acquisition (left) is composed of 2 subvolumes acquired over 2 consecutive cardiac cycles and has a lower volume rate and temporal resolution than a 7-beat 3D LV full volume acquisition (right). See 📹 Video 1.4 and 📹 Video 1.5.

Live 3D

- Live volume images generate real-time 3D acquisitions of the heart.
- This mode allows the generation of a 3D data set which is usually smaller than the full volume acquisition to achieve adequate frame rates.
- It is well suited to imaging during percutaneous interventions or closer inspection of valvular pathology, where a smaller volume of interest is being examined or during irregular cardiac rhythms (Fig. 1.25).

3D colour Doppler

- This combines grey scale volumetric data with colour Doppler and is useful for examination of regurgitant lesions or shunts (Fig. 1.26).

Applications and limitations of 3D echocardiography

Applications

- 3D echocardiography has been shown to be accurate for the assessment of left and right ventricular function and volumes.
- There has been research into whether 3D datasets provide novel indices for left ventricular dyssynchrony assessment.
- 3D echocardiography also allows for quantification of valvular abnormalities and also to guide cardiac interventions (e.g. PFO/ASD closure, TAVI and mitral clip implant).

Limitations

- Misalignment can occur when the subvolumes are merged together—called stitching artefacts, see Fig. 1.27.
- 3D image quality greatly depends on the quality of the 2D image.

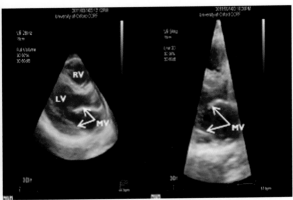

Fig. 1.25 Left: parasternal left ventricle (LV) 3D full volume acquisition. Right: live 3D parasternal acquisition of mitral valve (MV). RV = right ventricle. See 📹 Video 1.6 and 📹 Video 1.7.

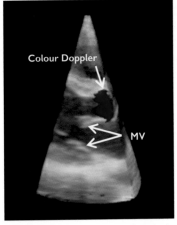

Fig. 1.26 3D full volume colour Doppler acquisition of mitral valve (MV) and aortic valve (AV). See 📹 Video 1.8.

3D artefacts

Stitch artefacts

- These occur during the acquisition of 3D full volume images where subvolumes are recorded and triggered by the cardiac cycle.
- Stitch artefacts are seen when subvolumes do not neatly merge together and instead the boundary between individual subvolumes can be identified (Fig. 1.27).
- Causes of stitch artefacts include an irregular cardiac rhythm, probe motion during acquisition or patient movement during acquisition (e.g. respiration).

Drop out artefacts

- These can occur when the volume of interest is acquired and a suboptimal gain setting used.
- For instance, when imaging the mitral valve, as the leaflets may be quite thin then if the gain setting is too low, a drop out may occur.
- Conversely if too high a gain setting is used this may lead to other imaging artefacts.

Attenuation artefacts

- As with 2D echocardiography, attenuation artefacts can occur. This is the process of a gradual deterioration of the signal intensity distal to the volume target due to reduced backscatter and absorption.

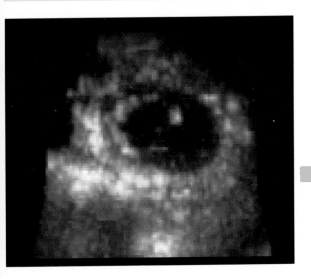

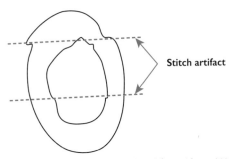

Stitch artifact

Fig. 1.27 2D short axis slice from a 3D full volume left ventricle acquisition. Cropping the ventricle in a short axis plane has revealed a stitch artefact.

Image display

- Following the acquisition of the 3D data sets, the advantages of 3D echocardiography become appreciated as all commercially available 3D echocardiography machines allow post processing.
- Post processing can be performed either directly on the same unit as that used for acquisition or indirectly via a stand alone software package.
- The use of post processing allows visualization of cardiac landmarks that would not have been possible with 2D echocardiography alone (e.g. surgical 'en face' view of the mitral valve).

Commercially available 3D software packages are able to perform post processing techniques (although the individual names of the techniques vary from vender to vender):

Cropping

- This allows the operator to remove unwanted information from the initial data set to focus solely on the target anatomy, e.g. cropping the ventricle to view the mitral valve looking from the apical position.
- Most commercially available 3D operating systems allow cropping (Fig. 1.28) to be performed either by rotating and removing unwanted data in a single plane through the image or using a 3-plane technique.

Following image cropping and rendering, the 3D acquisition can be displayed.

- There are several modes such as a volume rendered image, wire frame display, or multiplanar reformatting (MPR) slice display where three simultaneous orthogonal 2D-like slices can be presented.

Slice modes

- Most commercial 3D echocardiography systems offer a 'slice' format through which the data can be presented (e.g. Phillips iSlice; Fig. 1.29).
- Here, the 3D image volume can initially be optimized to avoid any foreshortening and then volume can be viewed as a number of uniformly spaced slices in the horizontal plane.

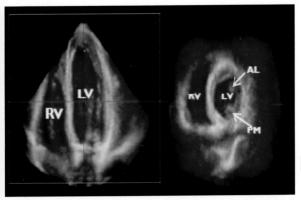

Fig. 1.28 Top 2 panels: full volume 3D acquisition of left ventricle (LV) from the apical view (left image) which has been rotated and cropped to show a short axis view of the left ventricle at papillary level (right image). AL = anterolateral papillary muscle; PM = posteromedial papillary muscle; RV = right ventricle.

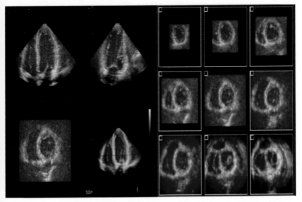

Fig. 1.29 3D full volume data sets of the left ventricle processed on Philips QLAB 7.1. Multiplanar reformatting (left) showing three orthogonal slices. Philips iSlice (right) allows the LV to be cut into 9 short axis slices.

3D image rendering

- Image rendering is vital to fully appreciate the target volume in detail. As with 2D echocardiography, it is a process which should begin prior to volume acquisition to ensure that the optimal image is acquired and can be completed post image acquisition to optimize the acquired image for visual presentation.
- Most commercial 3D echocardiography packages offer different image rendering capabilities, the main ones being:
  - *Smoothness*: this allows adjustment of image so that the finer detail at closer inspection is free from minor 'roughness',
  - *Gain adjustment*: it is particularly important during 3D image optimization to carefully adjust the overall gain of the image. High gain levels make the image appear more 2D like whereas lower gain reveals deeper tissue structure so that deeper tissues are more appreciated in the overall volume; see Fig. 1.30.
  - *Opacification/compression*: this determines how solid or transparent the final image is. Lowering the compression increases the image transparency and vice versa.
  - *Brightness*.
  - *3D vision/colour maps*: all 3D post processing systems offer a variety of colour maps or different '3D vision' which the operator can select from, each separate selection offering a combination of different colours to alter depth perception.
  - *Magnification*: allows the acquired image to be enlarged to appreciate finer structures in more detail.

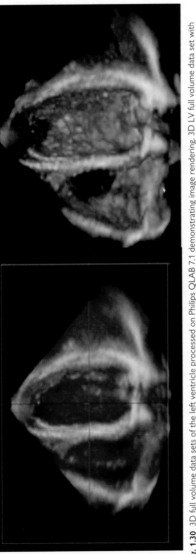

Fig. 1.30 3D full volume data sets of the left ventricle processed on Philips QLAB 7.1 demonstrating image rendering. 3D LV full volume data set with increased gain (left) and subsequently reduced gain (right) to allow deeper tissue structures to be appreciated. See ▣ Video 1.9 and ▣ Video 1.10.

Speckle tracking echocardiography

When imaging myocardial tissue, the ultrasound image of backscatter generated by the reflected ultrasound beam appears as a pattern of grey values. This is termed the 'speckle pattern'. The myocardial fibre orientation of the LV is complex. In healthy individuals myocardial fibres move in several different planes which can be detected by speckle tracking.

The speckle pattern is unique for each myocardial region. Speckle tracking software allows individual speckles within a region of interest to be tracked throughout the cardiac cycle, frame by frame. The scanner speckle tracking algorithm allows the displacement, velocity, strain, and strain rate for a myocardial region to be calculated.

Speckle tracking strain measurements

Peak strain values during systole are represented as a percentage of the final position of the speckles in relation to their original position. Longitudinal strain is measured from the LV apical views whereas radial and circumferential strains can also be obtained from LV short axis views (Fig. 1.31).

- *Longitudinal strain:* the motion from base to apex. During systole the contraction in this plane leads to fibre shortening, represented as a negative percentage value (i.e. the more negative the value—the greater the deformation which has occurred).
- *Radial strain:* the amount of thickening of the myocardium which occurs. During systole myocardial contraction leads to fibre thickening in the radial plane. This is represented as a positive percentage value (i.e. the more positive the value—the greater the deformation which has occurred).
- *Circumferential strain:* the change in radius in the short axis. During systole, myocardial contraction leads to fibre shortening. This is represented as a negative percentage value (i.e. the more negative the value, the greater the deformation which has occurred).

Cardiac twisting

During the cardiac cycle the left ventricle also undergoes a twisting motion. During systole the apex rotates counterclockwise whilst the base rotates in a clockwise fashion. These movements can also be estimated by speckle tracking:

- Rotation (degrees): the angular displacement of a myocardial segment in the short axis view.
- Twist or torsion (degrees): the net difference between apical short axis and basal short axis rotation.

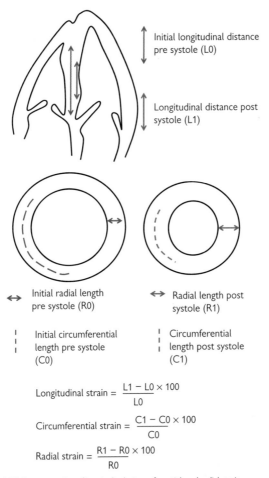

Fig. 1.31 Representation of longitudinal, circumferential, and radial strain.

2D vs. 3D speckle tracking (Fig. 1.32)

- All of the described strain parameters can be measured in 2D. In reality, speckles move through 3D space rather than remaining within the 2D sector (Fig. 1.32).
- Newer technology is now available allowing the measurement of 3D speckle tracking strain (Fig. 1.33). This has the advantage of tracking the motion of speckles within the scan volume, irrelevant of its direction.

Practical considerations for speckle tracking

- Unlike TDI, speckle tracking is an angle-independent technique and so the transducer can be placed off axis to obtain the optimal image.
- Clear delineation of the endocardial border is necessary for reliable tracking.
- To reduce through plane motion acquisitions should be made during breath hold.
- Drop out or reverberations if present are sometimes tracked, resulting in incorrect calculation of strain.
- The optimal frame rate for acquisition of images is around 50–90 frames per second (FPS), much lower than frame rates needed for TDI (>120 FPS). In patients with tachycardia or during rapid events in the cardiac cycle, these lower frame rates mean that there may be under sampling, with peak strain and strain rate values being lower than the true value.
- Higher frame rates will reduce the problem of under sampling but at the expense of spatial resolution. Lower frame rates are thus used to ensure optimal spatial resolution but care must be taken not to lower the frame rate too much otherwise the speckle will not be able to be tracked from frame to frame.
- A good balance between temporal and spatial resolution can be achieved by adjusting the sector width so that it is just wider than the myocardial wall.
- Whilst optimizing the image quality is important, it is also necessary to remember that speckle tracking is also dependent on the implemented vendor algorithm. Different vendor algorithms may produce different results.

Langranian and natural strain

There are two types of strain, *Lagranian* and *natural* strain. *Lagrangian* strain is defined on the basis of deformation from an original *length*. Whereas, *natural* strain is defined relative to deformation from a length at a previous *time*, which may not necessarily be the original length. *Natural* strain is more relevant to cardiac imaging as you may want to know how strain changes during the cardiac cycle rather than just relative to the start.

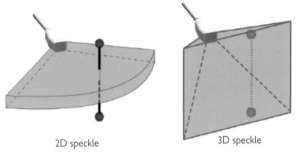

2D speckle   3D speckle

Fig. 1.32 Representation of 2D versus 3D speckle tracking. Individual speckles move in and out of the scan plane between the two blue dots. With 2D speckle tracking (left image) a narrow sector of speckles will be tracked (red dots). 3D speckle tracking (right image) tracks the motion of the speckles within the entire volume. Image courtesy of Toshiba Medical Systems, Europe.

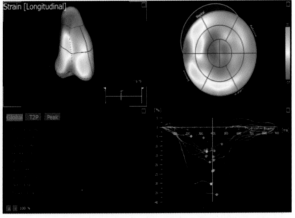

Fig. 1.33 Post processing (using TomTec, Germany) of a 3D LV full volume data set to show global 3D strain by speckle tracking. Strain curves during the cardiac cycle, colour coded for each of the LV myocardial segments, are displayed.

Second harmonic mode Doppler for contrast imaging

- Second harmonic imaging was originally developed in order to enhance signals from encapsulated contrast media (see Chapter 9).
- These are proprietary products and comprise very small (1–3μm) microspheres of gas contained within a hard outer shell.
- At very low ultrasound power levels, the microspheres act as conventional scatterers, but with slightly greater power (though still lower than normally used for imaging) the pressure waves distort them and they vibrate, emitting energy at the second harmonic frequency.
- A display derived from the second harmonic Doppler frequency thus selectively comes from the microspheres and not from surrounding tissue or blood.
- The addition of contrast greatly enhances the quality of both images of blood-filled cavities and of Doppler signals, giving a clear velocity profile for even very small jets.
- At higher ultrasound power levels, the microspheres shatter, releasing the contained gas, and generating a brief, but very intense, echo.

Power mode (amplitude) imaging

- As stated previously, the Doppler shift is determined by velocity, but the intensity of the Doppler signal relates to the number of scatterers within the ultrasound beam.
- If there are a lot of scatterers moving in random directions, the net velocity will be zero, but the amplitude of the Doppler signal quite high.
- A display showing the amplitude or power of the Doppler signal shows the density of scatterers, regardless of the velocities. This type of display is used, often in conjunction with harmonic mode, in contrast studies.

Basic fluid dynamics

Volumetric flow

- For steady-state flow (i.e. when velocity is constant) the volume of liquid flowing through a pipe for a given time period (T) is the product of the cross-sectional area of the pipe (A) and the mean velocity (V).

$$\text{Volume} = A \times V \times T$$

- If flow is pulsatile (e.g. blood flow in the circulation) then velocity increases and decreases over time. The product of velocity and time is replaced by use of the *velocity time integral* (VTI).

$$\text{VTI} = (\textstyle\int V \times dT)$$

Continuity equation (Fig. 1.34)

- If a fluid, which is not compressible, flows along a rigid-walled pipe, the amount entering one end of the pipe must be the same as that leaving the other end.
- If the diameter of the pipe is greater at the end than the start (i.e. cone-shaped) this still holds true.
- In order to maintain flow across a reduced cross-sectional area an increase in mean velocity of flow must occur.
- This is the explanation for the increased flow speed when squeezing the end of a hose pipe. This basic principle is described by the *continuity equation*:

$$A_1 \times V_1 = A_2 \times V_2$$

Where:
- A_1 is the cross sectional of area of the entrance to the tube.
- V_1 is the velocity of flow at position A_1.
- A_2 is cross sectional of area of the exit of the pipe.
- V_2 the velocity at position A_2.
- Providing that three of the terms in the equation are known, the fourth can be derived.
- The equation is used, for example, to determine the valve area in aortic stenosis:
  - Area of the left ventricular outflow tract (A_{LVOT}) is taken as the entrance to the tube (assumed to be circular and calculated from diameter as $\pi\, r_{LVOT}{}^2$)
- Entrance flow being pulsatile is replaced with velocity time integral measured with pulsed wave Doppler in the left ventricular outflow tract (VTI_{LVOT}).
- Exit flow is measured as the velocity time integral across the aortic valve (VTI_{AV}) with continuous wave Doppler, i.e.:

$$A_{LVOT} \times VTI_{LVOT} = A_{AV} \times VTI_{AV}$$

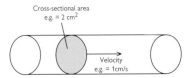

Cross-sectional area
e.g. = 2 cm^2

Velocity
e.g. = 1cm/s

Volume = cross-sectional area × velocity × time

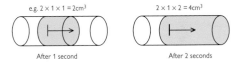

e.g. 2 × 1 × 1 = 2cm^3 2 × 1 × 2 = 4cm^3

After 1 second   After 2 seconds

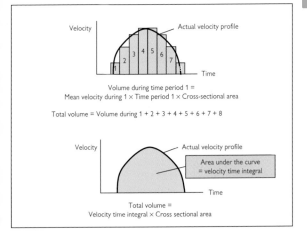

Velocity   Actual velocity profile

Time

Volume during time period 1 =
Mean velocity during 1 × Time period 1 × Cross-sectional area

Total volume = Volume during 1 + 2 + 3 + 4 + 5 + 6 + 7 + 8

Velocity   Actual velocity profile

Area under the curve
= velocity time integral

Time

Total volume =
Velocity time integral × Cross sectional area

Volume of blood that passes through pipe 1 in fixed time period
must equal volume that passes through pipe 2 in same time period
Area 1 × Velocity 1 = Area 2 × Velocity 2

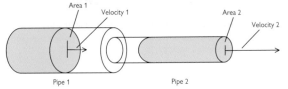

Area 1   Velocity 1   Area 2   Velocity 2

Pipe 1   Pipe 2

Fig. 1.34 Continuity equation.

Bernoulli equation (Fig. 1.35)
- The Bernoulli equation describes the relationship between pressure and velocity of a flow within a tube of fixed diameter.
- Liquid only flows along a pipe if there is a pressure difference between its ends.
- For a fixed pipe diameter, and steady-state flow, only a small pressure difference is required to overcome frictional losses.
- If the pipe becomes narrower in order to increase flow velocity (necessary to maintain flow) a higher pressure difference is required across the pipe. Again this is observed when putting your thumb on the end of a hose pipe, the pressure against your thumb increases as the velocity of water coming out of the narrowed end increases to maintain a steady state of flow through the pipe.

Neglecting the frictional losses, the relationship between pressure and velocity is:

$$P_1 - P_2 = \tfrac{1}{2}\, \rho\, (V_2{}^2 - V_1{}^2)$$

Where:
- V_1 is the velocity upstream to the narrowing.
- P_1 is the pressure at that point upstream to the narrowing.
- V_2 is the velocity after the narrowing.
- P_2 is the pressure after the narrowing.
- ρ is the density of the liquid.
- In most clinical cases of obstructed blood flow (e.g. aortic stenosis) the velocity before the narrowing (V_1) is small compared to that after the narrowing (V_2), for example 1m/s in the left ventricular outflow tract versus 4m/s across the aortic valve, and the difference is further magnified when the values are squared (i.e. $V_1 = 1$ and $V_2 = 16$) The equation simplifies by removing V_1 with little change in the pressure results and becomes:

$$P_1 - P_2 = \tfrac{1}{2}\, \rho\, V_2{}^2$$

- In echocardiography the pressure difference relates to blood (for which ρ is constant), the pressure is measured in mmHg and velocity in m/s. The equation can then be simplified further to:

$$P_1 - P_2 = 4\, V_2{}^2 \text{ or Pressure difference} = 4\, V_2{}^2$$

- If the upstream velocity is not small compared to the downstream for example in combined hypertrophic cardiomyopathy and aortic stenosis where a muscular subvalvular restriction can be combined with a valve stenosis then is not possible to omit V_1 from the Bernoulli equation.
- It is always worth remembering that a velocity of 2m/s across an aortic valve does not represent a pressure gradient of 16mmHg across the valve if the velocity in the outflow tract is 1.5m/s. In these cases (and for BSE exams) the full equation is:

$$P_1 - P_2 = 4\, (V_2{}^2 - V_1{}^2)$$

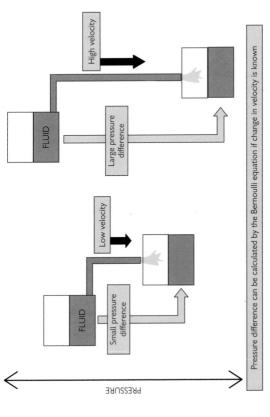

Fig. 1.35 Bernoulli equation.

Is ultrasound safe?

- No case of harm to a patient from diagnostic ultrasound has ever been documented in adult echocardiography. By any standards, the risk:benefit ratio of echocardiography is negligibly low, but there is no such thing as zero risk and to minimize it the user should always employ the 'ALARA' principle (As Low As Reasonably Achievable) for machine power levels and patient exposure times.
- Ultrasound at high power levels can be used to coagulate tissues, heat deep muscles, or clean dirty surgical instruments; however, commercially available ultrasound machines do not allow the transmission of power which may have potentially adverse bio-effects. Potential harmful effects are related to the beam intensity and ultrasound frequency.

Thermal index

- The energy lost through attenuation as the beam passes through tissues is largely converted to heat. The peak intensity as the ultrasound pulse passes may be quite high, but there are large gaps between pulses (pulse duration 2μs, interval between pulses 200μs) so the average heating is quite low.
- The term used to express this is *thermal index* and is the ratio of the actual beam power to that required to raise the temperature of a specific tissue by 1°C.

Temperature and transoesophageal echocardiography

A particular issue arises with transoesophageal scanning, where the transducer face is in contact with the oesophagus and local heating could, in the event of a fault within the transducer, cause tissue necrosis. For this reason, the probe tip temperature is monitored and there is an automatic thermal cut-out if it becomes too high.

Mechanical index

- Increasing transmitted power causes higher pressure fluctuations as the ultrasound waves travel through tissues.
- The potential for harm is quantified by the *mechanical index* (MI), a parameter derived by dividing the peak negative wave pressure by the square root of the ultrasound frequency. Most commercial cardiac scanners limit the maximum power to MI 1.1.

Contrast echocardiography

In contrast, echocardiography safety issues relate to the contrast itself and how it is broken down. Tissue bio-effects are negligible at the diagnostically recommended scanner settings. However, allergic or pseudo allergic reactions are possible but very rare (see 📖 p.570).

Transthoracic examination

Patient information

- Transthoracic echocardiography is a simple, non-invasive investigation. The patient can be given simple information on what is intended and how the pictures are created with sound waves.
- They should be aware that they will need to undress to the waist and lie on a bed on their side for around half an hour. If there is a sex discrepancy between echocardiographer and patient there should be the option of a chaperone.
- The operator should be alert to the fact that the patient may find lying in a fixed position on one side for a period of time uncomfortable (e.g. hip or knee problems) and give opportunities for the patient to move or consider alternative imaging positions. Furthermore the patient may find having the probe pressed against the chest uncomfortable.
- The operator should be aware of any complicating medical problems such as increased body mass index, chest deformities, lung disease, breast disease, or heart failure that may make imaging difficulty.

Patient preparation

- Ask the patient to undress to the waist and explain that this is *'so you can image the whole of the heart'*. A woman may appreciate a sheet or gown to cover them while preparations are in progress.
- Ask them to sit on the couch. The ideal position is with the patient sitting up at 45° supported by the raised head of the couch but rolled over onto their left side. Patients can find the concept of lying on their left side while sitting up confusing. They tend to slide down the bed on rolling over and end up lying down. Demonstrate the position if necessary and explain that they need to lie on their left side to *'bring the heart close to the chest wall'*. If the patient is more comfortable lying flat this is an acceptable alternative position.
- Ask them to raise their left arm and place their hand behind their head (some couches have a handle to hold onto). Explain that this is to *'make it easier to get to the heart'*.
- Make sure the patient is comfortable as they will need to stay in position for sometime.
- Attach ECG electrodes between patient and ultrasound machine and check there is a clear trace on the screen both to time images and trigger loop capture. Aim to have a large QRS complex without artefact. Usually the red electrode is placed by the right shoulder, yellow by left shoulder, and green on the lower chest (usually away from the apex to avoid the imaging window). Alternative positions are with the yellow electrode on the back and/or red in the centre of the chest. Consider more careful skin preparation or changing electrode stickers if the trace is not clear. Some machines allow you to rotate through lead combinations (e.g. I, II, III) to find the best trace. ECG gain can be changed to increase the size of the QRS complexes.
- Enter patient demographic details (and, ideally, details of body size) onto the machine.

Preparing machine and probe

- Set up an ergonomic orientation of machine, patient, and operator. This will depend on your preferred operator position. A standard way is to have the operator sitting behind the patient on the edge of the couch with their right arm holding the probe and wrapped over the patient. The machine is then operated with the left hand. Another standard method is to sit facing the patient holding the probe against the chest wall with the left hand (arm rested on the couch) and with machine operated by the right hand.
- Check transthoracic image settings on machine, with harmonic imaging (if available) and your preferred image post-processing options selected. Set overall gain, compress and transverse or lateral gain controls to standard positions.
- Make sure there is an ECG tracing on the echo machine and patient details are entered.
- Make sure image storage is possible (to magneto-optical disc, download to image server or videotape).
- Take the appropriate transthoracic probe, apply gel to transducer and start imaging.

Probe handling and image quality

- The probe should be held in one hand and pressed firmly against the chest wall. Varying the pressure will alter image quality. Ensure sufficient pressure to optimize the image but not too much to make it uncomfortable for the patient. The usual problem while learning is not to apply enough pressure to get good image quality.
- A layer of gel ensures good contact between probe and chest wall. It excludes any air (that would degrade image quality). However, too much gel makes it difficult to keep a stable position so, once a layer is established, try not to apply more gel as image quality will not improve.
- The probe has a dot on one side to orientate the probe in your hand with the image on the screen.
- The probe can be moved in multiple directions but the four key movements are (1) rotation around a point, (2) rocking back and forwards, (3) rocking side to side, and (4) sliding across the chest. Movements needed to improve image quality are usually quite small and with experience hand movements are almost subconscious.
- Remember that image quality may be improved by different patient or heart positions. These can be altered by physically rolling the patient, a little, one way or the other, readjusting the patient to ensure they are sitting up, or asking the patient to breathe in or out to move the diaphragm (and heart) up or down.
- Imaging well is hard work and requires concentration. If it is proving difficult to find, keep, or return to an image during a study remember a short break can help. Remove the probe from the chest, re-apply gel and start again.

2D image optimization

There are four things that can be altered to improve image quality. Check each when you change a view to ensure you have the optimal image. In certain situations a completely different approach is needed, e.g. contrast imaging.

- Contact between probe and chest—this minimizes acoustic loss between probe and heart. Ensure there is a sufficient layer of gel and that you are applying enough pressure on the probe (more pressure might be needed if there is significant fat or tissue under probe).
- Patient position—this can move the heart closer to the probe. Ensure the patient has not slipped out of position. See if rolling the patient slightly, one way or the other, improves the image.
- Cardiac and lung position—these two factors are altered by asking the patient to breath in or out. The heart moves up and down with the diaphragm and any lung tissue between the probe and heart (which contains air and therefore degrades the image) may also move out of the way. Ask the patient to breath in and out slowly. Watch the image. The best image may be at end inspiration or end expiration, or somewhere in between! Ask the patient to hold their breath when the image is at its best.
- Machine settings.
- Machines usually have *tissue harmonic imaging*, which should routinely be selected.
- Overall, as well as, transverse and lateral *gains* should be adjusted along with contrast controls (e.g. *compress*) to optimize contrast between blood and myocardium. Newer machines perform all these image optimization procedures automatically just by pressing an *optimization button*.

Maximize the frame rate (which determines resolution) while filling the screen with all required information. This can be done by adjusting *depth* to just behind the heart (or area of interest) and reducing *sector width* to the area being studied (particularly important for colour flow mapping and tissue Doppler, which reduce frame rate when switched on but, perversely, require relatively high frame rates to be useful.)

2D image acquisition

Standard acquisition

Images are acquired in a standard way—with a set sequence of views. The standard views should always be collected to ensure comprehensive data collection, with additional views when necessary. Even when there is a specific question a full dataset should be acquired to ensure nothing is missed.

Windows

There are 3 key areas or 'windows' on the chest and abdomen to collect standard images (with additional windows available if needed) (Fig. 2.1). It is normal to image through each window in turn starting with parasternal windows. However, it may be necessary to go back to windows as pathology is found that needs more detailed study.

1. Parasternal window

This window is usually just to the left of the sternum around the 3rd or 4th intercostal space. However, the best position for parasternal views varies with each patient. To find the best window move the probe up or down an intercostal space, and away from or towards the sternum.

2. Apical window

As the name suggests this is at the cardiac apex so normally will be at the bottom, left, lateral point of the chest. The apex beat may be felt under the probe. The window should, ideally, be from the true apex to avoid foreshortening. To optimize, ensure probe is lateral enough and move up or down an intercostal space.

3. Subcostal window

This lies below the xiphisternum in the epigastrium. Lie the patient on their back with stomach relaxed (may be easier if the patient bends their legs). Place probe on the abdomen, press it in and point it back up into the chest so that the image plane tucks under the ribs.

Additional windows

Suprasternal window

This is the suprasternal notch. Lie the patient on their back and raise the chin. Rest the probe in the notch and point it down into the chest.

Right parasternal window

This is often used to look at flow in the ascending aorta. A normal or a *stand alone* probe can be used. The patient should roll all the way over to lie on their right side. The window is on the right of the sternum usually slightly higher than the equivalent left parasternal window.

Supraclavicular window

This is rarely needed but can be used to look at vascular structures and the aorta. It lies above the clavicles.

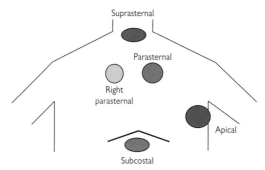

Fig. 2.1 Standard windows for transthoracic echocardiography.

Standard sequence of views

Parasternal windows
- Parasternal long axis view
- (Optional—parasternal right ventricle inflow)
- (Optional—parasternal right ventricle outflow)
- Parasternal short axis view (apex)
- Parasternal short axis view (papillary level)
- Parasternal short axis view (aortic level)
- (Optional—right parasternal window).

Apical window
- Apical four chamber
- Apical five chamber
- Apical two chamber
- Apical three chamber.

Subcostal window
- Subcostal long and short axis
- Inferior vena cava
- (Optional—aorta view).

Suprasternal window
- (Optional—aorta view).

3D image acquisition

3D acquisition differs in that it is used to supplement data collection to answer questions raised by 2D imaging. The windows selected are chosen to optimize data collection for a particular area of the heart. The probe is placed in the same positions on the chest as for 2D acquisition.

Windows

Apical window

The apical window is the main window used for 3D left and right ventricular acquisition. The setup of the image is nearly always the same as for 2D imaging with a need to identify the true apex. The probe can be altered to focus either on the right or left ventricle.

The apical window can also be used to evaluate the aortic, mitral, and tricuspid valves (Fig. 2.2).

Parasternal window

This is used in 3D echocardiography to acquire 3D datasets of the left ventricle, mitral, aortic, and tricuspid valves (Fig. 2.3). The window is found the same way as for 2D imaging as the 3D dataset is set up based on biplane 2D imaging. However, often modified parasternal windows are required in order to focus on a particular area of the heart, e.g. the tricuspid valve.

3D image optimization

When acquiring real-time 3D full volume datasets the following steps will help to optimize the final image:
- A good ECG signal with clear R wave is necessary to allow 3D full volume triggering.
- Adjust the scanner settings (as you would do for 2D imaging) to get the best 3D resolution:
  - Adjust gain setting.
  - Ensure the region of interest is within the 3D volume sector.
  - Minimize the sector (angle and depth) to focus on region of interest.
  - Maximize the number of subvolumes according to patient breath holding capability.
  - Select appropriate line density—the higher densities allow better resolution although at the expense of a narrower angle sector.
  - Optimize the volume size. All commercial scanners allow the final volume size to be adjusted slightly which may be beneficial in certain circumstances (e.g. dilated cardiomyopathy).
  - Acquire images with the probe maintained in a steady position and at end expiration.

Following acquisition, review image to look for any stitch artefacts. When happy with the image then accept the acquisition.

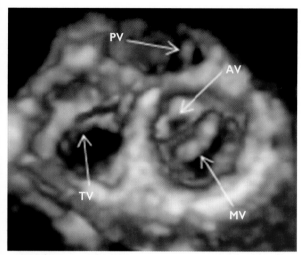

Fig. 2.2 3D full volume acquisition from the apical window. Subsequent rotation and cropping allows visualization of all 4 cardiac valves. AV = aortic valve; MV = mitral valve; PV = pulmonary valve; TV = tricuspid valve. See 🎞 Video 2.1.

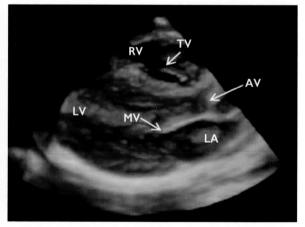

Fig. 2.3 Full volume 3D acquisition of the left ventricle (LV) imaged from the parasternal window. Rotation and cropping of the image shows the aortic valve (AV); left atrium (LA); mitral valve (MV); right ventricle (RV). With tilting the tricuspid valve (TV) is also seen. See 🎞 Video 2.2.

Multiplane image acquisition

Biplane imaging
- Commercial scanners allow the ability to view the image which is being acquired in two planes. Classically this has been used to assess left ventricular volumes and ejection fraction.
- Initially an optimal 4 chamber view of the left ventricle is acquired. When in biplane mode the orthogonal view (i.e. 2 chamber is shown in a split screen).
- Biplane has the advantage of maintaining the same probe position for the acquisition of both the 4 chamber and 2 chamber views thus reducing errors which may occur due to the use of different probe positions.
- Biplane echocardiography also has the advantage of viewing the target from 2 planes and so ensuring that foreshortening can be minimized.

Triplane imaging
- Recently, triplane imaging has allowed the target volume to be acquired and simultaneously viewed from 3 different orthogonal planes.
- When acquiring a 4 chamber view of the LV in triplane mode, the LV 2 chamber and 3 chamber views are simultaneously displayed (Fig. 2.4).

xPlane and iRotate
These modes available on Phillips echocardiography systems allow different planes selected by the operator to be imaged simultaneously from one acoustic window with a fixed probe position.
- *X-plane*: This has the advantage of being able to compare directly two individual planes side-by-side with the primary image displayed on the left and the secondary image selected by the operator (Fig. 2.5) displayed next to it.
- *iRotate*: In this technique the operator can alter the angle of the plane being viewed without moving the probe, using the controls on the machine, similar to changing the plane in TOE imaging.

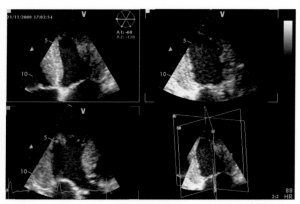

Fig. 2.4 Triplane acquisition of left ventricle: acquired 4 chamber apical view (top left); 2 chamber view (top right); 3 chamber view (bottom left) and representation of the acquired image planes (bottom right).

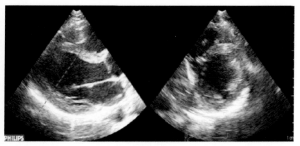

Fig. 2.5 xPlane mode (Phillips). The primary image (left) of parasternal LV view is acquired and a secondary imaging plane is selected (red dashed line) and secondary image of LV short axis is displayed on the right of the split screen. See 📹 Video 2.3.

Data acquisition

Techniques for each view

In each view, start the study with 2D imaging and then consider whether further echocardiography techniques are required to document the findings. Although a standard minimal dataset acquisition (📖 p.96) is vital, it is equally important that you analyse and interpret the images as you do the study. It is easy to save a standard set of images for later analysis but if you only notice pathology after the study you will not have acquired the right images. The preliminary analysis needed to search and identify pathology should be done during the study with detailed confirmation during later reporting. Consider in each view:

- Colour flow mapping
- M-mode
- CW Doppler
- PW Doppler
- Tissue Doppler imaging
- Speckle tracking imaging
- 3D imaging
- Contrast imaging.

In all views 2D and colour flow mapping are used. Most views also use CW and PW Doppler as well as occasional M-mode. In some views 3D, contrast and tissue Doppler imaging may be needed.

Image storage

- All images and data must be stored for future reference. With the current ease of storage it is no longer acceptable to perform an echocardiogram and only keep handwritten notes, even in emergencies.
- Images are usually stored and commonly then transferred directly to a main server. Digital storage is usually based on storing a single cardiac cycle loop, triggered off the ECG trace. If the patient has an arrhythmia with variable cardiac cycle length then it may be better to store 3–5 beats.
- It is desirable to have a digital laboratory to store all acquired views. Storage on digital media enables better post-processing and follow-up comparisons.

Formats

- The current preferred means of storage of studies is Digital Imaging and Communications in Medicine (DICOM). DICOM defines the way in which patient data is stored, transported, and retrieved.
- For movie storage image acquisitions can be stored commonly as AVI or MPEG formats.
- Widely used formats for still screen/non-movie storage for use in presentations include BMP, TIF, and JPEG.

Image compression

- In order to reduce overall storage requirements, image compression can be used.
- Image compression can either be *lossless or lossy*. Lossless image compression reduces the final file size by 2–5 times but allows an identical version of the original to be created if the compression is reversed. Lossy image compression reduces the final file size by a greater amount (up to 20 times) but this is at the potential expense of image degradation.

Parasternal long axis view

The first view. Gives an immediate over all impression of the major valves, left and right ventricle, aorta, and pericardium (Fig. 2.6).

Finding the view

- In the parasternal window hold the probe with the dot pointing to the right shoulder. Adjust probe with slight rotation and rocking.
- The optimal image cuts through the middle of mitral and aortic valves to display left ventricular inflow and outflow. Left ventricular walls lie parallel and straight across screen (anterior border of septum should be same distance from transducer as anterior wall of ascending aorta). Ascending aorta should be a tube with parallel walls.
- Sometimes not all structures can be aligned in a single view, in this situation record several views focused on each detail.

What to record?

- 2D images.
- Colour flow: aortic valve, left ventricle outflow tract, mitral valve.
- M-mode: aortic valve/left atrium, mitral valve, left ventricle.

What do you see?

Left ventricle: septum (anteroseptal portion), inferolateral (also sometimes called posterior) wall and cavity are seen. Use 2D (and M-mode) to assess left ventricle size, function, and hypertrophy. Also excellent for LV outflow tract size measurements and evidence of flow acceleration on colour flow. Septal defects may be seen with colour flow.

Aortic valve: right coronary cusp is at top and non-coronary cusp at bottom. 2D and M-mode can assess movement. Colour flow demonstrates regurgitation.

Aortic root: entire aortic root, including sinuses, sinotubular junction, and ascending aorta should be visible for measurement with 2D or M-mode.

Ascending aorta: slight adjustment by rocking the probe to one side can bring the proximal portion of the ascending aorta into view.

Descending aorta: seen in cross-section as a circle behind mitral valve. Use as landmark for studying pericardial and pleural fluid.

Mitral valve: A2 and P2 segments usually seen. 2D will pick up movement (prolapse, stenosis, etc.) and tip movement can be documented with M-mode. Use colour flow to identify regurgitation. Vena contracta or flow convergence may be evident.

Left atrium: left atrial size can be judged and measured with M-mode.

Right ventricle: the right ventricle lies near the probe and can be measured.

Pericardium: seen anteriorly in front of right heart and posteriorly behind heart. Good view to identify an effusion and measure size.

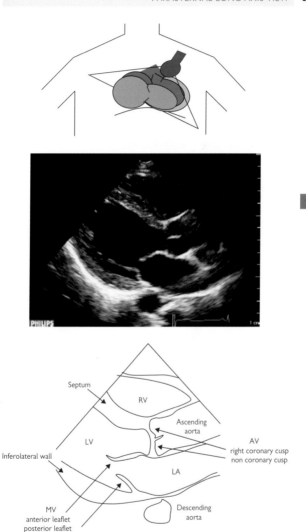

Fig. 2.6 Parasternal long axis view. See 🎬 Video 2.4.

Parasternal right ventricular inflow view

A useful extra view to look at tricuspid valve and right ventricular inflow (Fig. 2.7).

Finding the view

- From parasternal long axis view, rock probe slowly to point downwards. The tricuspid valve should come in to view. There usually needs to be some slight rotation to optimize the image.
- Optimal images demonstrate the tricuspid valve with right atrium behind and sometimes vena caval inflow.

What to record?

- 2D image.
- Colour flow across the tricuspid valve.
- CW and PW Doppler across the tricuspid valve.

What do you see?

- *Tricuspid valve:* main feature. Two leaflets seen in centre of screen. Use colour flow to document regurgitation. Jet may be aligned for Doppler measures of inflow and right ventricular systolic pressure.
- *Right atrium:* lies behind tricuspid valve and slight rotation may demonstrate right atrial appendage, Eustachian valve and inflow from vena cavae.
- *Right ventricle:* portion of right ventricle close to tricuspid valve seen.

Parasternal right ventricular outflow view

A useful extra view to look at pulmonary valve and artery (Fig. 2.7).

Finding the view

- From parasternal long axis view, rock probe slowly to point upwards. Pulmonary valve should come into view. Slight rotation will optimize image to include pulmonary artery.
- Optimal image demonstrates the pulmonary valve with pulmonary arterial trunk to bifurcation.

What to record?

- 2D image.
- Colour flow pulmonary valve.
- Continuous and pulsed wave Doppler across pulmonary valve.

What do you see?

- *Pulmonary valve:* main feature. Two leaflets seen in centre of screen. Use colour flow to document regurgitation. Jet normally aligned for Doppler measures of outflow and regurgitation.
- *Pulmonary artery:* in the far field. With slight adjustments can usually be followed to bifurcation. Can measure size and look for abnormal jets (patent ductus) or thrombus (pulmonary embolus).

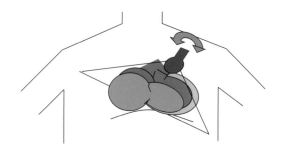

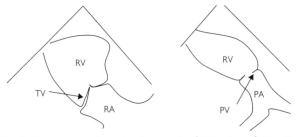

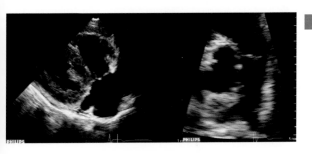

Fig. 2.7 Right ventricular inflow and outflow views. See Video 2.5 and Video 2.6.

Parasternal short axis (aortic) view

A series of parasternal short axis views are gathered in order to scan through the heart in cross-section. Together they give an impression of left ventricular function, aortic and mitral structure, and the right heart (Fig. 2.8).

Finding the view

• From the parasternal long axis view, rotate the probe around 90° so that the dot points to the left shoulder. Try and rotate from a long axis view with the aortic valve in the centre. Focus on keeping the valve in the centre and you should end up with the classic cross-section through the aortic valve.

• It can be difficult to get a true on-axis cut. To optimize the image try slight rotation around the point until the aortic valve appears circular with the right ventricle wrapped around the valve. Then rock the probe back and forward until the cut is straight.

• Optimal image should have a round aortic valve with 3 cusps evident. The tricuspid valve should be visible on the left and pulmonary valve on the right.

• If all structures are not seen remember to record several views focused on each detail.

What to record?

• 2D images.

• Colour flow: aortic, tricuspid, and pulmonary valve (also sometimes atrial septum).

• Doppler: pulmonary and tricuspid valve.

What do you see?

• *Aortic valve:* lies in centre with classic Y-shape: left coronary cusp on right, right towards the top, and non-coronary on the left. Use colour flow to identify regurgitation. Left main stem sometimes seen by left cusp.

• *Right ventricle:* basal right ventricle lies near the probe wrapped around aortic valve. Ventricle can be measured.

• *Tricuspid valve:* seen to left of aortic valve. Use colour flow to check for regurgitation. May be aligned for CW Doppler.

• *Pulmonary valve:* to right of aortic valve. Colour flow demonstrates regurgitation. CW and PW Doppler will document velocities.

• *Left atrium:* lies behind aortic valve.

• *Interatrial septum:* septum lies at 7 o'clock and view may be useful to identify septal defects with colour flow.

• *Pericardium:* seen anteriorly, in front of right heart.

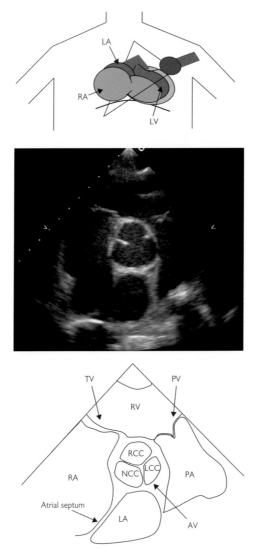

Fig. 2.8 Parasternal short axis (aortic) view. See 📹 Video 2.7.

Parasternal short axis (mitral) view

The classic *en face* or 'fish-mouth' view of the mitral valve (Fig. 2.9).

Finding the view
- From the parasternal short axis aortic view, rock the probe slightly towards the cardiac apex. By starting the parasternal cuts from the aortic valve the views tend to stay 'on-axis'.
- Optimal image should have a left ventricle with the 'fish mouth' mitral valve clearly seen.

What to record?
- 2D images. Consider 2D planimetry if stenosis.
- Consider colour flow across mitral valve, if regurgitation.

What do you see?
- *Mitral valve:* a classic *en face* view of the mitral valve to look at valve morphology (including the separate scallops) and movement. Consider colour flow or 3D imaging if abnormalities. Can also be used to measure valve opening with planimetry.

Parasternal short axis (ventricle) views

The classic short axis views of the left ventricle (Fig. 2.9).

Finding the view
- From the parasternal short axis mitral view, rock probe slightly more towards apex until left ventricle is in cross-section. The papillary level has the bodies of both papillary muscles evident.
- Further rocking towards apex creates an apical view distal to papillary muscles.
- Usually important to avoid off-axis images so that true assessment of left ventricle function is possible. Slight rotation helps bring out the circular ventricular shape. If it is proving very difficult to get a clear image consider moving the probe position slightly within the window.
- Optimal images should have a cross-section of the left ventricle.

What to record?
- 2D images at papillary level for measures: left ventricle size and mass.
- Consider a view recorded at apical level.
- Consider M-mode measures: left ventricle.
- Tissue Doppler imaging sometimes used in short axis.
- Speckle tracking imaging.

What do you see?
- *Left ventricle:* the short axis demonstrates septum, anterior, lateral, and inferior walls (in order clockwise). Use for measures of left ventricle size and thickness and to assess regional function of mid segments of walls.
- *Right ventricle:* right ventricle is seen as a crescent around the left ventricle. Use to judge right ventricle size, function, and haemodynamics.

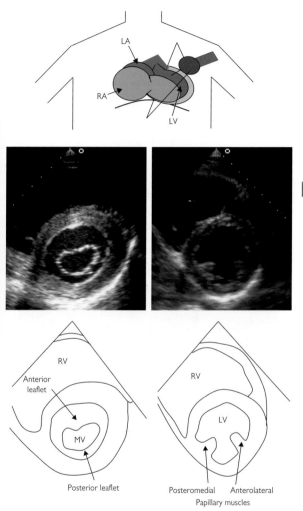

Fig. 2.9 Parasternal short axis (mitral and ventricle) views. See 📹 Video 2.8 and 📹 Video 2.9.

Parasternal 3D views

Finding the view

- The initial window is located in a similar fashion as for 2D acquisition with the probe marker pointing towards the right shoulder and the probe positioned in the 3rd or 4th intercostal space.
- Slight probe adjustment either laterally or medially to the sternum or manoeuvring the probe to an adjacent intercostal space will help identify the optimal position for acquisition.

What to record?

- Left ventricle full volume acquisition.
- Mitral valve full volume or live 3D acquisition.
- Mitral valve colour Doppler acquisition.
- Aortic valve full volume and/or live 3D acquisition.
- Aortic valve colour Doppler acquisition.

What do you see?

Similar anatomical landmarks can be appreciated as in the 2D view (Figs. 2.10 and 2.11). The advantage of 3D acquisition is appreciated following data collection when the dataset can be rotated to see anatomy (Fig. 2.12) and the spatial associations of different pathologies, e.g. mitral valve prolapse and the insertion of chordae.

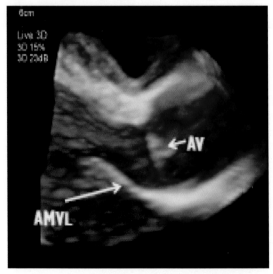

Fig. 2.10 3D live zoom acquisition of the aortic valve (AV) taken from the parasternal view. The anterior mitral valve leaflet is also seen (AMVL). See ♣ Video 2.10.

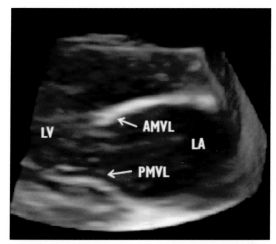

Fig. 2.11 3D live zoom acquisition of the mitral valve (MV) taken from the parasternal view. AMVL = anterior mitral valve leaflet; LA = left atrium; LV = left ventricle; PMVL = posterior mitral valve leaflet. See 📹 Video 2.11.

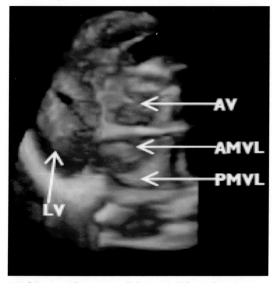

Fig. 2.12 Full volume 3D acquisition of left ventricle (LV) taken from the parasternal view. The image has been rotated and cropped to view from towards the left atrium. Image stopped in systole. The anterior mitral valve leaflet (AMVL) and posterior mitral valve leaflet (PMVL) and aortic valve (AV) position can be seen. See 📹 Video 2.12.

Apical four chamber view

Finding the view
- In the apical window, hold the probe with the dot pointing towards the couch.
- Probe needs to be as close to the left ventricular apex as possible so alter the image, focusing on obtaining the optimal left ventricular size and shape. The identifying characteristics of the apex are that it moves less than the other walls and is thinner. In a true apical view the left ventricle will be at its longest. Once you have identified the apex optimize the view with rotation and rocking to bring in the right ventricle, left and right atrium, as well as, mitral and tricuspid valves. Exclude the left ventricular outflow and aortic valve by tilting the probe.
- Optimal image should be at apex with both ventricles, both atria and both mitral and tricuspid valves visible. Septa should be straight down the centre of the image.

What to record?
- 2D images.
- Colour flow mapping: mitral and tricuspid valves.
- CW and PW Doppler: mitral and tricuspid valve.
- Consider Doppler of right upper pulmonary vein.
- Consider tissue Doppler imaging of right and left ventricle.
- Speckle tracking.
- 3D datasets.
- When appropriate use contrast.

What do you see ? (Fig. 2.13)
- *Mitral valve*: A2 and P2 segments of mitral valve are seen. 2D for movement. Colour flow mapping will show regurgitation (vena contracta, flow convergence, etc.) Doppler well aligned for stenosis and valve inflow. Tissue Doppler of lateral and septal sides of mitral ring may be possible.
- *Tricuspid valve:* lateral and septal leaflets displayed. As for mitral valve, colour flow, Doppler and tissue Doppler are possible.
- *Left and right atrium:* both atria and the interatrial septum can be seen. Pulmonary veins as well as vena cavae may be seen in far field. Use to measure atrial volumes.
- *Left ventricle:* key view to study global and regional left ventricle function. Septum, apex, and lateral wall are displayed. Good for 2D volume measures if endocardial border is clear. If assessing left ventricle function consider contrast and/or 3D to improve left ventricle data collection. Tissue Doppler of different wall segments is also possible.
- *Right ventricle:* a key view to look at right ventricle size and function. Usually compared relative to left but also tissue Doppler or M-mode of tricuspid free wall annulus can be considered.
- *Pericardium:* important view to see size and location of pericardial fluid. May also be used for ultrasound-guided pericardiocentesis.

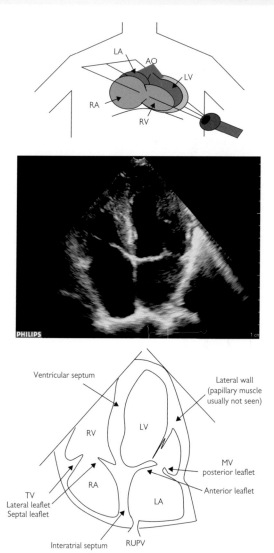

Fig. 2.13 Apical four chamber view. See ▣ Video 2.13.

Apical five chamber view

Used to look at left ventricular outflow and aortic valve (Fig. 2.14).

Finding the view

- From the apical four chamber view tilt the probe to bring the aortic valve and outflow tract into view.
- Sometimes a better alignment through aortic valve and ascending aorta is obtained by moving probe laterally on chest wall (more into axilla).
- This foreshortens left ventricle and alters alignment for other valves so use only to study the aortic valve.
- Optimal image looks similar to apical four chamber but with the aortic valve evident and ascending aorta in far field.

What to record?

- 2D images.
- Colour flow mapping: aortic valve.
- CW and PW Doppler: aortic valve and left ventricle outflow tract.

What do you see?

- *Aortic valve:* right and non-coronary cusps (although may not be easy to see). Colour flow demonstrates regurgitation. CW for stenosis and regurgitation.
- *Left ventricular outflow tract:* use colour flow mapping for aortic regurgitation or flow turbulence due to obstruction. Best view to place PW Doppler to assess outflow and obstruction.

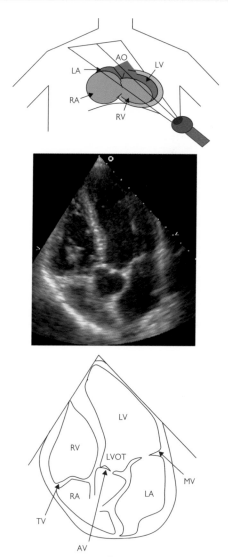

Fig. 2.14 Apical five chamber view. See 🎥 Video 2.14.

Apical two chamber view

An important view for global and regional left ventricular assessment (Fig. 2.15).

Finding the view

- From the apical four chamber view, rotate the probe around 90° anticlockwise. Watch the picture and try and keep the mitral valve in place. If the apex of the ventricle changes you were probably not at the apex and are foreshortening.
- Keep rotating until right ventricle disappears completely but before left ventricular outflow tract comes into view.
- Optimal image contains left ventricle (no right ventricle) from apex, centred in the image. Mitral valve is cut through the commissure. Left atrium is in far field and left atrial appendage may be visible.

What to record?

- 2D images.
- Consider Colour flow and Doppler measures across mitral valve.
- Consider tissue Doppler imaging of ventricle.

What do you see?

- **Left ventricle:** inferior wall on left, and anterior wall on right. Good for regional assessment. Use plane for ventricle volume measures and tissue Doppler of wall segments.
- **Mitral valve:** ideal image is of a commissural view with P3, A2, and P1 segments visible from left to right. Colour flow and Doppler measures are possible as well as assessment of the long axis of the mitral valve ring.
- **Left atrial appendage:** sometimes visible as a curved finger pointing towards probe around right side of mitral valve.
- **Coronary sinus:** the coronary sinus is usually seen in cross-section on the left of the mitral valve.

Adaptation of view

- *Right ventricle:* slight tilting of probe to point forwards can scan into a two chamber view of right ventricle (not a standard view).

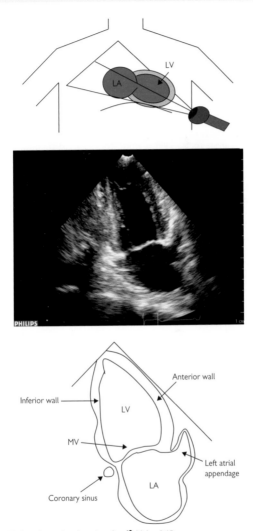

Fig. 2.15 Apical two chamber view. See 📹 Video 2.15.

Apical three chamber view

Similar to the parasternal long axis view but includes left ventricular apex (Fig. 2.16).

Finding the view

- From the apical two chamber view continue rotating the probe anticlockwise to around 135° from the four chamber view.
- Watch the picture and keep the mitral valve in place, rotating until the left ventricle outflow and aortic valve come into view. As for the translation from four to two chamber.
- Optimal image contains left ventricle from apex straight down the screen with mitral valve, left atrium, left ventricle outflow, and aortic valve in far field.

What to record?

- 2D images.
- Consider tissue Doppler and speckle tracking imaging of ventricle.
- Consider colour flow and Doppler measurements across aortic valve as may be well aligned.
- Consider colour flow and Doppler measures across mitral valve.

What do you see?

- *Left ventricle:* good view to assess septum on right of image, apex and inferolateral (posterior) wall on left of image.
- *Aortic valve:* right coronary cusp is on right and non-coronary cusp on left. Colour flow will demonstrate regurgitation and valve is usually aligned for Doppler measurements.
- *Mitral valve:* A2 and P2 segments of valve seen and can consider colour flow and other Doppler measures if not enough detail from other views.
- *Left atrium:* atrium lies behind mitral valve.

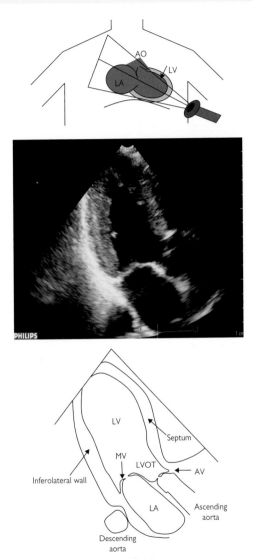

Fig. 2.16 Apical three chamber view. See 📹 Video 2.16.

Apical 3D views

Finding the view

- The initial window is located in a similar fashion as for 2D acquisition of the apical four chamber view (see 📖 p. 78).

What to record?

- Left ventricle full volume acquisition.
- Right ventricle full volume acquisition.
- Mitral valve full volume and live 3D acquisition.
- Mitral valve colour Doppler acquisition.
- Aortic valve full volume and live 3D acquisition.
- Aortic valve colour Doppler acquisition.
- Tricuspid valve full volume and live 3D acquisition.
- Tricuspid valve colour Doppler acquisition.

What do you see?

Similar anatomical landmarks can be appreciated as in the 2D view (Fig. 2.17). Following data acquisition, the 3D image can be rotated to make it easier to understand how any pathology relates to the different parts of the heart.

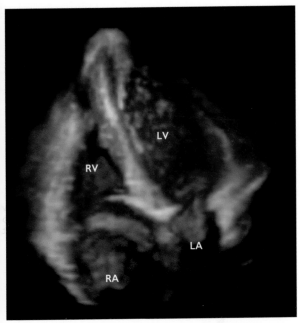

Fig. 2.17 Full volume 3D acquisition of the right ventricle (RV) imaged from the apical window. LA = left atrium; LV = left ventricle; RA = right atrium. See 🎞 Video 2.17.

Subcostal views

Very useful views to study pericardial effusions, assess right ventricular inflow, and screen for septal defects (Fig. 2.18). Also, alternative window for equivalent of parasternal views if parasternal window not possible.

Finding the view

- In the subcostal window have the probe flat and pressed into the stomach so that the imaging plane is directed upwards under the ribs.
- With slight rotation and tilting back and forward you will find the heart. You will need to increase the depth. If it is difficult to get an image, ask the patient to take a breath in. This drops the diaphragm and often brings the heart into view. Once you have found the heart optimize the image with gentle movements of the probe.
- Optimal image will look like a four chamber view but from the side. Both ventricles and both atria should be seen with the atrial and ventricular septa aligned horizontally across the screen. Both mitral and aortic valves should be evident.
- The probe can also be rotated 90° in this view to create a short axis subcostal view. By tilting back and forward this can be used to look at left and right ventricle and pulmonary valve.

What to record?

- 2D images.
- Colour flow mapping: tricuspid valve and septa (atrial and ventricular).

What do you see?

- *Right ventricle:* close to probe and both free wall and septum are seen. Wall thickness can be measured. The septum is flat across the screen so good alignment for colour flow mapping of septal defects.
- *Right atrium:* good view to look at right ventricle inflow as close to probe. May see Eustachian valve and entry of inferior vena cava. Because of horizontal alignment of interatrial septum an ideal view for colour flow mapping of atrial septal defects and Doppler alignment to quantify flow across defects.
- *Tricuspid valve:* close to probe and can be used for colour flow mapping of regurgitation.
- *Pericardium:* excellent view to assess size and depth of effusion when planning pericardiocentesis as probe in position of a subxiphisternum approach.
- *Left ventricle:* in far field. Septum and lateral wall are seen.
- *Mitral valve:* in far field and little extra information provided.
- *Left atrium:* little extra information provided about left atrium.

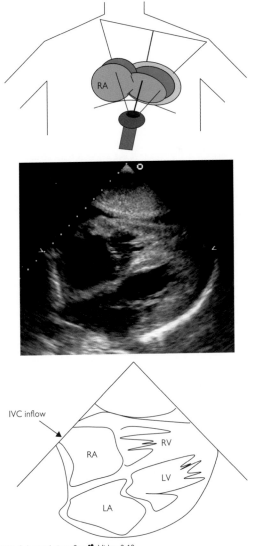

Fig. 2.18 Subcostal view. See 📹 Video 2.18.

Inferior vena cava view

Essential to assess right atrial pressure (Fig. 2.19).

Finding the view
- From the subcostal view rotate the probe anti-clockwise.
- Keep the right atrium in the centre of the image and focus on the atrium as you rotate the probe. The opening of the inferior vena cava should become more obvious. As you rotate the probe the vena cava should open out into a long tubular structure horizontally across the screen. If you are worried it may be the aorta, not the vena cava, use pulsed wave Doppler to demonstrate continuous, low velocity venous flow rather than pulsatile, high velocity aortic flow.
- Optimal image is of the vena cava like a railway track across the screen perhaps seen opening into right atrium. Hepatic veins emptying into vena cava may also be seen.

What to record?
- 2D images with inspiration and expiration (a 5-beat loop may be required).
- M-mode measures with respiration.
- Consider pulsed wave Doppler in aligned hepatic veins.

What do you see?
- *Inferior vena cava:* use to measure diameter and whether it reduces in size with inspiration (normally should do).
- *Liver and hepatic veins:* these can be seen draining into the vena cava and may be aligned for Doppler measures. If right atrial pressures are high they may be dilated.

Abdominal aorta view

Not an essential view but interesting (Fig. 2.19)! A simple screening test for aortic aneurysm.

Finding the view
- From the subcostal inferior vena cava view tilt the probe out of the plane of the inferior vena cava. The aorta should come into view and look very similar to the vena cava. It usually lies to the left of the vena cava and slightly deeper. Confirm it is aorta with PW Doppler to demonstrate arterial flow.
- Optimal image is of the aorta like a 'railway track' across the screen.

What to record?
- 2D images.

What do you see?
- *Aorta:* may see wall thickening, aneurysm or even gross mobile thrombus and plaque.

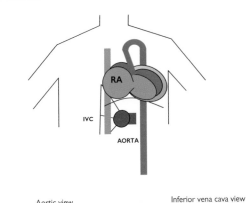

Aortic view   Inferior vena cava view

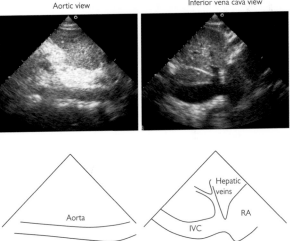

Fig. 2.19 Subcostal abdominal aorta view (left) and inferior vena cava view (right). See 📷 Video 2.19.

Suprasternal view

A view to look at size of aorta and aortic flow for coarctation or aortic regurgitation (Fig. 2.20).

Finding the view

- In the suprasternal window have the probe pointing, slightly rotated, into the chest behind the sternum. The dot on the probe should be towards the left shoulder. Use light pressure (with extra gel to maintain contact between probe and skin if necessary) as it can be uncomfortable.
- Tilt probe back and forward until the arch comes into view then rotate to maximize the curve of the arch. Colour flow may help identify flow in the aorta.
- Optimal image has distal ascending aorta, arch, and proximal descending aorta with origin of the left subclavian on the right, and potentially origin of left carotid and brachiocephalic.

What to record?

- 2D images.
- Doppler of flow in ascending and descending aorta.
- Consider colour flow mapping around arch and subclavian artery (looking for jets associated with patent ductus arteriosus, coarctation or obstruction).

What do you see?

- *Aortic arch:* curves through picture and can be measured.
- *Ascending aorta:* can be difficult to see clearly but can provide alignment for CW Doppler measures in aortic stenosis.
- *Descending aorta:* usually better seen than ascending aorta. Size can be measured and is aligned for Doppler studies of aortic flow to grade aortic regurgitation or coarctations.
- *Left subclavian artery:* easiest branch to see and important landmark for isthmus (common site of dissection and coarctation).

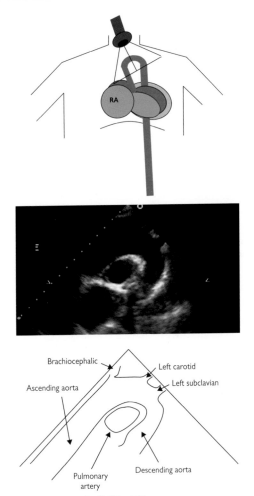

Fig. 2.20 Suprasternal view. See 📹 Video 2.20.

Right parasternal view

An extra view to look at ascending aorta and judge severity of aortic stenosis but can be difficult to find (Fig. 2.21).

Finding the view
- Roll patient over onto right side. Place probe on right side of sternum pointing down and under sternum (both stand alone and 2D probes can be used).
- Adjust probe in all directions looking for Doppler across aortic valve and up ascending aorta. If using stand alone Doppler probe look for the aortic spectral pattern and if using a 2D probe use colour flow mapping to identify ascending aorta. Once a signal has been found keep adjusting probe position until maximal Doppler signal.
- Optimal image has ascending aortic flow aligned with probe.

What to record?
- 2D images with colour flow to demonstrate aorta.
- CW Doppler of flow through aortic valve.

What do you see?
- *Ascending aorta:* often little to see but can be very useful for a second measure of an aortic gradient if there is concern that it is being underestimated. The alignment of flow through the aortic valve for Doppler measures is often better in the right parasternal view than the apical or suprasternal views.

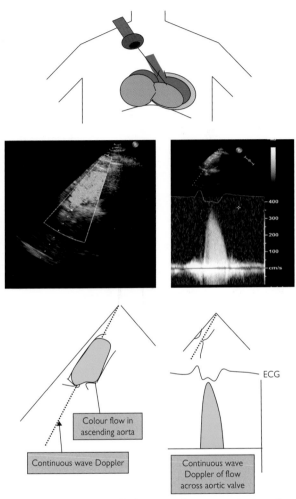

Fig. 2.21 Right parasternal view. Used to measure flow across aortic valve and in ascending aorta.

Standard examination

The minimal sequence of views and measurements needed to perform a study can be standardized to ensure collection of a *minimal dataset*. Minimal datasets are published by bodies of experts as a guide to what information should be collected.

A graphic description of a standard examination in the order of data collection is given in Figs. 2.22–2.29.

Quality of echocardiographic recordings

The quality of echocardiographic recordings is based on:
- Is the dataset complete i.e. a full standard examination and minimal dataset?
- Are all the recordings obtained from the appropriate imaging points, i.e. correct apical position etc.?
- Is image quality good, i.e. are the views appropriately recorded, correct gain and depth, etc.?

Image quality

2D/3D imaging is best judged on endocardial border definition. Look at the proportion of the border that is clearly seen in the 3 apical views. Judge image quality as:
- Good if >80% of the border is seen in the 3 apical views.
- Poor if the endocardium is not visible.
- Image quality is moderate if endocardial border is visible but <80%. For stress echocardiography good image quality is required and there should be a maximum of 2 segments not seen in any view.

Spectral Doppler should be judged as:
- Good if the cursor position is displayed, there is good alignment (with the angle between flow and beam <30°) and the spectrum has a clear envelope.
- Poor if the angle between flow and beam is >30° or the spectrum is incomplete.
- Only good spectral Doppler tracing should be used for quantitative analysis.

Colour flow mapping should be judged as:
- Good if the flow of interest is aligned with the probe and gain settings are correct (just below the level that produces background noise). If for flow convergence, the baseline has been shifted.
- Poor if the flow is not aligned or gain settings are incorrect.
- For assessment of regurgitation colour flow mapping must be good.

When used to align spectral Doppler then suboptimal settings may be sufficient.

Parasternal long axis view

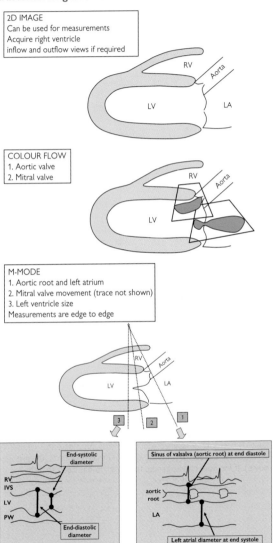

2D IMAGE
Can be used for measurements
Acquire right ventricle
inflow and outflow views if required

RV
Aorta
LV
LA

COLOUR FLOW
1. Aortic valve
2. Mitral valve

RV
Aorta
LV

M-MODE
1. Aortic root and left atrium
2. Mitral valve movement (trace not shown)
3. Left ventricle size
Measurements are edge to edge

RV
Aorta
LV
LA

3   2   1

End-systolic diameter
RV
IVS
LV
PW
End-diastolic diameter

Sinus of valsalva (aortic root) at end diastole
aortic root
LA
Left atrial diameter at end systole

Fig. 2.22 Summary of parasternal long axis view.

Parasternal short axis view—ventricle and mitral valve

2D IMAGE
Assess LV function and regional abnormalities
Assess RV
Can be used for M-mode or 2D measures of LV size and function

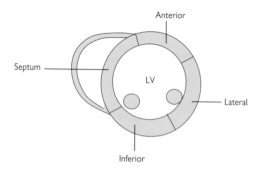

2D IMAGE
Assess mitral valve morphology
Consider colour flow across mitral valve and planimetry

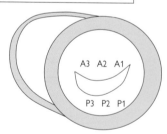

Fig. 2.23 Summary of parasternal short axis view.

Parasternal short axis view—aortic valve level

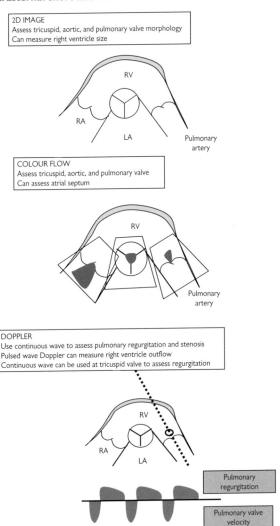

Fig. 2.24 Summary of short axis view—aortic valve level.

Apical views—four chamber

2D IMAGE
Assess LV size, thickness, function, and regional wall motion
Assess RV size and function
Look at mitral and tricuspid morphology

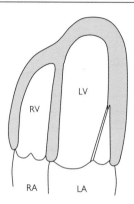

COLOUR FLOW
Assess mitral and tricuspid valves

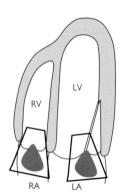

Fig. 2.25 Summary of apical four chamber view.

Apical views—four chamber: Doppler

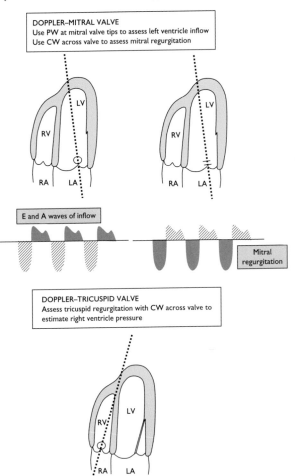

DOPPLER–MITRAL VALVE
Use PW at mitral valve tips to assess left ventricle inflow
Use CW across valve to assess mitral regurgitation

E and A waves of inflow

Mitral regurgitation

DOPPLER–TRICUSPID VALVE
Assess tricuspid regurgitation with CW across valve to estimate right ventricle pressure

Tricuspid regurgitation velocity

Fig. 2.26 Summary of apical four chamber view—Doppler.

Apical views—five chamber

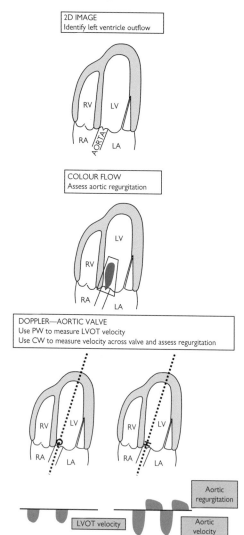

Fig. 2.27 Summary of apical five chamber view.

Apical views—two and three chamber

2D IMAGE
Assess LV function and regional abnormalities
Assess mitral valve morphology

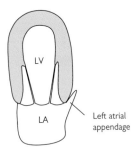

2D IMAGE
Assess LV function and regional abnormalities
Assess mitral and aortic valve morphology
Can use Doppler at aortic and mitral valves

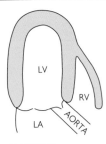

Fig. 2.28 Summary of apical two chamber view.

Subcostal and suprasternal views

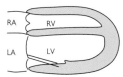

2D IMAGE
Assess right heart and look for pericardial effusion

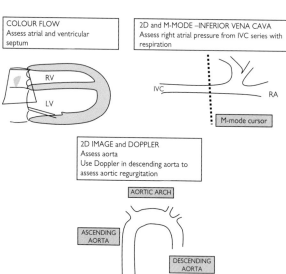

COLOUR FLOW
Assess atrial and ventricular septum

2D and M-MODE –INFERIOR VENA CAVA
Assess right atrial pressure from IVC series with respiration

2D IMAGE and DOPPLER
Assess aorta
Use Doppler in descending aorta to assess aortic regurgitation

Fig. 2.29 Summary of subcostal and suprasternal views.

Transthoracic anatomy and pathology: valves

Mitral valve

Normal anatomy

The mitral valve has two leaflets (anterior and posterior). The posterior is long and thin, and forms a crescent around the wider anterior leaflet. The surface area of both leaflets is approximately equal but the distance between mitral ring and coaption line is shorter on the posterior leaflet. Each leaflet has 3 scallops which meet each other along the coaption line. They are named: A1, A2, A3 (anterior) and P1, P2, P3 (posterior). P1 and A1 are adjacent to the anterolateral commissure and A3 and P3 nearest the right heart. Below the valve are two papillary muscles: a larger antero-lateral (usually a single trunk) and a smaller posteromedial (often 2–3 distinct trunks). These support chordae tendinae: 1st order attached to leaflet tips, 2nd order to undersurface of leaflets, and 3rd order run directly from ventricular wall to leaflet undersurface. Chordae from both papillary muscle attach to both leaflets. The valve leaflets are supported by the mitral valve annulus, which divides the left atrium and ventricle, and is a fibrous elliptical structure.

Normal findings

2D views

- The mitral valve can be seen in most views (Fig. 3.1). Parasternal long axis and parasternal short axis (mitral valve level) are particularly useful to look at valve motion and structure.
- The 3 apical views offer the ability to scan through the mitral valve in multiple planes and do Doppler measurements.

2D findings

- Parasternal long axis: segments of the anterior leaflet (A2—nearest the left ventricular outflow tract) and posterior leaflet (P2) are seen as thin structures uniform in echogenicity. The posteromedial papillary muscle may be seen attached to the posterior wall.
- Parasternal short axis: at the mitral valve level, all three segments of each leaflet are seen and the 2 commissures. This creates the classic 'fish mouth' appearance. At the mid level of the left ventricle the bodies of the two papillary muscles can be seen.
- Apical 4-chamber view: the A2 and A1 segments of the anterior leaflet are shown on the left and the P1 segment of the posterior leaflet on the right. The mitral valve annulus is usually slightly out of line with the tricuspid valve annulus (the tricuspid annulus is normally up to 1cm closer to the right ventricular apex).
- Apical 2-chamber view: the P1 and P3 segments are seen either side of the A2 segment of the anterior mitral valve leaflet.
- Apical 3-chamber view: the A2 and P2 segments are visualized similar to the parasternal long axis view.

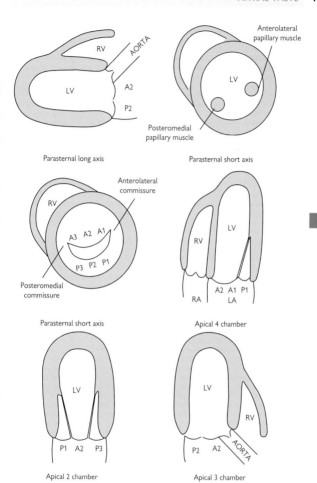

Fig. 3.1 Standard echocardiography views of mitral valve.

3D views

- Real-time 3D transthoracic imaging is now available and is an excellent tool in assessment of the mitral valve. Biplane 2D live images are optimized to ensure accurate probe position to assess the lesion in question before full volume acquisition.
- The parasternal long axis, parasternal short axis basal ventricular level and apical 4-chamber views are the most suitable for imaging the mitral valve in 3D.
- All the 3D acquisitions modes (📖 p.34) can be used: full volume datasets/live 3D imaging (Fig. 3.2)/live 3D zoom and 3D colour Doppler imaging.
- 3D echocardiography findings are enhanced by rotation and cropping of the 3D volume either after acquisition or during live monitoring.
- This rotation allows the mitral valve to be viewed from multiple angles and allows for the generation of specialized views such as the 'surgeons view'. i.e. a view of the mitral valve from the left atrium with the left atrial appendage on the left and the aorta at the top of the image.

3D findings

- Use the surgeon's view to assess all 3 scallops of the anterior and posterior leaflets.
- 3D mitral valve reconstruction and post-processing also allows the unique shaped curvature of the mitral valve to be modelled for precise measures of annulus size, extent of prolapse, etc.

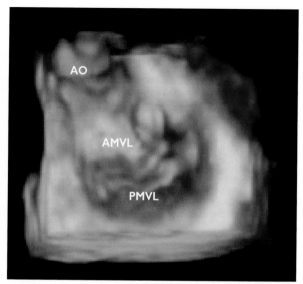

Fig. 3.2 Live 3D acquisition of mitral valve. Subsequent rotation and cropping to allow visualization of the valve from the LV apex. AMVL = anterior mitral valve leaflet; PMVL = posterior mitral valve leaflet and aorta (AO). See 🎬 Video 3.1.

Mitral stenosis

General

The commonest cause of mitral stenosis is still rheumatic disease. Systemic lupus erythematosus is a rare cause and congenital mitral stenosis is very rare. Clinically, atrial myxoma and cor triatriatum may mimic mitral stenosis. Mitral annular calcification is common in the elderly and can involve the entire posterior part of the annulus. Occasionally annular calcification can extend to the base of the leaflets leading to stenosis but more commonly leads to regurgitation.

Assessment

- Echocardiography should be used to diagnose stenosis and describe probable aetiology based on appearance.
- Severity should be graded according to: valve area; pressure gradient across the valve; changes to left atrium, left ventricle, and right heart.
- The examination should also be used to look for associated valvular lesions (in particular rheumatic aortic disease) and complications such as endocarditis.

Appearance

Comment on the valve:

- Mobility of base of leaflet compared to tips. In rheumatic disease the tips tend to be restricted so the valve appears to 'dome'. This may also be referred to as a 'hockey stick' or'elbowing' appearance (Fig. 3.3).
- Thickening or calcification of leaflets, annulus and subvalvular apparatus.
- Evidence of fusion of the commissures. Use a short axis view.
- Chordae—thickening, shortening, calcification.

Comment on associated features:

- Associated valvular lesions (aortic rheumatic disease).
- Left atrium:
  - Usually grossly enlarged. Give measurement.
  - Spontaneous left atrial contrast (associated with significant stenosis and suggests very slow atrial blood flow or stasis).
- Right heart:
  - Tricuspid regurgitation and right ventricular pressure.
  - Right ventricle and atrial size.
- Left ventricular function.

Differentiation of rheumatic mitral stenosis from calcification

In rheumatic disease (in contrast to degenerative mitral valve disease):
- Thickening comes first with calcification later.
- Leaflet thickening affects the commissures and leaflet edges whereas mitral annular calcification tends to spare the leaflet tips.
- There is subvalvular involvement with shortening of chordae.
- Combination of loss of leaflet mobility due to commissural fusion and chordal shortening and tethering leads to 'doming' or 'hockey-stick' appearance of, in particular, the anterior leaflet.

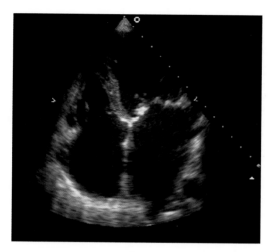

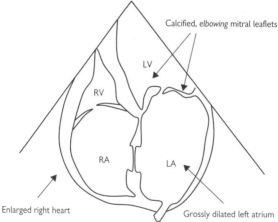

Fig. 3.3 Apical 4-chamber view demonstrating rheumatic mitral stenosis with doming, calcified valve. The left atrium is grossly dilated. See 🎞 Video 3.2.

Grading of mitral stenosis

- Grade stenosis as mild, moderate, or severe based on *valve area* (Table 3.1). Use *planimetered* measurements and *pressure half-time* across the valve. Also, report the actual measures.
- Back this up with assessment of *pressure gradient* across the valve.
- Comment on associated changes that support your assessment. Include changes to the *left atrium* and *right-sided pressures*.

Planimetry: 2D

- In parasternal short axis view, angle the probe to the mitral valve level.
- Move the probe back and forth until you are sure you are at the level of the *leaflet tips*. If the plane is too basal, stenosis will be underestimated.
- Record a loop and scroll through to find the maximum opening in diastole (Fig. 3.4).
- Trace along the *inner edge* of the leaflets. This may be difficult in heavily calcified valves so comment if there is a lot of calcification.
- Report the surface area of the orifice.

3D in assessment of mitral stenosis

3D transthoracic echocardiography (Fig. 3.5) is more accurate, quicker and reproducible than 2D for planimetered measures because it is easier to be confident you have the smallest area. To planimeter mitral valve area in 3D:

- Optimize a 3D view from the parasternal short axis mitral valve level. Using this view reduces distance between probe and valve, so will improve resolution.
- Ensure the volume includes the 'mouth' of the mitral valve to ensure planimetry of the stenosis is possible.
- Acquire a volume dataset and then use postprocessing software such as QLAB (Philips) to identify the 2D plane that cuts through the mitral leaflet tips. Then trace around the inner edge of the leaflets as for 2D imaging.
- Report the surface area of the orifice.

Problems with planimetry

- Planimetered mitral area methods are useful as they are not affected by haemodynamic changes but can overestimate size if the tips of the leaflets are not identified.
- It is important when estimating the planimetered area that the optimal plane is used to ensure that the smallest area from the leaflets free edge is traced.

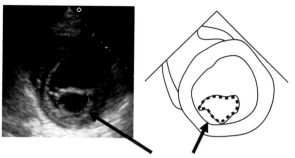

Planimetered orifice

Fig. 3.4 2D planimetered mitral valve orifice in parasternal short axis.

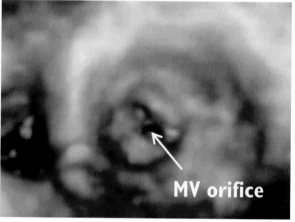

MV orifice

Fig. 3.5 Full volume acquisition of mitral valve taken from apical 4-chamber view. Subsequent rotation and cropping to view this valve of a patient with mitral stenosis from the atrial side. Image shown at end diastole. See ⛶ Video 3.3.

Pressure half-time

- In the apical 4-chamber view get a good view of the mitral valve.
- Align continuous wave Doppler with the inflow jet through the stenosis. Try and minimize any angle between the beam and the jet.
- Record a spectral trace and measure the slope of the diastolic flow across the valve (Fig. 3.6).
- Use the E-wave if both E-wave (diastolic filling) and A-wave (atrial systole) are present (often there is no A-wave because the patient is in atrial fibrillation). If the trace is slightly curved with a steep start (a 'ski-slope'). Ignore the start and use the flatter portion.
- The machine automatically reports pressure half-time and mitral valve area. The relation between these measures is simple:

$$\text{Mitral valve area} \left(\text{in cm}^2\right) = 220/\text{pressure half-time} \left(\text{in ms}\right)$$

Mean transmitral valve diastolic pressure gradient

- Use the same technique/recording as used for pressure half-time.
- Trace the Doppler profile of the transmitral diastolic flow. The machine automatically reports the mean pressure gradient.
- Pressure gradient varies significantly with the filling time. If the patient is in atrial fibrillation this will vary so report the mean of 2–3 beats.

Problems with pressure half-time and pressure gradient

- Quantification based on pressure half-time assumes normal left ventricle pathophysiology. Significant changes in left ventricular compliance (e.g. left ventricular hypertrophy) or pathology that increases left ventricular pressure during diastole (e.g. aortic regurgitation) shorten the pressure half time. Valve area is overestimated.
- Normal atrial pathophysiology is also assumed. An atrial septal defect with left-to-right shunt shortens the pressure half time (as blood also leaves from left to right atrium) and valve area is overestimated. Conversely a right-to-left shunt will lengthen the pressure half time.

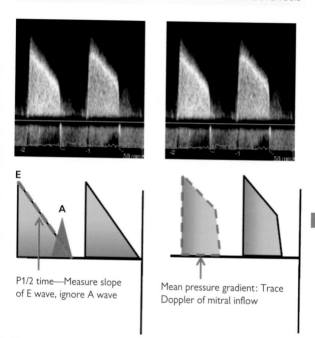

Fig. 3.6 Pressure half-time and mean pressure gradient.

Table 3.1 Parameters to determine severity of mitral stenosis

	Mild	Moderate	Severe
MV area (cm²)	2.2–1.5	1.5–1.0	<1.0
MV pressure half-time (ms)	100–150	150–220	>220
Mean pressure gradient (mmHg)	<5	Variable	>10
Tricuspid regurgitant velocity (m/s)	<2.7	Variable	>3
Pulmonary artery pressure (mmHg)	<30	Variable	>50

Mitral regurgitation

General
Mitral regurgitation is common. A trace of 'physiological' mitral regurgitation is seen in up to 50% of people with normal cardiac anatomy. Pathological mitral regurgitation can be caused by changes in the leaflets (e.g. endocarditis, myxomatous change), subvalvular apparatus (e.g. papillary muscle rupture) or mitral annulus (e.g. left ventricular dilatation).

Assessment
- Mitral regurgitation is easily identified with colour flow placed over the mitral valve and left atrium in parasternal long axis and apical views.
- Once identified a wider study of the appearance of the valve, subvalvular apparatus, and left ventricle should be used to determine aetiology and impact on cardiac function.
- Severity should be judged by combining measurements from all main Doppler modalities (colour flow, continuous and pulsed wave) and 2D echocardiography.

Appearance
- Map the *regurgitant jet* with colour flow in parasternal and apical views (Fig. 3.7). Establish the shape and pattern. Comment on:
  - Where the regurgitation passes through the valve, e.g. central, by a commissure, or through a perforation.
  - The direction of eccentric jets (anterior or posterior). Anteriorly-directed suggests a posterior leaflet problem and posteriorly-directed suggests an anterior leaflet problem. Note which left atrial wall the jet entrains against and how far back it goes.
  - If there are several jets, comment on each one.
  - Spectral Doppler and colour M-mode can define the timing of regurgitation e.g. confined to a short period after valve closure (closing volume) or to late systole (often found in mitral valve prolapse).
- In parasternal and apical views use M-mode and 2D to look at both *valve leaflets*. Comment on:
  - Movement, evidence of prolapse, calcification, masses, vegetations.
- Look at *subvalvular apparatus*. Comment on:
  - Papillary muscle and chordae with reference to shortening, rupture.
- Report associated features:
  - Left atrial size, left ventricular size and function—important when considering surgery, any changes to right heart and right ventricular systolic pressure.

Physiological, mild, or trace (trivial) regurgitation

It is reasonable to decide mitral regurgitation is *mild* if:
- Jet is small (jet area <4 cm^2 or <20% left atrial area) and central.
- No flow convergence zone is displayed.
- Trace regurgitation is a qualitative description that implies 'not as severe as mild.'

To call mitral regurgitation *physiological* make sure:
- Valve morphology is normal.
- The regurgitation has a short duration (typically post valve closure).
- It is mild or trivial.

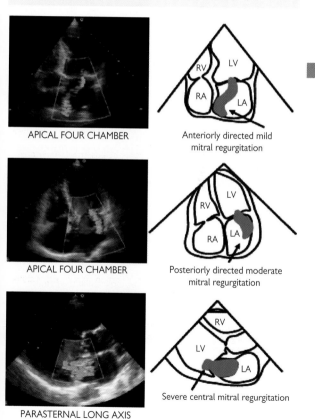

APICAL FOUR CHAMBER

Anteriorly directed mild mitral regurgitation

APICAL FOUR CHAMBER

Posteriorly directed moderate mitral regurgitation

PARASTERNAL LONG AXIS

Severe central mitral regurgitation

Fig. 3.7 Colour flow mapping of mitral regurgitation with eccentric and central jets. See 📹 Video 3.4, 📹 Video 3.5, 📹 Video 3.6.

Grading severity

- Gauge severity as mild, moderate or severe based on the combination of *jet area, vena contracta, flow convergence (PISA)* and changes in *systolic pulmonary vein flow* (if technically possible) (Table 3.2).
- Gross pathology, e.g. a flail leaflet, points to severe regurgitation.
- Once you have an impression of severity use *CW Doppler waveform density*, changes in left ventricular *mitral inflow*, and left ventricular function to support your assessment.
- You can provide further quantification of regurgitation with measurement of *effective regurgitant orifice* area (EROA), *regurgitant volume*, and *regurgitant fraction*.

Colour Doppler jet area

- Establish an apical image that includes the whole left atrium.
- Using colour flow mapping, optimize the image to include the whole regurgitant jet. Set Nyquist limit at 50–60cm/s.
- Record a loop and scroll through to reach the frame with the maximum jet size.
- Trace the regurgitant jet. Trace the border of the left atrium (Fig. 3.8). If there are multiple jets add the separate jet areas together.
- Report the absolute size of the jet and the size relative to the size of the left atrium (percentage).
- Grade the severity but bear in mind:
  - If the jet area relative to left atrium suggests the regurgitation is mild or moderate but the left atrium is very large (>70mm^2) then grade it as moderate or severe respectively.
  - If the jet area suggests the regurgitation is severe but the regurgitation is not pansystolic then overall regurgitation may be moderate.

Problems with jet area to gauge severity

Correlation between jet area and severity of mitral regurgitation is poor and the measurement should be used only in combination with the other methods. This is because:

- The regurgitant jet area includes turbulent (aliased) flow signals as well as laminar velocities in the same direction as the mitral regurgitation jet. Movement of blood already in the left atrium that moves with the regurgitant jet (entrainment) is therefore included.
- Jet area can be artificially changed. Reducing the scale increases the area because the lower filter setting means lower velocities are displayed. Try and use average scale settings (50–60 cm/s) and ensure the same setting on follow up scans.
- Eccentric jets are underestimated as they flatten out against walls and go out of plane.

Table 3.2 Assessment of severity of mitral regurgitation

Specific signs of severity

	Mild	Severe
Jet (Nyquist 50–60cm/s)	<4cm^2 or <20% left atrium; small & central	40% or 10cm^2 large & central or wall impinging and swirling
Vena contracta	<0.3cm	>0.7cm
PISA r (Nyquist 40cm/s)	None/minimal (<0.4cm)	Large (>1cm)
Pulmonary vein flow	–	Systolic reversal
Valve structure	–	Flail or rupture

Supportive signs of severity

	Mild	Severe
Pulmonary vein flow	Systolic dominant	
Mitral inflow	A-wave dominant	E-wave dominant (>1.2 m/s)
CW trace	Soft & parabolic	Dense & triangular
LV and LA	Normal size LV if chronic MR	Enlarged LV & LA if no other cause

Report as **moderate** if signs of regurgitation are greater than **mild** but there are no features of **severe** regurgitation.

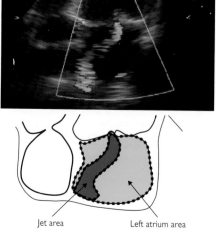

Jet area   Left atrium area

Fig. 3.8 Colour jet area and area of left atrium as marker of severity.

Vena contracta

- Obtain a clear view of the colour flow through the mitral valve in parasternal long axis or apical 4-chamber views.
- If necessary, scan along the commissural line to ensure you have the point of regurgitation through the valve.
- Zoom in on the colour flow through the mitral valve.
- Record a loop and scroll through to identify the image with maximal flow through the valve.
- The vena contracta is the narrowest region of the regurgitant jet (usually just below the valve in the left atrium).
- Report the diameter. >0.7cm suggests severe regurgitation.
- A parasternal short axis view just below the mitral valve level can be used and cross-sectional area of the regurgitant jet recorded. The cross sectional area is one way of measuring the EROA.

Problems with vena contracta as marker of severity

This method is simple and thought to be independent of haemodynamics, driving pressure, and flow rate. However, low colour gain, poor acoustic windows, or failure to assess multiple jets can underestimate the vena contracta. A high colour gain, irregular shape of jet, or atrial fibrillation can lead to overestimation.

Flow convergence (PISA—proximal isovelocity surface area) (see 📖 p.126)
Pulmonary venous flow

Normally blood flows from the pulmonary veins throughout the cardiac cycle. As mitral regurgitation becomes more severe left atrial pressure increases more rapidly during systole and reduces the amount of blood that can flow from the pulmonary vein (blunted systolic pulmonary vein flow). With severe regurgitation atrial pressures are high and blood starts to be forced back into the veins (reversed systolic pulmonary flow).

- Obtain an apical 4-chamber view with enough depth to see the back of the left atrium.
- Try to identify the pulmonary vein orifices on the back of the left atrium. With transthoracic echocardiography, often only the right upper pulmonary vein (by the atrial septum) is seen and can be aligned.
- Place the PW sample volume ~1cm into the ostium of the vein (Fig. 3.9).
- A good spectral tracing confirms you are in the right place.
- Look at the systolic and diastolic components.
    - If they are in opposite directions with the systolic component going away from the probe report *reversed systolic flow*.
    - If in the same direction, measure the height of the two waves and comment if the systolic wave is *blunted* relative to diastolic or the relation is normal (systolic slightly larger—*systolic dominant*).

Problems with pulmonary venous flow

Any pathology that increases left atrial pressure can blunt pulmonary vein flow. If systolic flow reversal is present then this is very specific but not very sensitive for severe regurgitation.

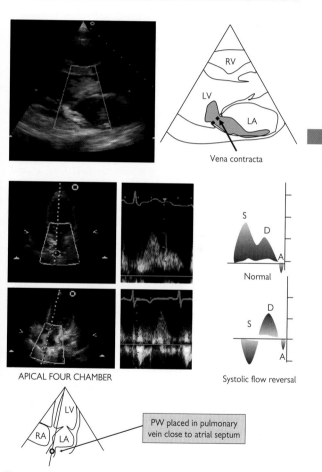

Fig. 3.9 Measuring pulmonary vein flow.

Supportive measures
Mitral inflow
As regurgitation becomes more severe the amount of blood forced into the left atrium during systole increases. This increased volume of blood increases left atrial pressure. Therefore, blood leaves the atrium more quickly at the start of diastole i.e. *peak early diastolic velocity* increases.
- In an apical 4-chamber view place the PW Doppler cursor at the mitral valve tips.
- E wave >1.2m/s is indicative of severe mitral regurgitation (Fig. 3.10).
- However, a hyperdynamic circulation or even minor degrees of mitral stenosis can also increase E wave amplitude. If the A wave is dominant, severe mitral regurgitation is virtually ruled out.

Continuous wave Doppler intensity/shape
- In an apical 4-chamber view place the CW Doppler through the mitral valve orifice and record a spectral trace (Fig. 3.11).
- Make a qualitative judgement about the density of the systolic regurgitant waveform relative to the mitral inflow density. If they are the same this suggests there is as much blood flow into the atrium during systole as back into the ventricle during diastole and regurgitation is severe. (Peak velocity allows calculation of *regurgitant orifice area* (📖 p.126).)

Regurgitant volume/regurgitant fraction
The principle behind the *regurgitant volume* is that the amount of blood that flows through the mitral valve into the left ventricle during diastole (assuming there is no aortic regurgitation to fill the ventricle as well) should equal the amount of blood that leaves the left ventricle during systole. The amount of blood leaving through the aortic valve in systole can be calculated and subtracted from the amount flowing across the mitral valve in diastole. The difference is the volume flowing back through the incompetent mitral valve. *Regurgitant volume* is not usually calculated as accuracy depends on accurate measures of the outflow tract and mitral valve area. The mitral ring is difficult to assess because it is not circular and changes throughout the cardiac cycle. To measure:
- In apical 4-chamber view record PW at the mitral valve (it is controversial whether the sample volume should be at annulus or valve tip level). Trace the vti. Estimate mitral valve cross-sectional area (CSA). Use annulus width and assume a circular orifice (alternatively measure the annulus in two perpendicular planes and calculate area as an oval).

$$\text{Mitral inflow volume} = \text{vti} \times \text{CSA mitral valve}$$

- In apical 5-chamber view record PW in left ventricular outflow and measure vti. Measure outflow tract diameter in parasternal long axis and estimate CSA (assuming it is circular).

$$\text{Left ventrication outflow} = \text{vti} \times \text{CSA left ventricular outflow}$$

- Mitral regurgitant volume is:

$$\text{Mitral inflow volume} - \text{left ventricular outflow volume}$$

- Regurgitant fraction is: (<20% mild, >50% severe regurgitation)

$$\text{Mitral regurgitant volume} / \text{mitral inflow volume}$$

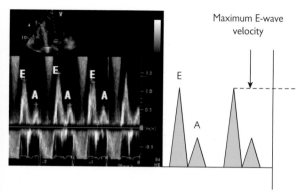

Fig. 3.10 Pulsed wave Doppler trace of a patient with severe mitral regurgitation. Maximum E-wave velocity >1.2 m/s indicating severe regurgitation. E = early diastolic filling velocity; A = velocity during atrial contraction.

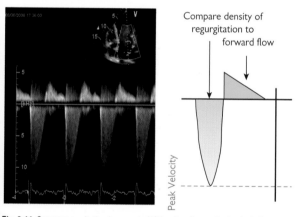

Fig. 3.11 Severe regurgitation is suggested if density of regurgitation is similar to forward flow. Peak velocity can be used with PISA to calculate effective regurgitant orifice area (📖 p.126).

3D in assessment of mitral regurgitation?

3D colour flow imaging may be useful for:

Qualitative assessment of regurgitant jet

- 3D colour flow mapping of mitral regurgitation allows the mitral regurgitation to be assessed in all planes, proving useful in the analysis of eccentric mitral regurgitation or visualization of multiple jets (Fig. 3.12).

Quantitative assessment of regurgitant jet

3D can also be used to measure the same parameters that have been measured by 2D. There is no unique, additional 3D parameter but 3D can be particularly useful to ensure accuracy of measures. For example:

- Estimation of the PISA value by the operator assumes that flow acceleration is symmetrical towards the regurgitant orifice. This geometric assumption is not always true and can be evaluated in 3D as the entire flow convergence area can be displayed and viewed from the left atrium. Thus 3D allows for a better judgement of the likely accuracy of 2D PISA values. Theoretically, it would be possible to measure the area in 3 dimensions to obtain a very accurate PISA.
- 3D echocardiography also allows the anatomic regurgitant orifice area to be measured directly using planimetry of the regurgitant orifice or regurgitant jet where it passes through the valve. This has been shown to correlate well with the EROA calculated by the proximal convergence method.

Remember that acquisition of 3D colour flow often requires more cycles to be captured than for anatomical images. Therefore reconstruction can be difficult as there may be problems with artefacts, especially with atrial fibrillation. However, advancing technology is heading towards clinically useful real-time 3D colour flow mapping.

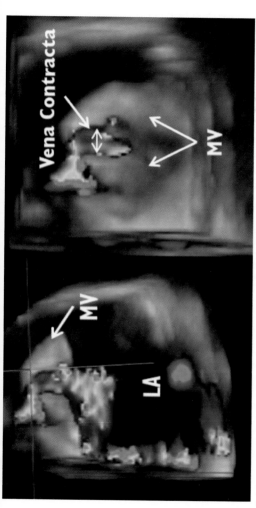

Fig. 3.12 3D full volume colour Doppler acquisition of a patient with mitral regurgitation (MR). Images were initially acquired from the apical window. Left: cropping towards the mitral valve (MV) leaflet tips to find the level of the vena contracta. Right: the vena contracta is then tilted to give an *'en face'* view allowing its measurement. LA = left atrium. See ▣ Video 3.7 and ▣ Video 3.8.

PISA (proximal isovelocity surface area)

PISA or *flow convergence zone* is a measurement of how much blood travels through a valve. It has been applied in several situations (e.g. aortic regurgitation, mitral stenosis) but is validated for assessment of mitral regurgitation. If regurgitation is mild, only blood near the valve moves towards the atrium. With severe regurgitation blood further away in the ventricle moves backwards. An impression of how far this *flow convergence zone* extends into the ventricle is obtained by looking at the velocity of blood flow in the ventricle with colour flow mapping. To quantify the distance you use the principle that at a certain velocity the colour flow will alias (change colour). The further away this change in colour, the more blood is being funnelled back through the mitral valve, and the more severe the regurgitation. In 3D the aliasing layer is a coloured hemisphere sitting on the mitral valve. The *PISA* refers to the surface area of the hemisphere (Fig. 3.11) and correlates to the *regurgitant flow*.

Assessment

- Get a good image of the mitral valve (usually the apical 4-chamber view is best) and ensure you are in the plane of the regurgitant jet.
- Check what the colour scale is set to, i.e. aliasing velocity, $V_{aliasing}$. You can use this velocity if the flow convergence is obvious but to optimize the colour contrast at the boundary it is normal to shift the zero of the baseline so that the aliasing velocity is 40cm/s.
- Acquire a loop of the cardiac cycle and scroll through to identify the mid-systolic hemisphere shell. (Fig. 3.13).
- Measure the radius (r) from valve orifice to point of colour change. If the colour flow is obscuring the valve orifice on your loop, place a caliper at the aliasing zone then suppress the colour flow and position the second cursor on the valve.
- Report severity based on the parameters listed in 📖 'Grading severity', p. 126.

Grading severity

Radius (r):
A simple approach is just to record r with the aliasing velocity set at 40cm/s. Severe mitral regurgitation is present if r >1cm and mild if <0.4cm.

Regurgitant flow:
Regurgitant flow is calculated as: $2\pi r^2 \times V_{aliasing}$ and has been validated against angiographic grades of regurgitation. Clinically it is normally used with the continuous wave Doppler velocity to measure orifice area.

Effective regurgitant orifice area:
Regurgitant flow can be combined with the peak continuous wave velocity (📖 p.122) to calculate effective regurgitant orifice area (EROA).

$$EROA = \frac{regurgitant\ flow}{peak\ velocity\ on\ CW}$$

0–20 mm^2: mild; 20–40 mm^2: moderate; >40 mm^2: severe.

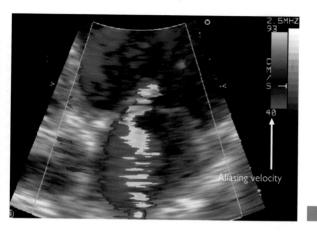

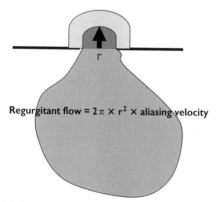

Regurgitant flow = $2\pi \times r^2 \times$ aliasing velocity

Fig. 3.13 Calculation of regurgitant flow in mitral regurgitation using the principle of proximal isovelocity surface area. Note the zero baseline shift to get an aliasing velocity of 40cm/s and measurement of radius from valve orifice to edge of aliasing boundary.

Mitral valve prolapse

Early studies suggested a high prevalence of up to 20% for mitral valve prolapse but revised criteria for diagnosis have lead to more conservative estimates of around 2%. The key to the change is the differentiation of an anatomically normal valve that bows more than normal from a thickened valve, classically with myxomatous degeneration, that truly prolapses. This is important because it is only the latter patients who have clinical complications. Prolapse can be seen with M-mode but 2D is usually preferred to identify the condition. 3D echocardiography allows detailed anatomical assessment of all mitral valve scallops, the geometry of the mitral valve annulus, and the anatomy of the subvalvular apparatus. Studies have shown that when image quality is adequate, 3D transthoracic echocardiography has a similar accuracy for identifying segmental prolapse as transoesophageal 2D echocardiography.

Assessment

- Study the valve in the parasternal long axis view.
- Comment on leaflet thickening or abnormal appearance.
- Report mitral valve *prolapse* if one or both leaflets entirely crosses the plane of the mitral valve annulus back into the left atrium during systole and the tip is >2mm into the left atrium. If the tip is within the plane of the annulus and there is no more than trivial regurgitation then this can be reported as *bowing,* without prolapse (Fig. 3.14).
- The leaflet position relative to the valve plane is determined precisely by drawing a line between each side of the annulus.
- Comment on which leaflets (and scallops if possible) prolapse and check if any part of the prolapsing leaflet is flail (see 📖 p. 130).
- Report any associated changes in the subvalvular apparatus (papillary muscle or chordae rupture).
- Report degree of regurgitation (remember anterior leaflet prolapse will be related with posteriorly-directed regurgitation and vice versa).

3D in assessment of mitral prolapse?

3D echocardiography allows the mitral valve anatomy to be viewed from multiple planes from different directions, thus increasing the operator's understanding of the mechanism of the mitral valve prolapse.

- Obtain a 3D view from the parasternal rather than apical windows as this improves imaging with the probe closer to the valve.
- Rotate the image to obtain an *en face* or 'surgeon's view' looking from the left atrium.
- Report prolapsed position and extent.
- Use the reconstructed full volume dataset to demonstrate and measure the maximal position of prolapse (Fig. 3.15).
- Use 3D colour flow to confirm the direction, number and extent of eccentric jets.

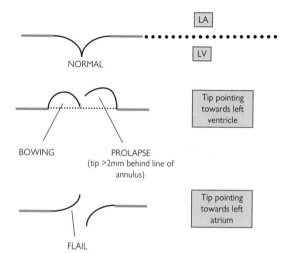

Fig. 3.14 Definitions of normal, prolapsing and flail.

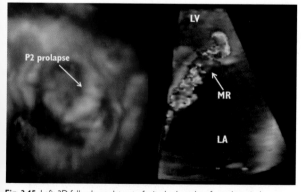

Fig. 3.15 Left: 3D full volume dataset of mitral valve taken from the apical window. Subsequent cropping and rotation to show an *en face* view of the valve demonstrating P2 mitral valve leaflet prolapse. Right: 3D full volume colour Doppler acquisition of mitral valve from the apical view. LA = left atrium; LV = left ventricle; MR = mitral regurgitation. See 🎬 Video 3.9 and 🎬 Video 3.10.

Flail leaflets

Flail leaflets (Fig. 3.16) usually occur due to damage to the subvalvular apparatus. This can be secondary to degeneration, destruction by endocarditis, or ischaemia associated with myocardial infarction. The extent of the flail can vary from just the leaflet tip (due to chordae failure) through to the whole valve (usually papillary muscle rupture). The degree of flail associates with the severity of the associated regurgitation. This can vary from mild to severe and clinically from asymptomatic to haemodynamically unstable.

- Report a flail leaflet/leaflet scallop/leaflet tip if part of the leaflet points back into the left atrium in systole rather than towards the ventricle.
- Comment on which leaflet is affected. If you can see, mention how extensive and which scallop.
- There will be regurgitation so report severity.
- Assess both papillary muscles and the chordae to look for ruptures. To look at the subvalvular apparatus use a combination of views—parasternal long and short axis, all the apical views (2-chamber view can be good to see both papillary muscles) and subcostal views.
- Report related findings according to suspected clinical aetiology, e.g. regional wall motion abnormalities and left ventricle function in myocardial infarction, vegetations in endocarditis.

Transthoracic assessment for mitral valve repair

When assessing the echocardiographic suitability for mitral valve repair, note:

Leaflet motion and structure
- Record whether the leaflet motion appears normal, excessive due to prolapse, or restricted.
- The anatomy of each leaflet and its integrity should be noted. Normal leaflet thickness is <5mm.

Annulus size
- Accurate annulus size measurement should be performed and documented.

Calcification
- The presence and degree of calcification should be accurately documented at the annulus, leaflets, and subvalvar apparatus.

Mitral regurgitation severity and mechanism
- The MR jet direction, severity and mechanism should be reported.

If there is a question over the MR severity/mechanism or the quality of transthoracic images obtained then TOE is indicated.

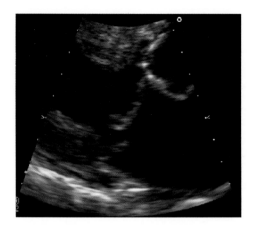

Posterior leaflet prolapse behind line of annulus

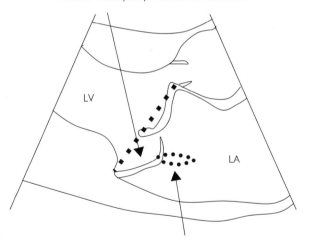

Flail leaflet would point back into atrium

Fig. 3.16 Example of a prolapsing posterior mitral leaflet seen in a parasternal long axis view with superimposed figure of a flail element. See ⚏ Video 3.11.

Aortic valve

Normal anatomy

The aortic valve has 3 cusps of similar size, which close to form a Y shape. Each cusp tip has a small thickened nodule (*nodule of Arantius*). The cusp edges usually overlap by 2–3mm and the lines where they meet are called *commissures*. Closure of the cusps is referred to as *coaption* and opening as *excursion*. Around each cusp are outpouchings of the aortic root called the *sinuses of Valsalva*. The sinuses create a pool of blood above the valve in diastole that improves blood flow down the coronaries and ensures a tight seal. Cusps and associated sinuses are named according to the coronary artery that originates from the sinus (right, left, and non). Above the valves the bulging sinuses merge into the tubular ascending aorta at the *sinotubular junction*. Below the valve is the *left ventricular outflow tract* made up of the *membranous interventricular septum*, *anterior mitral valve leaflet*, and *anterior left ventricular wall*.

Normal findings (Fig. 3.17)

2D views

- The minimal views are: parasternal long axis, parasternal short axis (aortic valve level), and apical 5-chamber.
- Aortic valve velocities are also obtained from the *right* parasternal view, which can be used for detailed assessment of aortic stenosis.
- Apical 3-chamber and subcostal views can also be used.
- Suprasternal view allows measurement of flow in the aorta for assessment of aortic regurgitation.

2D findings

Aortic valve

- Parasternal long axis: 2 cusps are seen (usually right coronary by septum and non-coronary by mitral valve). The leaflets open to lie parallel to the aorta and close to form 2 curved lines.
- Parasternal short axis (aortic valve level): all 3 cusps are seen (left cusp on the right, right cusp at the top, and non-coronary cusp on the right). This is the classic Y-shape view. The left main coronary artery may be seen and helps identify the left coronary cusp.
- Apical 5- and 3-chamber: the valve is aligned for Doppler measures and 2 cusps are seen (usually non-coronary cusp next to atrium and right coronary cusp next to septum).

Sinuses of Valsalva and sinotubular junction

- Parasternal long axis: the sinuses bulge to the right of the valve and the sinotubular junction is the point where the ascending aorta starts.
- Parasternal short axis (aortic valve level): sinuses surround each cusp.

Left ventricular outflow tract

- Best seen in parasternal long axis. Formed by septum and anterior mitral valve leaflet. Usually around 2cm wide and roughly circular.

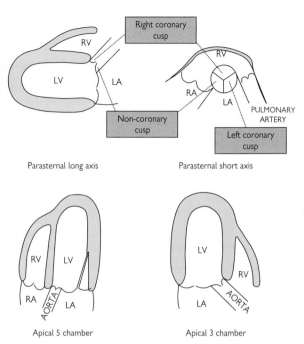

Parasternal long axis

Parasternal short axis

Apical 5 chamber

Apical 3 chamber

Fig. 3.17 Key views to study the aortic valve.

3D views and findings

- 3D datasets are best obtained from the parasternal window and can be used to assess valve pathology. Detailed evaluation can be limited by image quality but can be very useful to perform measures of size.

Aortic stenosis

General

Aortic stenosis is common. Aortic valve thickening occurs in 25% of people aged >65 and severe stenosis occurs in 3% aged >75. In the West, the predominant cause is calcific degenerative disease. A bicuspid valve occurs in 2% of the population. Rheumatic disease is now uncommon.

Assessment

The echocardiographic study is aimed at determining the appearance of the valve, the grade of stenosis, the effect on the left ventricle, and the presence of associated disease.

Appearance

Comment on:

- Degree and distribution of thickening. The term *aortic sclerosis* describes valve leaflet thickening (>2mm) without significant stenosis (Vmax < 2.5m/s).
- How many functional cusps (2 in a bicuspid valve, 3 in rheumatic or calcific degenerative disease)? (Fig. 3.18)
- Is the closure line central (calcific degenerative or rheumatic disease) or eccentric (bicuspid valve)?
- Motion: normal or reduced? Systolic bowing (bicuspid or rheumatic)?
- Commissural fusion (rheumatic disease).
- Associated rheumatic mitral stenosis suggests a rheumatic aetiology.

Grading severity

Grade stenosis from peak *velocity* across the valve, mean *pressure gradient*, and *effective orifice area* (calculated from the *continuity equation*) (Table 3.3). Sometimes further supportive measures can be used such as direct planimetry of the aortic valve area using 2D or 3D.

Aortic peak velocity

- In apical 5-chamber view (or 3-chamber) align the continuous wave Doppler, from the apex, through the aortic valve into the aorta. Spend some time looking for the maximum velocity. Always repeat this measurement with the stand alone CW probe from the apex.
- Record several beats and measure the peak velocity on the spectral trace with the greatest velocity. This can be affected by the filling time so ignore ectopic or post-ectopic beats and in atrial fibrillation average 2 or 3 beats. (Fig. 3.19)
- Repeat the measurement in at least one other approach (e.g. suprasternal or right parasternal) and report the maximum velocity found from all measures.

Table 3.3 Parameters to assess severity of aortic stenosis

	Mild	Moderate	Severe
Peak velocity (m/s)	2.5–2.9	3.0–4.0	>4.0
Peak gradient (mmHg)	<35	35–65	>65
Mean gradient (mmHg)	<20	20–40	>40
Valve area (cm²)	>1.5	1.0–1.5	<1.0

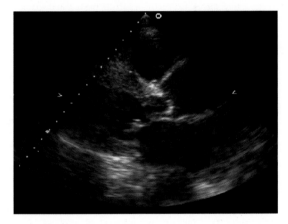

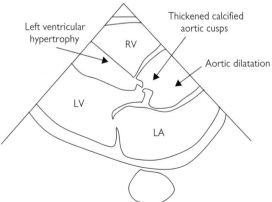

Fig. 3.18 Parasternal long axis demonstrating calcified aortic valve.
See 📷 Video 3.12.

Peak pressure gradient

The peak gradient is usually automatically calculated by the machine from the *peak velocity*. The relation between the two is very simple (the simplified Bernouli equation).

$$\text{Peak gradient} = 4 \times \text{peak velocity}^2$$

The equation is less accurate if the peak velocity is <3.0m/s and the long form of the Bernoulli equation can be used:

$$\text{Peak gradient} = 4 \times \left(V_2^2 - V_1^2\right)$$

where v_2 = peak aortic velocity and v_1 = peak left ventricular outflow tract velocity.

Mean pressure gradient

To obtain the mean pressure gradient trace the continuous wave spectral trace of flow through the aortic valve (Fig. 3.19) and the machine will automatically calculate the *vti* (velocity time integral) and *mean pressure gradient* (mean pressure across the valve during systole).

Effective orifice area/valve area

The continuity equation is based on the principle that the volume of blood that flows through the left ventricle outflow tract during 1sec must equal the blood through the aortic valve during 1sec.

- Obtain the continuous wave Doppler trace through the aortic valve (Fig. 3.19) and record the *peak velocity* and *vti*$_{(VALVE)}$.
- In an apical view, record PW Doppler in the left ventricle outflow tract (LVOT). Trace the waveform and record *peak velocity* and *vti*$_{(LVOT)}$. (Fig. 3.20).
- In the parasternal long axis view zoom in on the LVOT and measure the diameter. Record the maximum edge-to-edge diameter just below the insertion of the aortic valve leaflets.
- Calculate the CSA of the LVOT:

$$\text{Area LVOT} = \pi \times \left(\text{LVOT diameter} / 2\right)^2$$

- Put the figures into the rearranged continuity equation:

$$\text{Valve area} = \text{Area LVOT} \times \text{vti}_{(LVOT)} / \text{vti}_{(VALVE)}$$

The equation can be calculated with peak velocity substituted for vti.

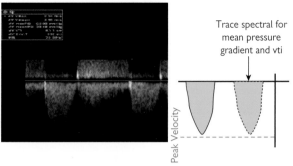

Fig. 3.19 Continuous wave in an apical view to measure velocities.

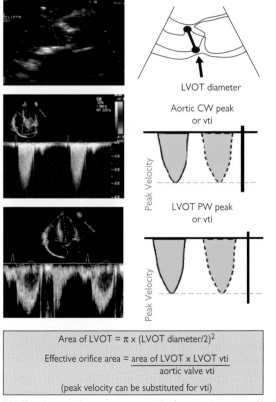

$$\text{Area of LVOT} = \pi \times (\text{LVOT diameter}/2)^2$$

$$\text{Effective orifice area} = \frac{\text{area of LVOT} \times \text{LVOT vti}}{\text{aortic valve vti}}$$

(peak velocity can be substituted for vti)

Fig. 3.20 Two views and three measures are needed for continuity equation. Use a parasternal long axis view to measure left ventricular outflow tract diameter using zoom (top). In an apical 5-chamber view measure continuous wave Doppler across the aortic valve (middle) and PW Doppler in the left ventricle outflow tract (bottom).

3D in assessment of aortic stenosis?

Planimetry of the aortic valve area can be undertaken on 2D images although this can be inaccurate. As with 3D transthoracic imaging of mitral stenosis, a combination of live 3D and full volume acquisitions has been employed to estimate aortic valve area by planimetry using 3D. Recent papers suggest assessment of aortic stenosis by planimetry of transthoracic 3D images has good agreement with standard 2D transoesophageal imaging. However, planimetry is limited due to limited spatial resolution and to be accurate requires excellent image quality. Valvular calcification related to the aortic stenosis can be problematic as it causes drop-out artefacts distal to the probe. Sometimes, apical windows (Fig. 3.21) may provide a more effective window as drop-out from the calcification extends into the aorta rather than across the posterior part of the valve. However, resolution may be reduced because of the increased distance between probe and valve. If you want to use 3D to support suspicions of severity gathered by 2D imaging then do the following:

- Obtain a 3D volume of the aortic valve, ideally from a parasternal window as this is closest to the valve.
- Use post-processing analysis software to align a 2D plane accurately through the tips of the aortic valve.
- Trace around the inner edge of the valve and calcifications and report planimetered valve area.

Effect of other diseases on diagnosing and grading stenosis

- Moderate or severe aortic regurgitation will increase transaortic flow and may lead to overestimation of the grade of stenosis if using gradient alone. The continuity equation remains valid and should be used.
- Left ventricular dysfunction can be associated with lower transaortic and LVOT velocities and therefore underestimation of gradient. The continuity equation remains valid and should be used.
- A subaortic membrane or septal hypertrophy may occasionally be mistaken for valvular stenosis. Use PW Doppler in different positions in the LVOT to identify whether the blood starts to accelerate below or at the level of the valve.
- Examine the aorta for dilatation of the ascending aorta (commonly associated with bicuspid aortic valve, but also with calcific degenerative disease). If a bicuspid valve is suspected, use the suprasternal window to look for associated aortic coarctation.
- Pulmonary hypertension is common in severe aortic stenosis and is associated with a high operative risk. Estimate pulmonary artery pressure and assess the right ventricle.

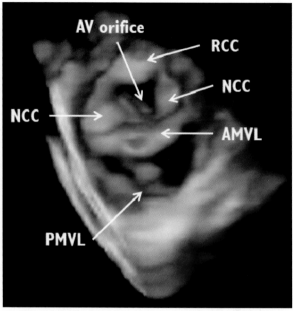

Fig. 3.21 3D full volume apical 3D dataset obtained from an apical window. Subsequent cropping and rotation reveals the aortic valve (AV) orifice and the right (RCC), left (LCC), and non-coronary cusps of the aortic valve. Image seen at peak systole. AMVL = anterior mitral valve leaflet; PMVL = posterior mitral valve leaflet. See ⬛ Video 3.13.

Effect on the left ventricle

Left ventricular hypertrophy or concentric remodelling (relative wall thickness >0.45 without hypertrophy (see 📖 p.218) are usual in compensated severe aortic stenosis. The left ventricle can also dilate if there is high wall stress as a result of severe pressure load, excessive fibrosis, or another cause of left ventricle dysfunction (e.g. myocardial infarction).

- During assessment of aortic stenosis also report a full evaluation of the left ventricle (for function, see 📖 p.226 and for hypertrophy, see 📖 p.218).

A common dilemma in the relation between the left ventricle and aortic stenosis is whether any left ventricular dysfunction is secondary to the stenosis or another pathology (e.g. ischaemia). Also, an apparently small gradient or a decline in gradient may be secondary to impaired left ventricle function. The continuity equation remains accurate and should be used to assess valve area.

- If the mean gradient is <30mmHg (suggesting mild to moderate stenosis) but the valve area calculated by the continuity equation is <1.0cm^2 (suggesting severe stenosis) then a dobutamine stress echocardiogram can be considered to differentiate:
  - End-stage severe aortic stenosis.
  - Moderate aortic stenosis associated with left ventricle dysfunction from another cause (e.g. myocardial infarction or myocarditis).

Dobutamine stress echocardiography

Give low-dose dobutamine intravenously (5 then 10, if necessary 20 micrograms/kg/min in 5-min stages). Aim for a 10% increase in heart rate or 20% increase in LVOT or aortic valve vti (Fig. 3.22). If the patient also has coronary artery disease, ischaemia may occur at very low levels of stress in the presence of aortic stenosis.Therefore carefully monitor wall motion and left ventricle size to look for evidence of ischaemia during the study (see Chapter 10).

There are two things to look for during the study. The first is to determine whether severe aortic stenosis is present or not. The second is to determine whether the impaired left ventricle is able to increase output (*ventricular reserve* is present). This is important because the risk of mortality following aortic valve replacement for severe aortic stenosis is approximately 5% if contractile reserve is present and 35% if absent.

- Severe aortic stenosis is defined by:
  - Mean gradient >30 mmHg at any time during dobutamine stress.
  - Valve area <1.2 cm^2 throughout the infusion.
- Ventricular reserve is present if there is:
  - A rise in LVOT vti by >20% during the study.

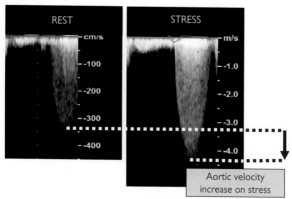

Fig. 3.22 Stress echocardiography in a patient with aortic stenosis and impaired left ventricle function. Velocities during stress are consistent with a mean gradient of >30mmHg (severe aortic stenosis) and the increase in vti is >20%, suggesting preserved ventricular contractile reserve.

Aortic regurgitation

General

Aortic regurgitation (AR) is usually seen easily with colour flow Doppler imaging over the aortic valve, which has 95% sensitivity and 100% specificity. Traces of central regurgitation are seen more frequently with increasing age (<1% below 40 years; 10–20% at 60 years; and in the majority >80 years), but are not clinically significant.

Causes of AR are listed in Box 3.1; changes in either the aortic root or the valve itself can be the underlying pathology.

Assessment

Use colour flow mapping to identify and describe any AR (Fig. 3.23). The study should then look for probable aetiology, grade severity, and check for associated problems.

Appearance

- Map the regurgitation with colour flow. Use colour flow mapping to identify and describe any AR. The study should then look for probable aetiology, grade severity, and check for associated problems.
  - Visualize the regurgitation with colour flow.
  - Look at the jet in all views and establish the shape and pattern of the regurgitation.
  - Comment on whether it is central, eccentric, along a commissure, or even through a perforation (often easiest to see in parasternal short axis views).
- Use a systematic approach to establish cause based on the clinical situation:
  - Aortic root: in the parasternal long axis, measure aortic root dimension, look for a dissection flap. In parasternal short axis look at the aortic root for evidence of thickening or abscess.
  - Aortic valve: parasternal long axis—abnormal valve motion/prolapse, vegetations, calcification/rheumatic changes. Parasternal short axis—number of cusps.
  - Look at the rest of heart: Evidence of congenital abnormalities that may relate to AR, e.g. ventricular septal defect?
- For prosthetic valve regurgitation, comment on whether the regurgitation is through the valve (valvular) or around the side (paravalvular), and document any degree of valve motion relative to the annulus ('rocking').

Box 3.1 Causes of aortic regurgitation

Aortic valve
- Degeneration: calcific
- Infectious: endocarditis, post rheumatic fever
- Congenital:
  • Bicuspid valve
  • Associated with other congenital abnormalities.

Aortic root dilatation
- Hypertension
- Dissection/aneurysm
- Trauma
- Congenital (e.g. Marfan's, Ehlers–Danlos)
- Osteogenesis imperfecta
- Inflammatory:
  • Rheumatoid arthritis
  • Systemic lupus erythematosus
  • Syphilis, Reiter's syndrome
  • Giant cell arteritis, ankylosing spondylitis.

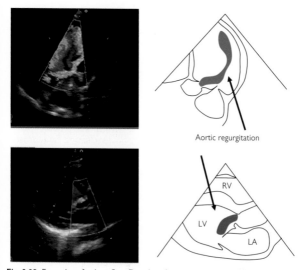

Fig. 3.23 Examples of colour flow Doppler of aortic regurgitation. Top: apical 5-chamber view demonstrating severe regurgitation with a long, broad jet. Bottom: parasternal long axis view showing mild regurgitation. See 📹 Video 3.14.

Grading severity

Assess the severity of AR using jet width, vena contracta and descending aortic flow (Table 3.4). Once you have an impression of the severity use pressure half-time and LV function to further your assessment.

Vena contracta

- The vena contracta is the narrowest part of the colour Doppler jet, where flow convergence occurs. Best seen in parasternal long axis view.
- Measure the vena contracta width perpendicular to the jet direction with calipers and report the absolute measurement. Severe regurgitation is associated with width >0.6cm (Fig. 3.24).
- The same measurement can be done in cross-section in the parasternal short axis view, though it is difficult to be sure you are at the correct level (at the narrowest point).

Jet width as proportion of outflow tract

- Measure the *vena contracta* (jet width).
- Suppress the colour and measure the width of the LVOT at the same point.
- Report the jet width as a percentage of LVOT. Severe regurgitation is suggested by a jet that is >65% of outflow tract.
- Jet size assessed in parasternal short axis can also be used (although technically more difficult and does not supply more information). Report area relative to left ventricle outflow tract area in the same view.

Problems using jet width to assess AR

- Eccentric jets tend to 'flatten out' along the outflow tract wall and are no longer circular in cross-section, so will have different widths depending on the orientation of the image plane.
- Changes in gain and colour scale will affect jet width, so control settings should be kept constant (50–60cm/s), especially for F/U.

Descending aorta flow

- In the suprasternal view, obtain a view of the aortic arch and descending aorta (Fig. 3.25).
- Place the PW Doppler cursor in the centre of the descending aorta and look at the spectral trace.
- Flow down the descending aorta is normally away from the probe (below the line) for virtually all of the cardiac cycle.
- Examine diastolic flow—a small amount of flow reversal (above the line) may be seen at the start of diastole. However, in severe regurgitation, all flow during diastole is reversed (back towards the heart) as a large volume of blood flows back into the ventricle. If this is seen, report *holodiastolic aortic flow reversal* (Fig. 3.25).

Table 3.4 Parameters to determine severity of aortic regurgitation

	Mild	Severe
Specific signs of severity		
Vena contracta	<0.3cm	>0.6cm
Jet (Nyquist 50–60cm/s)	central, <25% of LVOT	central, >65% of LVOT
Descending aorta	No or brief early-diastolic flow reversal	Holodiastolic flow reversal
Supportive signs of severity		
Pressure half time	>500ms	<200ms
Left ventricle (only for chronic lesions)	Normal LV size	Moderate or greater LV enlargement (no other cause)

Report as **moderate** if signs of regurgitation are greater than **mild** but there are no features of **severe** regurgitation.

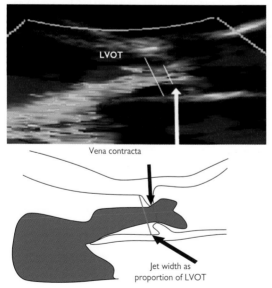

Vena contracta

Jet width as proportion of LVOT

Fig. 3.24 Parasternal long axis with vena contracta and left ventricular outflow tract diameter marked. See ♻ Video 3.15.

Supportive signs

Pressure half time

Obtaining the spectral Doppler trace

- In the apical 5-chamber (or 3-chamber) view, align the CW Doppler through the AR jet (identified with colour flow mapping). Try and ensure the Doppler passes through the regurgitant orifice of the valve and is in line with the jet direction (for eccentric jets the view may need to be adjusted).
- On the spectral trace, the regurgitant jet will be seen as a broad trace with a flat, sloped top, above the baseline that coincides with diastole on the ECG (Fig. 3.26).
- Measure the slope of the flat part of the curve. The *deceleration slope* (the slope of the curve) and *pressure half-time* (time for pressure to fall by a half) are usually calculated automatically. The two measures are generally correlated.

Parameters to assess

- Density of the waveform compared to the systolic waveform. Similar density suggests severe regurgitation.
- Peak diastolic velocity (usually 4–6m/s).
- The *pressure half-time:* <200ms indicates the pressure between the aorta and left ventricle equalizes very quickly in diastole (usually due to a large regurgitant volume) and suggests severe regurgitation. See also 📖 p.150.
- The *deceleration slope:* >400cm/s^2 indicates severe AR (the larger the number, the steeper the slope).

Left ventricle

- Serial studies of changes in left ventricular size are useful in monitoring progression of AR and help decide the timing for intervention.
- Assessment can be based on standard measures of LV size (📖 p.196).
- A LV end-diastolic dimension of >7cm and/or LV end-systolic dimension of >4.5 cm are markers of severe LV dilation ± dysfunction 2° to chronic AR.

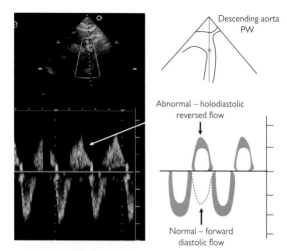

Fig. 3.25 A suprasternal view with pulsed wave Doppler placed in the descending aorta. The spectral trace shows reversed holodiastolic flow.

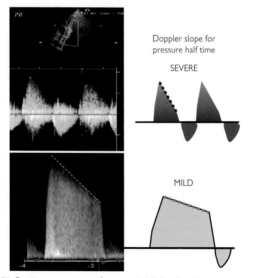

Fig. 3.26 Continuous wave traces from an apical 5-chamber view to measure pressure half-time.

Other possible measures of AR severity

Length of the jet

A rough estimation of the severity of AR can be made on the length of the jet: if the jet reaches the end of the anterior mitral valve leaflet (moderate) or extends into the body of the LV (severe); Fig. 3.27. Originally this was performed using PW Doppler to identify the jet, but this has been extrapolated to colour flow jets which are highly dependent on control settings due to the low velocities at the boundary layers.

Jet area

Judging the severity of AR by the size (area) of the regurgitant jet is inaccurate—it is susceptible to loading conditions, angles of the jet and image plane, and colour flow settings, and should not be relied upon. In addition, eccentric jets may be long and thin as they track along structures and the severity is easily underestimated.

Colour M-mode

If the M-mode cursor is placed below the valve in a parasternal long axis view with colour flow (Fig. 3.27), the position of the regurgitation within the outflow tract and timing during diastole can be studied (e.g. late diastole due to aortic leaflet prolapse or mild regurgitation in early diastole). Measurements of jet width and left ventricular outflow tract can also theoretically be done with the same tracing.

3D assessment of aortic regurgitation?

3D echocardiography modes (full volume datasets, live 3D or colour Doppler imaging) can be used to aid quantification of the severity of aortic regurgitation. The same parameters as developed in 2D are used but the 3D datasets allow better alignment for assessment. This is because the pyramidal datasets can be cropped in any plane so even eccentric jets can have accurate plane alignment. Studies have demonstrated that the measurement of vena contracta width and vena contracta area show good correlation with the angiographic grading of the aortic regurgitation severity.

- To measure vena contracta use the parasternal window to obtain a 3D dataset.
- To measure vena contracta *area* use postprocessing to create an *en face* 2D view of the regurgitation jet as it passes through the aortic valve and LVOT. Then scan up and down the jet to identify the narrowest past and trace around the vena contracta. Report the area relative to the outflow tract area at that level.
- For the vena contracta *width* postprocess the 3D dataset as for area but this time create an imaging plane that lies parallel to the regurgitant jet. Then scan through the jet to identify the plane that cuts through the narrowest point. Measure the jet width and report the value relative to the outflow tract width.

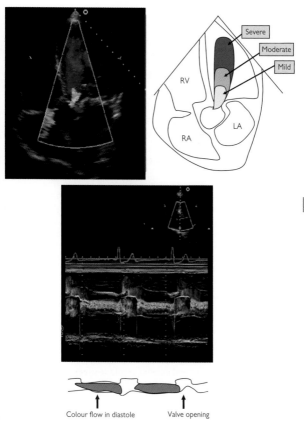

Fig. 3.27 Additional measures to assess aortic regurgitation: length of jet extending into the ventricle based on an apical 4-chamber view (top figure) and colour M-mode in a parasternal long axis view to demonstrate the regurgitant flow in the outflow tract during diastole (bottom figure).

Quantifying regurgitant volume

This can be calculated because blood flow across the aortic valve in systole should be the same as the blood flow into the LV during diastole. The diastolic component comprises blood flow across the mitral valve plus any AR. Both flow across the aortic valve in systole and mitral inflow can be calculated and the aortic regurgitant flow will be the difference between the two:

Regurgitant volume = LVOT flow − mitral valve inflow

The principle is the same as that used for determining regurgitant volume in mitral regurgitation, and the same measures (mitral valve inflow and LV outflow tract flow) are used (see 📖 p.122 for how to measure these).

Interestingly, the stroke volume should be the same at any valve in the heart if it is competent and there is no shunt, so if measurements are difficult at the mitral valve, the pulmonary or tricuspid could be used. Theoretically, the *proximal isovelocity surface area* (PISA) method (📖 p.126) can be used at any regurgitant valve, although it is usually only practical and validated for the mitral valve.

However, the calculation has several potential areas of inaccuracy:
- Measuring LVOT flow and mitral inflow involves significant assumptions and calculations, and these may be inaccurate. Calculating a third measurement from these 2 derived parameters carries a high risk of further inaccuracy.

Significant mitral regurgitation reduces systole aortic flow and distorts the measurement.

Acute or chronic regurgitation?

- In acute severe AR, the LV is usually of normal dimension and thickness, with vigorous function. In chronic severe AR there has been time for dilatation and possibly eccentric hypertrophy.
- Acute severe AR is usually poorly tolerated by patients, due to the lack of time for LV compensation, and they are very symptomatic, often in heart failure.
- Cause: dissection and endocarditis are likely causes of acute AR.
- Pressure half-time is particularly useful as a marker of severity in acute regurgitation. With chronic regurgitation left ventricular function and aortic compliance change to accommodate larger regurgitant volumes. This slows down the equalization in pressure and leads to a longer pressure half-time.

Bicuspid and quadricuspid valves

The aortic valve can occur with fewer or more than 3 cusps. Bicuspid valves are seen in 2% of the population and quadricuspid valves in 0.04% of the population (Fig. 3.28). 5 cusps have also been reported although this may often be secondary to endocarditis. Sometimes valves have 3 cusps but are functionally bicuspid because of fusion of 2 cusps along a commissure. Bicuspid valves are often associated with aortic stenosis and multiple cusps with aortic regurgitation.

It is very easy to make a tricuspid valve appear bicuspid in a parasternal short axis view if the plane is slightly off axis. If you suspect a bicuspid valve make sure this is consistent in several views. Clues to a valve being truly bicuspid include:

- Leaflets of unequal size. True congenital bicuspid valves occur because of failure of separation of the right and non-coronary cusp or failure of separation of the right and left coronary cusps.
- An atypical orientation of the commissure in the parasternal short axis. This will either lie roughly horizontal (between 10 and 4 o'clock) or roughly vertical.
- Abnormal valve motion (best seen in a parasternal long axis view). The valve typically domes with the valve opening off centre.

When assessing a bicuspid valve report the suspected cause, e.g. true congenital or due to valve fusion, degree of calcification (they are more prone to degeneration), associated functional problems (regurgitation and stenosis), associated congenital problems (they are linked with coarctation of the aorta), and associated changes to the aorta (e.g. dilatation or dissection).

Lambl's excresences

These are thin strands attached to the aortic cusps several millimetres long. They are also seen on the mitral valve. They are not clinically significant although their relevance will depend on the clinical situation as it is important not to miss endocarditis vegetations.

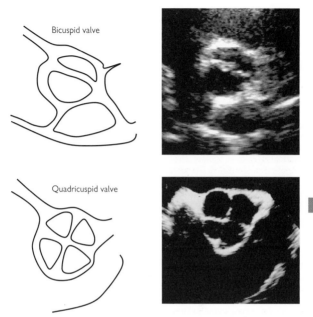

Bicuspid valve

Quadricuspid valve

Fig. 3.28 Examples of bicuspid and quadricuspid aortic valves. See 🎬 Video 3.16, 🎬 Video 3.17, 🎬 Video 3.18, 🎬 Video 3.19, 🎬 Video 3.20.

Tricuspid valve

Normal anatomy

The tricuspid valve has 3 cusps of unequal size: anterior (largest) extends from infundibulum anteriorly to the inferolateral wall posteriorly. The posterior leaflet arises along the posterior margin of the annulus from the septum to the inferolateral wall and the septal (smallest) leaflet extends from the interventricular septum to the posterior ventricular border (Fig. 3.29). Their anatomy is very variable. The free margins of the cusps are attached to chordae tendinae which are, in turn, attached in groups to three papillary muscles (anterior, posterior, and septal) that project from the septum and right ventricular free wall. Chordae from each papillary muscle attach to all leaflets. The valve has an annulus and valve ring with a normal area of 5–8cm^2. The valve allows free flow of blood from the right atrium during diastole but closes as systole increases the intraventricular pressure. Abnormalities of the tricuspid valve must not be overlooked, especially in mitral valve disease.

Normal findings

2D views

- The best views are: parasternal short-axis (aortic valve level), right ventricular inflow, apical 4-chamber, and subcostal views.

2D findings

- Parasternal short axis (aortic valve level): the tricuspid valve lies to the right of the aorta. The anterior leaflet is seen on the left and septal is closest to the atrial septum. In all views the tricuspid leaflets demonstrate wide diastolic opening and a normal coaptation in systole.
- Right ventricular inflow: this gives a very good view of the posterior (on the left) and anterior (on the right) leaflets as well as the right atrium, right ventricle and, sometimes, the inferior vena cava, coronary sinus and Eustachian valve.
- Apical 4-chamber: the anterior and septal leaflets are seen (septal nearest the septum). In this view the tricuspid annulus (normal adult 28 ± 5mm) should lie closer to the apex (up to 1cm) than the mitral annulus. This plane also provides a good view of the right heart.
- Subcostal 4-chamber: this view allows good access to images of the right atrium, atrial septum and inferior vena cava. The tricuspid valve (anterior and septal leaflets) is usually clearly seen similar to the apical 4-chamber view.

3D views and findings

- 3D datasets are best obtained from the apical position. However, it is possible to use a modified position within the parasternal window that lies close to the tricuspid valve, or sometimes a subcostal window.
- The tricuspid valve and apparatus has a complex geometrical shape and 3D views can be used for a more detailed quantitative assessment of the anatomy prior to surgical intervention.

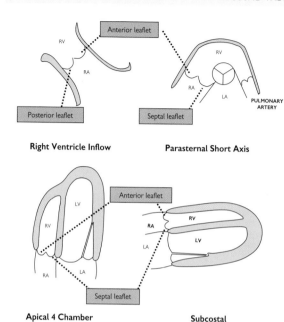

Right Ventricle Inflow

Parasternal Short Axis

Apical 4 Chamber

Subcostal

Fig. 3.29 Key views to study the tricuspid valve.

Tricuspid regurgitation

General

Tricuspid regurgitation is common. Because the leaflets are irregular a small amount of central, physiological regurgitation is seen in up to 70% of normal individuals. Physiological regurgitation is associated with normal valvular anatomy and no dilatation of the RV. Pathological regurgitation is usually secondary to right ventricular and tricuspid annular dilatation. Primary causes of tricuspid regurgitation are due to changes to the valve or subvalvular apparatus (Box 3.2).

Tricuspid regurgitation is usually seen in patients with multiple valve lesions, including aortic and mitral.

Assessment

'Physiological' regurgitation should be commented upon (<1cm adjacent to valve closure). Transthoracic echocardiography should aim to establish the aetiology of pathological tricuspid regurgitation and provide a quantitative estimate of severity. The assessment must also include evaluation of the right-sided chambers (Table 3.5).

Appearance

- Anatomy: assess for prolapsing (usually septal and anterior), flail, or billowing valve. An apical 3D full-volume set enables detailed assessment of tricuspid valve apparatus from multiple views and commissural fusion/leaflet coaptation can be assessed using the '*en face*' view.
- Look at the regurgitant jet with colour flow Doppler in several views and comment on the direction and size of the jet.
- Report abnormal valve appearance (restricted motion and thickening of carcinoid, vegetations of endocarditis or valve rupture).
- Report tricuspid valve annulus size.
- Report right heart size and function (📖 p.264) and assess right ventricular systolic pressure (📖 p.162).

Pacemakers and tricuspid regurgitation

Tricuspid regurgitation is more common with a pacemaker lead (both temporary and permanent) because it disrupts leaflet coaption. Tricuspid valve velocity however will not be affected as this is determined by right ventricular systolic pressure.

Box 3.2 Causes of tricuspid regurgitation

Valve and apparatus
- Infection
  - Endocarditis
  - Rheumatic heart disease
- Congenital: Ebstein's anomoly
- Metabolic: carcinoid
- Connective tissue disease
- Subvalvular
  - Chordal rupture
  - Papillary muscle dysfunction
- Infiltration
- Malignancy
- Non-penetrating trauma.

Right heart
- Pulmonary hypertension
- Right heart failure with lung pathology
- Ischaemic heart disease
- Pulmonary valve disease
- Cardiomyopathy
- Volume overload
- Pacing lead

Table 3.5 Parameters to assess severity of tricuspid regurgitation

	Mild	Severe
Qualitative		
Valve structure	Normal	Abnormal
Jet (Nyquist 50–60cm/s)	<5cm^2	>10cm^2
CW trace	Soft & parabolic	Dense & triangular
Semi-quantitative		
Vena contracta	–	>0.7cm
PISA r (Nyquist 40cm/s)	<0.5cm	>0.9cm
Tricuspid inflow	Normal	E wave dominant >1m/s
Hepatic vein flow	Normal	Systolic reversal
Quantitative		
EROA	Not defined	≥40mm^2
R vol	Not defined	>45mL
RV/RA/IVC	Normal size	Usually dilated

Report as **moderate** if signs of regurgitation are greater than **mild** but there are few features of **severe** regurgitation.

Grading severity

- The methods to grade severity are borrowed directly from those used for mitral regurgitation. Assessment of tricuspid regurgitation tends to be more subjective with less clinical need for accuracy. Colour flow imaging should be used to diagnose TR. Quantitative assessment is performed using *vena contracta*, *flow convergence* (PISA), *continuous wave density*, and *contour*. There are also changes in *hepatic vein flow* which are equivalent to changes in pulmonary vein flow seen in mitral regurgitation (see Table 3.5). It is essential to use multiple views to assess severity.

Vena contracta

- In the apical 4-chamber view place colour flow over the tricuspid valve and obtain a plane that demonstrates the regurgitant orifice.
- Zoom in on the valve and measure the vena contracta (narrowest diameter of the colour flow jet as it passes through the valve)—>7mm suggests severe regurgitation, see Fig. 3.30.

Continuous wave Doppler waveform

- In the apical 4-chamber, parasternal short axis or right ventricular inflow views drop the continuous wave through the tricuspid valve aligned with the regurgitant jet.
- Report the signal intensity relative to the antegrade flow and comment on the waveform (parabolic or triangular). Triangular and dense suggests severe regurgitation, see Fig. 3.31.
- Use TR jet to determine RV or pulmonary artery systolic pressure (📖 p.162)

Jet area

- In the apical 4-chamber view obtain an image that includes the entire right atrium and the main plane of the regurgitant jet.
- Record a loop and scroll through to a frame with the largest jet. Trace around the jet and report the area. >10cm^2 suggests severe regurgitation.

Right ventricular inflow

- Flow of blood into the right ventricle can be used as a guide to severity (equivalent to measurement of E wave velocity in mitral regurgitation). Peak E velocity at the tricuspid valve of ≥1m/s suggests severe tricuspid regurgitation.

Hepatic vein flow

- In a subcostal view place the PW Doppler cursor in a hepatic vein that aligns with the probe and record a spectral tracing of flow. Normally flow through both systole and diastole is towards the right atrium. In severe tricuspid regurgitation the rise in right atrial pressure leads to flow away from the right heart during systole. Report systolic flow reversal if seen.

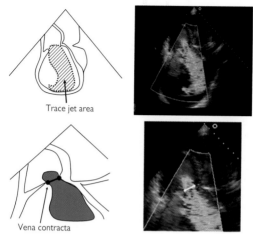

Trace jet area

Vena contracta

Fig. 3.30 Measurement of jet area (top) and quantify your assessment with a vena contracta (bottom) or PISA measurement.

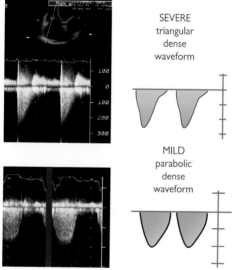

SEVERE
triangular
dense
waveform

MILD
parabolic
dense
waveform

Fig. 3.31 Density and shape of Doppler can give clues to severity.

3D for assessment of tricuspid regurgitation?

3D echocardiography can be used to help quantify tricuspid regurgitation severity and also the mechanism, in particular the annulus size (Fig. 3.33).

Colour flow mapping

- As with 3D the assessment of mitral regurgitation, full volume colour Doppler imaging permits the regurgitant jet to be rotated and cropped to ensure that the vena contracta is being measured in a plane that is parallel to the jet and also at the narrowest point during maximal flow (Fig. 3.32).
- 3D echocardiography allows the valve to be assessed from the 'en face' view to help identify prolapsing valve segments accurately.

Tricuspid annulus

- Real-time 3D transthoracic echocardiography is routinely available and allows simultaneous assessment of the morphology, movement of the three leaflets and attachment to the tricuspid annulus.
- It has been shown that 3D echocardiography allows visualization and measurement of the entire oval-shaped annulus in patients with dilated or normal sized annuluss, something which was underestimated by 2D echocardiography.

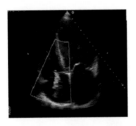
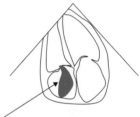

Mild and severe tricuspid regurgitation

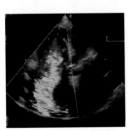
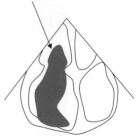

Fig. 3.32 Colour flow mapping of tricuspid regurgitation in apical 4-chamber views with examples of mild (top) and severe (bottom) regurgitation. See ▣ Video 3.21.

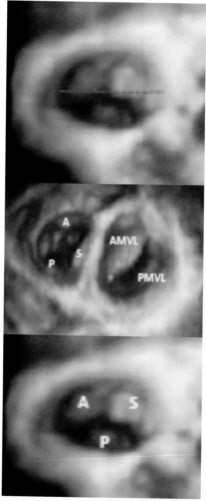

Fig. 3.33 3D full volume acquisition of the tricuspid valve. The initial image was taken from apical 4-chamber view. Top: subsequent rotation and cropping to reveal the TV from the ventricular side and show the anterior leaflet (A), septal leaflet (S), and posterior leaflet (P). Anterior (AMVL) and posterior (PMVL) mitral valve leaflets also seen. Bottom: TV rotated and leaflets seen from the right atrial view. Full volume 3D acquisition of the tricuspid valve. The oval shape of the annulus is appreciated. See 📹 Video 3.22.

Right heart haemodynamics

The most widely reported haemodynamic measure in echocardiography is *right ventricular systolic pressure*. This is partly because it has a broad clinical relevance and partly because it is easy to measure as it uses tricuspid regurgitation—found in 70% of individuals.

Measurement is based on velocity of regurgitation across the tricuspid valve. This is used to calculate pressure across the valve—the higher the pressure in the right ventricle relative to the right atrium, the higher the velocity of regurgitant blood. To calculate right ventricular systolic pressure *right atrial pressure* must be added to this pressure. Fortunately, there are clinical (jugular venous pressure [JVP]) and echocardiographic methods (inferior vena cava [IVC] and right atrial size) to estimate right atrial pressure.

Right atrial pressure

- JVP can be used but requires accurate clinical assessment with the patient lying at 45°. The measure lacks accuracy if very low or very high and is directly affected by moderate to severe tricuspid regurgitation.
- A floating constant of 5, 10, or 15 mmHg can be used based on the pattern of changes in *right atrial size*, *inferior vena cava*, and *tricuspid regurgitation severity* (Table 3.6).
  - Assess right atrial size from an apical four chamber view (📖 p.284). Report as normal, dilated, or very dilated. Measure IVC diameter from a subcostal view (<1.7 cm is normal, except in athletes when diameter can be 2–3cm) and check for respiratory variation (ask the patient to sniff). IVC should reduce in size by around 50% (Fig. 3.34). Tricuspid regurgitation severity is assessed routinely (📖 p.158).
- If accurate assessment of right atrial pressure is not possible then a constant of 10mmHg (or 14mmHg) can be used but this will systematically overestimate right systolic ventricular pressures (RSVP) at low levels and underestimate it at high levels.
- Recently, an alternative approach has been suggested based on IVC diameter and response to sniff. If IVC <2.1cm and collapses >50% then RA pressure is 3mmHg. If IVC >2.1cm and collapses <50% then RA pressure is 15mmHg. Otherwise assume pressure is 8mmHg.

Tricuspid velocity and right ventricular systolic pressure

- In apical four chamber, parasternal short axis or right ventricular inflow view, align continuous wave through the tricuspid valve regurgitation.
- Record a spectral trace and measure the peak velocity (Fig. 3.35). Based on the simplified Bernoulli equation:

$$\text{Pressure gradient} = 4 \times \text{peak velocity}^2$$

- Report *right ventricular systolic pressure* as the tricuspid *pressure gradient* plus the estimate of *right atrial pressure*.

Pulmonary artery systolic pressure

- By subtracting the pressure gradient across the pulmonary valve (📖 p.174) from *right ventricular systolic pressure* you can calculate *pulmonary artery systolic pressure*. Because the gradient is usually small and right atrial pressure is estimated, *right ventricular systolic pressure* is often reported as *pulmonary artery systolic pressure*.

Table 3.6 Parameters to help identify fluid status

	Suggests hypovolaemia	Normal range	Suggests volume overload
IVC diameter and response	<1cm and collapsing	1–2.5cm, collapsing 25–75%	>2.5cm, no response to respiration
LVIDd/BSA (cm/m²)	<2.4 women	2.4–3.2	>3.2
	<2.2 men	2.2–3.1	>3.1
LVEDAI (short axis)	<5.5	5.5–10	>10
End point septal separation	<0.5m	>0.5cm	–
LVESD	Papillary apposition	2.0–4.0cm	–
RV internal dimensions	–	See below	RVIDd >LVIDd
Interventricular septum	–	No flattening	Diastolic flattening
Right atrium	–	<20cm²	>30cm²

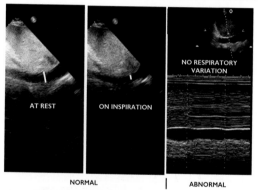

NORMAL | ABNORMAL

Fig. 3.34 The 2D images demonstrate normal respiratory variation of the inferior vena cava and the M-mode trace lack of variation.

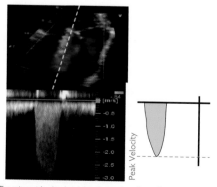

Fig. 3.35 The tricuspid valve has been focused on from the apical 4-chamber view to obtain a continuous wave Doppler trace across the tricuspid valve to measure peak velocity and derive a pressure gradient.

Tricuspid stenosis

General
Tricuspid stenosis is rare. The commonest cause is rheumatic heart disease with coexistent mitral stenosis. Other causes include: carcinoid (Fig. 3.36), lupus valvulitis, pacemaker or valvular endocarditis, right atrial tumour, and obstruction of right ventricle inflow tract (large atrial thrombus or large vegetations). It is usually associated with tricuspid regurgitation.

Appearance
Comment on:
- Leaflet thickening or calcification.
- Leaflet motion: classically restricted with diastolic doming of 1 or more leaflets (especially the anterior leaflet).
- Right atrial enlargement.
- Dilated IVC.
- 3D echocardiography provides anatomical detail of leaflets and orifice area.

Grading severity
- Determine severity on the transvalvular gradient (Table 3.7):
  - Use CW Doppler aligned across the tricuspid valve in an apical 4-chamber view (averaged throughout the respiratory cycle).
  - Measure peak velocity (Fig. 3.37) and calculate peak gradient using the Bernoulli equation.
- Severe tricuspid stenosis is associated with a valve area of <1cm^2 or a peak gradient of >7mmHg (mean >5mmHg) and an inflow time-velocity integral >60cm.
- Pressure half time can not be used to measure valve area as the appropriate constant for the tricuspid valve has not been determined.
- Severity can also be assessed from valve area. This can be calculated using the continuity equation. A PW Doppler vti can be taken at the level of the valve annulus and the CSA of the tricuspid annulus calculated based on the annulus diameter and the assumption that the orifice is circular. These measurements can then be combined with the continuous wave vti across the valve.

Tricuspid valve area = (Annulus PW vti × area of annulus)/valve CW vti

3D for assessment of tricuspid stenosis?
- In mitral stenosis it is possible to accurately planimeter the valve orifice area in the short axis view with 2D imaging. Due to the complex geometry of the tricuspid valve it is not possible to accurately assess the valve orifice area with 2D short axis views.
- 3D echocardiography allows the tricuspid valve to be rotated and cropped in any plane and to appreciate the morphology from short axis views and to also see the valve *en face* and delineate the individual leaflets. Both of these 3D tools can be used to planimeter the orifice.

Table 3.7 Parameters of TS

	Mild	Moderate	Severe
Mean gradient (mmHg)	<4	4–7	>7
Valve area (cm^2)	–	–	<1

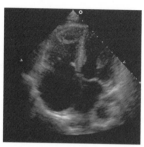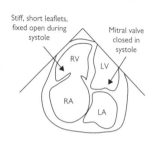

Stiff, short leaflets, fixed open during systole

Mitral valve closed in systole

RV

LV

RA

LA

Fig. 3.36 An apical 4-chamber view demonstrating carcinoid heart disease causing tricuspid stenosis. See ▣ Video 3.23.

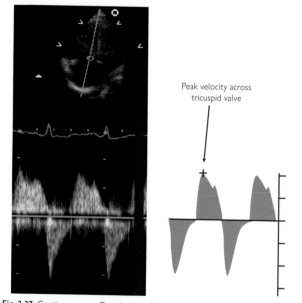

Peak velocity across tricuspid valve

Fig. 3.37 Continuous wave Doppler is used in an apical 4-chamber view to record peak velocity across the tricuspid valve. This can be used to estimate a gradient in tricuspid stenosis.

Tricuspid valve surgery

Tricuspid valve surgery—replacement or annuloplasty—is considered in severe tricuspid regurgitation with haemodynamic consequences or when associated with mitral valve disease.

Carcinoid syndrome

Characterized by the release of 5-hydroxytryptamine from a metastasizing tumour resulting in thickened and shortened tricuspid leaflets with severe tricuspid regurgitation. The pulmonary valve may also be involved and the right atrium and right ventricle are frequently dilated.

Infective endocarditis

Right-sided endocarditis is uncommon except in intravenous drug users, patients with indwelling catheters, or those with ventricular septal defects. Vegetations usually occur on the tricuspid valve (Fig. 3.38) in intravenous drug use, but many have associated left-sided lesions.

Ebstein anomaly

A congenital anomaly of the tricuspid valve with apical displacement of 1 or more leaflets. This diagnosis should be considered when the distance between the mitral and tricuspid valve planes is >1cm. There is enlargement of the right atrium and tricuspid regurgitation.

3D transthoracic echocardiography provides detailed anatomical and functional images prior to surgical intervention.

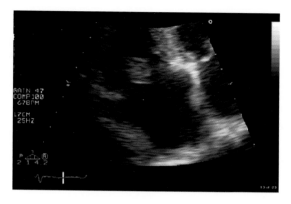

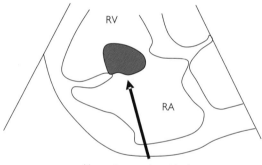

Vegetation on tricuspid valve

Fig. 3.38 A zoomed apical 4-chamber view to highlight a vegetation on the tricuspid valve. See ⚏ Video 3.24.

Pulmonary valve

Normal anatomy
The pulmonary valve consists of 3 leaflets: anterior, left, and right. It develops alongside the aortic valve and then the right heart and pulmonary artery twists around the left heart and aorta. The valve lies at the junction of the right ventricular outflow tract and the pulmonary trunk. It is thinner than the aortic valve as a result of the lower right heart pressures.

Normal findings
Views
- There are limited views of the pulmonary valve (Fig. 3.39). The best views are the parasternal short axis (aortic valve level) and the right ventricular outflow. Subcostal short-axis views (at the aortic valve level) can also be used but are similar to the parasternal short axis view.

Findings
- Parasternal short axis (aortic valve level): this provides a view of the tricuspid valve, right ventricle, and pulmonary valve wrapped around the aortic valve. The pulmonary valve lies on the right and this view can be used to align Doppler through the right ventricle outflow, pulmonary valve, and pulmonary artery.
- Right ventricular outflow: in some people this provides excellent views of the pulmonary valve, pulmonary artery, and bifurcation. This view can also be used for alignment of Doppler.

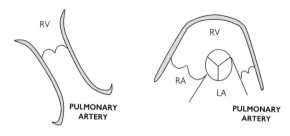

Right ventricle outflow   **Parasternal short axis**

Fig. 3.39 Key views to assess the pulmonary valve.

Pulmonary regurgitation

General

Colour flow mapping of the pulmonary valve identifies small regurgitant jets in most people (Fig. 3.40). These can often be quite eccentric. Pathological causes of regurgitation are similar to those for tricuspid regurgitation (Table 3.5, Box 3.2).

Primary valve problems include: rheumatic heart disease, infective endocarditis, carcinoid, iatrogenic (post-valvuloplasty), congenital (following surgery for tetralogy of Fallot, leaflet absence). Secondary causes are due to dilatation of the pulmonary artery (e.g. pulmonary hypertension, Marfan's).

Appearance

- Examine for anatomic abnormalities to identify mechanism of regurgitation including anomalies of cusp number, structure or movement. Comment on any visible valve pathology (e.g. thickening, vegetation).
- Map the regurgitation with colour flow in the parasternal short axis and right ventricular outflow views. Comment on size, site of regurgitation, and direction.
- Pulmonary regurgitation is commonly at one edge of a commissure and can appear to lie next to the aorta. This should not be confused with an aorta–pulmonary communication which would have flow throughout the cardiac cycle instead of just during diastole.

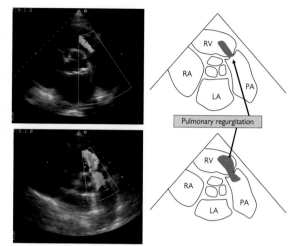

Fig. 3.40 Colour flow mapping of pulmonary regurgitation in parasternal short axis views. Mild (top) and severe (lower) regurgitation. See ⚎ Video 3.25.

Grading severity
- Criteria for assessment are borrowed from aortic regurgitation but assessment is more qualitative (Table 3.8).
- Grade severity as *mild*, *moderate* or *severe* based on:
  - Jet length and width relative to outflow tract: Jet diameter is measured at pulmonary valve leaflets level during early diastole: jet diameter >0.98cm indicates significant regurgitation. Jet width >65% of right ventricular outflow tract indicates severe pulmonary regurgitation.
  - Pulmonary regurgitation index (PR Index) is the ratio between pulmonary regurgitation time and total diastole. An index <0.77 suggests severe PR. The lower the value, the more severe the regurgitation.
  - Vena contracta width lacks validation. 3D vena contracta provides more quantitative assessment of PR. EROA values mild <20mm^2, moderate 21–115 mm^2, and severe >115mm^2 have been proposed.[1]
  - Continuous wave regurgitation intensity and shape. Increased intensity and slope of the Doppler signal (deceleration time) suggests severe (Fig. 3.41).
  - (Abnormal pulmonary artery anatomy suggests more severe regurgitation.)
  - Flow across pulmonary valve relative to systemic circulation and evidence of right ventricle dilatation.
  - Holodiastolic flow reversal in the main pulmonary artery (equivalent to aortic flow reversal) suggests severe regurgitation.
- Comment on changes to the right heart—with severe PR, patients often develop RV dilatation from volume overload and tricuspid annulus dilatation and tricuspid regurgitation.

Pulmonary artery diastolic pressure
- The velocity of the regurgitant jet can be used to quantify the pressure gradient (using the Bernoulli equation) between the pulmonary artery and right ventricle during diastole.
- Add right ventricular diastolic pressure (assumed to be *right atrial pressure*, see Table 3.6) to the pulmonary valve pressure gradient to calculate *pulmonary artery end diastolic pressure*.
- To calculate *mean pulmonary artery end pressure* use pulmonary artery systolic pressure (📖 p.162) in the equation:

$$\frac{diatolic\ pressure + systolic\ pressure}{3}$$

Table 3.8 Parameters to assess pulmonary regurgitation

	Mild	Severe
Pulmonary valve anatomy	Normal	Abnormal
Jet size on colour flow	<10mm long	Large with wide origin
CW density and shape	Soft and slow	Dense and steep
PR Index		<0.77
Jet width of RVOT		>65%
Pulmonary artery flow compared to systemic	Increased	Greatly increased
Right ventricle size	Normal	Dilated

If features suggest more than **mild** regurgitation but no features of **severe** grade as **moderate**.

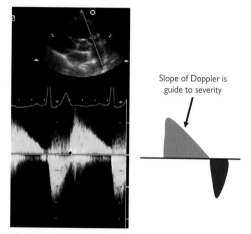

Slope of Doppler is guide to severity

Fig. 3.41 Doppler features to assess pulmonary regurgitation.

Reference

1 Pothineni KR et al. Live/real time three dimensional transthoracic echocardiographic assessment of pulmonary regurgitation. *Echocardiography* 2008; **26**(8):911–17.

Pulmonary stenosis

General

Pulmonary stenosis is usually valvular and congenital (e.g. related to rubella, Noonan's, or tetralogy of Fallot). The valve usually has fusion of several cusps to form a funnel. Pulmonary stenosis can also occur due to stenosis of the main pulmonary artery (e.g. following rubella, post-surgical banding of the pulmonary artery) or subvalvular problems (e.g. congenital in association with valvular stenosis, tetralogy of Fallot, and transposition of the great arteries).

Rheumatic pulmonary stenosis is rare. Carcinoid disease is the commonest cause of acquired pulmonary stenosis. Functional pulmonary stenosis may arise from RV outflow tract compression by tumours.

Appearance
- Comment on the valve:
  - Number of leaflets.
  - Thickened, dysplastic, calcified leaflets.
  - Motion: doming of valve leaflets in systole and restricted motion.
  - Measure size of pulmonary annulus.
- Comment on associated structures:
  - Right ventricular outflow tract and evidence of narrowing, e.g. infundibular/subvalvar stenosis.
  - Post-stenotic dilatation of the pulmonary artery.
  - Right ventricular hypertrophy.
  - Functional tricuspid regurgitation secondary to pressure overload.

Grading severity

Grade severity based on the peak gradient. This can be supported by calculating the valve effective orifice area (Table 3.9).
- In the parasternal short axis (aortic valve level) or right ventricular outflow view measure the velocity across the pulmonary valve with CW Doppler aligned through the right ventricular outflow tract, pulmonary valve and common pulmonary artery.
- Report velocity and gradient across the valve (calculated with the simplified Bernoulli equation). Mean gradient and pulmonary valve vti can be obtained by tracing the spectral waveform (Fig. 3.42).
- Measure right ventricular systolic pressure.
- The continuity equation can be used to measure effective orifice area of the pulmonary valve. In the parasternal short axis view record a right ventricular outflow tract (RVOT) PW Doppler peak velocity or vti (velocity$_{(RVOT)}$). Measure the outflow tract diameter at this point and calculate a CSA assuming it is circular (cross sectional area$_{(RVOT)}$). Then use the continuity equation including these measures and the peak velocity or vti from CW across the valve (velocity$_{(pulmonary\ valve)}$). Pulmonary valve CSA equals:

$$\left[\text{velocity}_{(RVOT)} \times \text{cross-sectional area}_{(RVOT)} \right] / \text{velocity}_{(pulmonary\ value)}$$

Table 3.9 Parameters to determine severity of pulmonary stenosis

	Mild	Moderate	Severe
Peak velocity (m/s)	<3	3–4	>4
Peak gradient (mmHg)	<36	36–64	>64
Valve area (cm^2)	>1.0	0.5–1.0	<0.5

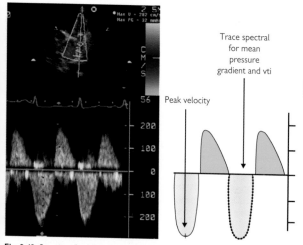

Fig. 3.42 Severity of pulmonary stenosis can be assessed in a similar way to assessment of aortic stenosis. In this example a continuous wave Doppler trace has been obtained from a parasternal short axis view. The peak velocity can used to calculate a gradient or be used in the continuity equation.

Mechanical prosthetic valves (Fig. 3.43)

All mechanical valves consist of a mobile component (occluder), the restraining system (to restrict occluder motion), and the sewing ring (attaches prosthesis to vessel). Blood flow is restricted through these and normal pressure gradients are therefore higher across mechanical, compared to native, valves. Valve components are metallic or plastic coated, with a carbon layer. These cause shadows and reverberations so scanning from different positions is required to assess the valve. In particular, mitral prosthesis regurgitation is masked on transthoracic images and if valve dysfunction is suspected transoesophageal imaging maybe required.

Ball and cage (Starr Edwards)

The ball and cage valve consists of a sewing ring attached to a cage made of 3 or 4 struts. The blood flows on all sides around a Silastic ball occluder, which moves within the cage. Blood flow is directed laterally within the valve and converges downstream (Fig. 3.44, upper image).

Assessment

Use all standard imaging planes adjusted where necessary with slight rotation or tilting to minimize shadows.

Normal appearances

Whether valve is open or closed there will be significant shadows from the sewing ring and reverberation from the ball. Structures and flows behind the valve are masked. Physiologic regurgitation is a trivial central jet.

Tilting disc (e.g. Medtronic-Hall, Omniscience)

A single circular disc suspended within a frame, with an off-centre hinge point. Opening therefore creates 2 orifices, 1 large (major) and 1 small (minor).

Assessment

Use standard imaging planes with slight rotation or tilting as necessary. Images are usually best when through the central hinge point or perpendicular to the closed disc. For mitral prostheses use apical windows for assessment. For aortic prostheses use apical windows for Doppler and parasternal to differentiate valvular from perivalvular regurgitation.

Normal appearances

There are shadows from the sewing ring and reverberations from the disc throughout the cardiac cycle.

- *Valve closed:* structures and flow behind the valve are masked. Physiologic regurgitation is 2 small jets between disc and ring. Some may have a jet associated with the central strut and some a very long central jet.
- *Valve open:* disc opens to 55–75°. The strut can be seen in a central position underneath the sewing ring. 2 colour jets can be displayed. CW Doppler velocities are similar through minor and major orifice.

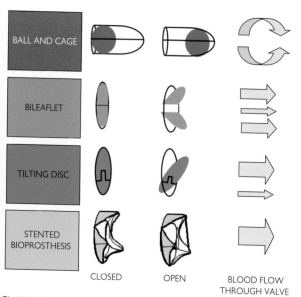

Fig. 3.43 Diagram of mechanical prosthesis design and blood flow.

When to use transoesophageal echocardiography?

Transthoracic echocardiography usually provides good alignment with the transprosthetic flow. Therefore detection of prosthesis stenosis is not a problem. However, transthoracic assessment of regurgitation is limited by shadowing and distance to the transducer. Haemodynamic assessment or an aortic valve prothesis is usually better with a transthoracic study. Indications for transoesophageal imaging are:

- Transthoracic imaging is inconclusive or non-diagnostic.
- Transthoracic findings not in agreement with clinical findings.
- Suspected problems of mitral mechanical valve prosthesis.
- Suspected prosthetic valve endocarditis.
- Suspected prosthetic valve thrombosis.
- Intraoperative use (to guide repair, assess success, complications).

Bileaflet (e.g. Carbomedics, St. Jude)

These consist of 2 leaflets, separately hinged in the centre of the prosthesis. 3 orifices are created in the open position: 2 large lateral orifices and 1 small central orifice (Fig. 3.44, lower image). If used in the aortic position a supra-annular placement is often possible and may be used in double valve replacement in order to achieve greater separation of the valves.

Assessment

As for single tilting disc, use standard imaging planes, mainly apical for mitral prostheses and both apical and parasternal for aortic valves. Before making diagnosis of impaired motion of one or both discs, ensure transducer has been rotated thoroughly to obtain a position in which the cursor (ultrasound beam) is aligned perpendicularly to the central line of the disc coaptation.

Normal appearances

There will be shadows from the sewing ring and reverberation from discs throughout the cardiac cycle.

- *Valve closed:* discs close at about 25° and mask structures and flow behind the valve. Physiologic regurgitation is up to 4 jets originating at pivot points near the edge of the valve.
- *Valve open:* discs open to 55–75° and 2 separate discs are often seen. There is more flow acceleration through the narrow central orifice. Therefore CW measures through the centre may overestimate the overall pressure gradient, especially for small aortic prosthetic valves. Use mean rather than peak gradient.

Physiologic regurgitation

Physiologic regurgitation is normal with tilting disc and bileaflet prostheses. There are 2 components: (1) an initial backward flow during valve closure (2) holosystolic flow designed to 'wash' the valves and reduce risk of valve thrombosis. These are referred to as 'wash' or 'closing' jets.

Differentiation of closing and physiologic jets from pathological regurgitation?

Physiologic jets:

- Flow is contained within the sewing ring.
- Colour flow pattern is usually thin and laminar.
- Jet length usually less <2–3cm.

Pathologic jets:

- Any perivalvular jets (outside the sewing ring).
- Different from the expected signature of the physiologic pattern for the valve.

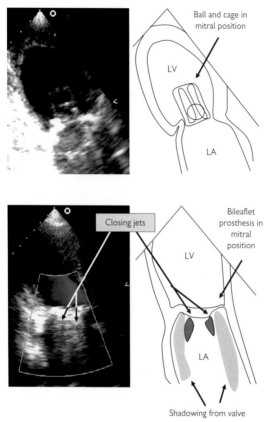

Fig. 3.44 Examples of apical views of mitral mechanical prostheses. The top figure demonstrates a ball and cage valve and the lower figure a bileaflet prosthesis with two closing jets. Note shadows behind the sewing ring. See 📹 Video 3.26 and 📹 Video 3.27.

Bioprosthetic valves

Bioprosthetic valves are made from porcine aortic valve or bovine pericardium. The leaflets are stiffer than native valve leaflets. Bioprostheses may be stented or stentless. Stents or struts support the cusps and protrude downstream (into the aorta with aortic bioprostheses or left ventricle with mitral bioprostheses). Struts and the ring are metallic so cause shadowing (although less than mechanical prostheses). Some models can be implanted in a supravalvular position. Although their flow profile is similar to native valves, there is still an increased pressure gradient across the prosthetic valves, particularly stented bioprostheses.

Stented bioprosthesis (Fig. 3.45)

Assessment
Use standard scan planes. Image prostheses through apical windows with the beam perpendicular to the closed leaflets. Rotate transducer whilst using colour flow mapping to assess perivalvular regurgitation.

Normal appearance
There will be shadows from the sewing ring and stents protruding downstream throughout the cardiac cycle. In the apical view usually 2 struts are displayed and, in the short axis, the ring and 3 struts are visible. If the aortic root is dilated there may be free space between sewing ring and root.
- *Valve closed:* leaflets appear thin like a native valve. Physiologic regurgitation may be present as small central jet (usually early postoperatively).
- *Valve open:* valve opens widely with leaflets parallel to the stent (2–4mm distance).

Stentless bioprosthesis

Assessment
Use standard scan planes. Usually no shadowing.

Normal appearance
Usually very similar to native aortic valve. Leaflets may appear thickened and junction between valve and annulus may be thickened due to sutures. Pulmonary valve homografts may have supravalvular thickening and stenosis. Ideally, no regurgitant jet but sometimes minor distortion during implantation or due to mismatch of prosthesis causes mild central regurgitation. Jet may be eccentric if due to distortion.

Homografts and autografts

May be used in endocarditis or as an autograft in young patients in aortic valve disease (Ross procedure: native pulmonary valve is used for aortic valve replacement and a bioprosthesis is implanted as pulmonary valve). Scan planes and appearances are as for stentless bioprosthesis.

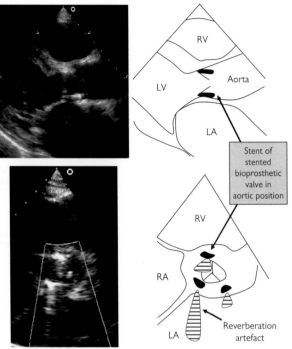

Fig. 3.45 Examples of stented bioprosthetic valves. The top figure shows a parasternal long axis view of an aortic prosthesis and the lower figure a parasternal short axis view. Note the bright struts with artefacts extending away. See 📽 Video 3.28 and 📽 Video 3.29.

Prosthetic valve abnormalities

Vegetation, thrombus, pannus

Extended masses on a prosthesis. Pannus is excessive endothelial proliferation causing obstruction and/or failure in complete valve closure. Pannus is sometimes difficult to distinguish from thrombus. Both may be present. No specific texture differentiates masses so to differentiate use:

- Appearance: thrombi usually larger, protrude from the sewing ring and less echocardiographically dense.
- Clinical information: suboptimal anticoagulation makes thrombus more likely, bacteraemia makes vegetation more likely.
- Associated abnormalities: vegetations may be associated with paravalvular abscesses, leaks.

Bioprosthetic valve degeneration

Observed in most prostheses after several years. Infrequent in first 3 years. Leaflet calcification results in irregular thickening (usually >3mm in thickness). Rigid leaflets have decreased cusp motion, cause stenoses and may rupture resulting in prolapse (or flail cusp) and valvular regurgitation.

Prosthetic valve dehiscence—'rocking' valve (Fig. 3.46)

Exaggerated mobility of valve ring indicates dehiscence. Assess with 2D. Usually associated with severe paravalvular regurgitation. Valve dehiscence is usually preceded by paravalvular leaks.

Valve prolapse In bioprostheses, prolapse of leaflet tissue is possible and is seen in standard views. Usually leaflets are degenerated (irregular thickening and calcification) and valvular regurgitation will be present.

Structural damage For example, broken occluder or restraining system, will be combined with intravalvular regurgitation.

Sutures Seen as immobile, dense structures within the ring. Can be difficult to differentiate from focal fibrosis. They will be mobile if dehisced.

Strands Mobile, filamentous strands on normal and abnormal valves (rarely seen adjacent to native valve). Thought to be fibrin strands (they can disappear after thrombolysis of thrombosed prostheses). Poor reproducibility in imaging these structures as visualization is highly dependent on machine settings.

Pseudo-microbubbles (Fig. 3.47) Look like single contrast microbubbles. Probably due to micro-cavitation. Found with normal valves but more often if valve dysfunction. Appear as dots, moving away from prosthesis, visible only shortly after valve closure (unless valvular or paravalvular leak). In contrast, spontaneous echo contrast is seen only in areas of low blood velocity (therefore not at orifices or leakages of prosthetic valves) and is smoke-like in appearance with swirling patterns.

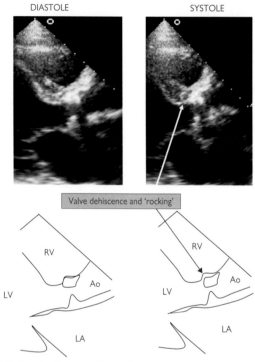

Fig. 3.46 Example of aortic prosthesis rocking.

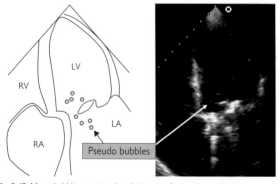

Fig. 3.47 Micro-bubbles associated with closure of a mitral prosthesis.

Prosthestic valve stenosis

Prosthetic valve stenosis suggests an acceleration of blood through the prosthetic valve because of some pathology. Pressure gradients may go up with thrombus/pannus and, rarely, vegetations or degeneration.

Assessment

General

If stenosis is suspected, initial assessment should be to look for pathology that might explain stenosis (thrombus, vegetation, valve dysfunction) and check the level of any obstruction (outflow tract, valve level). Then gather supportive information about severity of any stenosis.

Grading severity

Pressure gradient and velocity (Fig. 3.48)

Techniques are as for native valves (CW Doppler) but mechanical prostheses can have 2 or 3 different-sized orifices so application of Bernoulli equation is not straightforward and calculations can vary depending on Doppler alignment. With cage-and-ball prostheses it is almost impossible to get optimal Doppler alignment. In clinical practice, calculation of effective orifice area is useful.

Orifice area—aortic valve prostheses

Use same technique as for native valve (CW, PW, and LVOT diameter). Reporting orifice area also avoids problems with variation in cardiac output. For St. Jude bileaflet aortic prosthesis a Doppler velocity index has been validated:

vti across LVOT/vti across aortic valve <0.23 suggests severe stenosis

Orifice area—mitral valve prostheses

Use techniques as for native valves. The pressure half-time tends to underestimate effective orifice area but can be used. Width of the forward flow may be an alternative, if measured in 2 orthogonal planes.

What is abnormal for prosthetic valves?

Normal mechanical and stented bioprostheses have a pressure gradient equivalent to mild or moderate stenosis. Normal ranges vary between manufacturers and valves so refer to published information to give clinical advice. Pressure gradients also vary with haemodynamics, such as cardiac output, so there is considerable interpatient variability. General principles about what might need investigation are best based on calculated orifice area:

- Aortic prostheses may be stenotic if calculated valve area is <1cm^2 or there has been a >30% change from last follow-up.
- Mitral prostheses may be stenotic if pressure half-time >200ms and peak diastolic velocity >2.5m/s (if only mild regurgitation).
- Tricuspid prostheses may be stenotic if peak diastolic velocity >2.5ms (if only mild regurgitation).

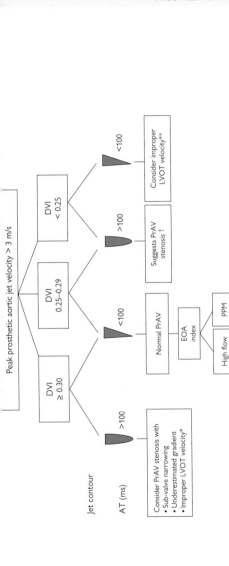

Fig 3.48 Algorithm for evaluation of elevated peak prosthetic aortic jet velocity incorporating DVI, jet contour, and acceleration time (AT). *Pulse wave (PW) Doppler sample too close to the valve (particularly when jet velocity by continuous wave (CW) Doppler is ≥ 4m/s). ** PW Doppler sample too far (apical) from the valve (particularly when jet velocity is 3-3.9m/s). † Stenosis further substantiated by estimated orifice area (ERO) derivation compared with reference values if valve type and size are known. Fluoroscopy and trans esophageal echocardi-ography (TEE) are helpful for further assessment, particularly in bileaf-let valves. Aortic valve replacement (AVR). Doppler velocity index (DVI) is the ratio of the proximal velocity in the left ventricle out flow tract to that of flow velocity proximal to the stenosis. Adapted from Figure 10, Recommendations for Evaluation of Prosthetic Valves With Echocardiography and Doppler Ultrasound. *American Society of Echocardiography* 2009, **22**(0):975–1014.

Prosthetic valve regurgitation

- *Transvalvular regurgitation* describes regurgitation within the sewing ring. This can be caused by leaflet prolapse (bioprostheses), incomplete disc closure due to clot, pannus (mechanical prostheses) or structural damage (broken retainment system, dislodged disc).
- *Paravalvular regurgitation* has its origin outside the sewing ring. This can occur immediately after surgery (usually trivial and resolves after protamine or with endothelialization during first few postoperative weeks), be due to dehiscence of the sewing ring, or secondary to endocarditis.

Assessment

Decide if regurgitation is *transvalvular* or *paravalvular* (Fig. 3.48). When jet is easily displayed it is often *paravalvular*, as physiologic and *transvalvular* regurgitation is shadowed by valve.

Use multiple views and look at jet position with colour flow (use systematic approach similar to identification of mitral leaflet scallop prolapse). Short axis views of rings are very useful to position jets. 3D echocardiography may give further information. If *paravalvular*, report extent and localization with figure or reference to 'clock face' in parasternal short axis view (for mitral valve, area adjacent to aortic valve is 12 o'clock).

Transoesophageal echocardiography provides a comprehensive assessment of severity and cause. It should always be performed if transthoracic screening suggests there may be clinically significant regurgitation.

Grading severity

Pathological regurgitant jets are usually eccentric and often multiple. Shadowing from sewing ring, struts or disc limit field of view. Therefore, colour flow area, PISA and vena contracta are not reliable. Assessment of severity is often qualitative, in which case indirect supportive measures should also be provided and transoesophageal echocardiography advised.

Supportive measures

- Increase in cavity diameters compared to previous studies.
- If no prosthetic stenosis, an increase in forward flow velocity (due to volume overload). For mitral prostheses moderate to severe regurgitation is suggested by a peak velocity >1.9m/s and mean gradient >5mmHg. If no aortic stenosis and only mild regurgitation then a ratio of vti mitral prothesis/vti aortic valve >2.5 suggests moderate to severe regurgitation.
- Pulmonary venous flow for mitral regurgitation (systolic flow reversal). If left ventricle function is impaired a blunted pulmonary vein flow pattern is 'normal' after mitral valve replacement.
- Aortic flow pattern for aortic regurgitation (diastolic flow reversal).

Other techniques

With *transvalvular* regurgitation (both mitral and aortic) one option is to measure the proportional area of the sewing ring occupied by the jet in a short axis view: <10% is mild, 10–25% is moderate, and >25% is severe.

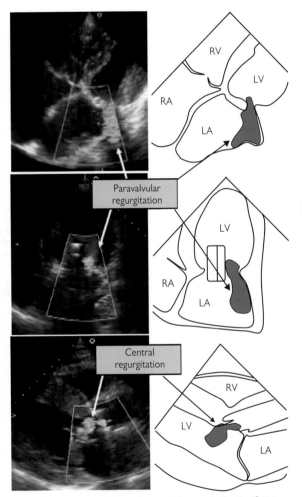

Fig. 3.49 Examples of paravalvular and transvalvular regurgitation. See 🎬 Video 3.30.

Endocarditis

Diagnosis of endocarditis is based on clinical factors (positive blood cultures with appropriate organisms, predisposing factors, new valve dysfunction, peripheral stigmata) supported by echocardiographic abnormalities (Duke's criteria are widely used). A normal echocardiogram never excludes endocarditis and, if clinical suspicion is high, transoesophageal echocardiography should always be performed. If normal, repeat imaging can be considered to monitor for developing pathology.

Assessment

For diagnosis use a full systematic examination with focus on valves (main site). Bear in mind clinical situation: right-sided valves if intravenous infection (drugs, lines), known abnormal valves (prosthetic or degenerative), previous endocarditis (old vegetations). For monitoring use full examination and make sure you comment on change from previous findings.

For all studies report on: vegetations (location, number, size), abscess (particularly valve rings), fistulae (e.g. aorta to right heart), valve dysfunction (including severity, dehiscence, rupture), pericardial effusion.

Vegetation (Fig. 3.49)

Key features to help diagnose: (1) attachment to upstream-side valve; (2) irregular shape; (3) oscillating motion distinct from valve; (3) related valve dysfunction. Comment on number of vegetations, attachments, size (measure in at least 2 directions and provide overall assessment—small, moderate, large).

Abscess (Fig. 3.50)

Abscesses can be perivalvular or valvular. Appearances initially are often of a thickening and 'spongy' appearance to valve ring (particularly aortic root) or valve leaflet. An echo-free, fluid-filled centre may develop. Abscesses may open into adjacent cardiac chambers (technically the space is then no longer an abscess).

For each abscess comment on location with reference to position around valve (e.g. annulus right coronary cusp). Measure size in different planes and judge as small, moderate or large. Comment on functional effects of abscess (e.g. outflow tract or valve distortion).

Fistula

Fistulae usually develop following an abscess and describe an abnormal connection between 2 cardiac chambers. Use colour flow mapping to track fistulae and identify jets in cardiac chambers. If aligned, use Doppler to quantify flow direction and size.

Comment on physical size (length and width) and which chambers are connected. Give an estimate of haemodynamic significance (e.g. size of shunt left-to-right heart, change in ventricle size and function, degree of regurgitation if fistula across valve).

Severity of valvular lesion (see individual valve sections)

Pericardial effusion (see 📖 p.298)

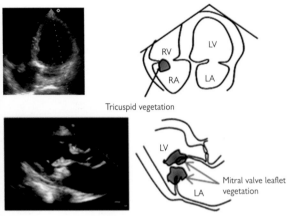

Tricuspid vegetation

Mitral valve leaflet vegetation

Fig. 3.50 Top: apical 4-chamber views of tricuspid valve vegetation. Bottom: parasternal view showing mitral valve vegetation. Note irregular appearance and valve leaflet attachment. See 📹 Video 3.31 and 📹 Video 3.32.

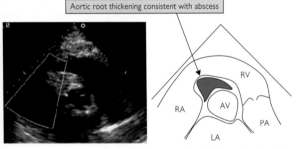

Aortic root thickening consistent with abscess

Fig. 3.51 Parasternal short axis view that demonstrates thickening of aortic root in 10 o'clock position consistent with an aortic root abscess.

Transthoracic anatomy and pathology: chambers and vessels

Left ventricle

Normal anatomy

The left ventricle is a cavity with muscular walls that contains the papillary muscles and their chordal attachments. The anatomic characteristics of the chamber size and thickness can vary significantly with pathology, and many cardiac and systemic processes are associated with cardiac dilatation or hypertrophy.

Normal findings

2D views

The left ventricle is seen in virtually all windows. The minimal views are parasternal long and short axis and the apical 4-, 2-, and 3-chamber views (Fig. 4.1).

2D findings

- Parasternal long axis: the basal and mid segments of the septum and posterior wall (in some publications it is also referred to as the inferolateral wall) are visible. This view is used for linear measures of wall thickness and cavity dimensions. The left ventricular outflow tract can also be assessed.
- Parasternal short axis: by angling the probe back and forth, the whole of the left ventricle can be scanned in cross-section. The key ventricle views are mid-ventricle (mid-papillary) and apical. The mid-ventricle level is used for linear and area measures of walls and cavity. Regional wall motion abnormalities can also be assessed in (in clockwise order) septum, anterior, lateral, and inferior walls.
- Apical 4-chamber: provides best views of apex, septum (on left) and lateral (on right) walls for regional assessment. Suitable for tracing ventricle area and left ventricle length.
- Apical 2-chamber: focuses on inferior (on left) and anterior walls (on right).
- Apical 3-chamber: the parasternal long axis view but from the apex. Looks at posterior (inferolateral) wall and septum.
- Subcostal provides an alternative view of the left ventricle but is not essential.

3D views and findings

- 3D acquisitions of the left ventricle can be obtained from either the parasternal or apical window.
- 3D full volume acquisition mode is preferably used to ensure that the entire left ventricle is imaged.
- Following acquisition, the 3D image can be rotated and cut through any plane to examine any region of interest.
- Good 2D endocardial definition is important when deciding on suitability for 3D LV assessment.
- See Chapter 2.

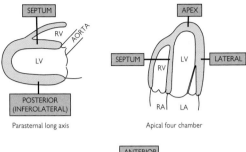

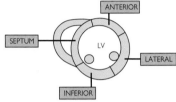

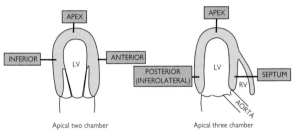

Fig. 4.1 Key views to assess the left ventricle with walls marked.

Left ventricular assessment

General

Accurate left ventricular assessment (diameters, volumes, wall thickness, mass, and function) is critical in clinical practice. Measurements can be altered by virtually all cardiovascular pathologies. The most common indication for echocardiography is evaluation of left ventricular function, with ejection fraction being the most sought parameter. Assessments are frequently visually estimated but there is significant interobserver variability and dependence on interpreter skill. Quantitative measures are recommended to ensure diagnostic accuracy.

Assessment

- Start with an overview of the ventricle in all views (parasternal and apical) and gather an impression of appearance, size, and function.
- Comment on obvious structural changes:
  - Ventricular shape, aneurysms, wall thinning, wall hypertrophy, wall character ('speckling' etc.).
- Report quantitative measures of size (□ p.196) and a general summary: *normal, mild, moderate,* or *severe* dilatation; *normal, mild, moderate,* or *severe* hypertrophy. If hypertrophy, give an idea of the pattern based on appearance and *relative wall thickness,* i.e. *eccentric, concentric, asymmetric (septal, apical)* (□ p.218).
  - 2D and M-mode quantification of left ventricular size and mass has been well validated but both have advantages and disadvantages.
  - M-mode measures in parasternal views are widely used. They are very dependent on M-mode alignment and take no account of left ventricle shape or regional wall motion abnormalities. The alignment problem is reduced with 2D guided or direct 2D measures.
  - In general, left ventricle shape changes are best accounted for by using the volumetric *biplane Simpson's* method for volumes and the *truncated ellipsoid* method for left ventricle mass. These methods should therefore be used to provide accurate assessment of left ventricle volume and mass respectively.
  - Reference ranges are dependent on gender and body habitus. Ideally, height and weight should be recorded and body surface area used to correct left ventricular dimensions.
- Using the measures of left ventricular size, report a quantitative assessment of systolic function (e.g. *ejection fraction*) and summarize as *normal* systolic function or *mild, moderate,* or *severe* systolic dysfunction (□ p.226).
- From apical and parasternal views look at changes in regional wall motion (*normal, hypokinesis, akinesis, dyskinesis, aneurysmal*). Report abnormalities (□ p.234).
- When relevant, assess and report *left ventricular diastolic function* from changes in mitral valve inflow and tissue Doppler imaging (□ p.246).
- Finally, ensure you have reported fully pathologies that might relate to the changes you have identified in the left ventricle (e.g. valve disease).

Left ventricular size

Because it is difficult to quantify a 3D structure using 2D imaging, the techniques that developed with 2D echocardiography rely on measuring the ventricle in standard places. The measures are then reported directly (*linear methods*) or used in mathematical equations to model an assumed shape for the ventricle (*volumetric measures*). In principle, the more measures of the left ventricle in the more planes the more accurate the assessment. Conversely, the fewer measures the more assumptions have to be made and the more likely that regional pathology is overlooked. Sometimes—such as in a normal heart—simple linear measures are adequate. However, if there is pathology accuracy is required. More recently, collection of 3D datasets has enabled much more accurate chamber size quantification.

Linear measures

M-mode

This is based on change in size in a single plane at the mid ventricle level in a parasternal view (Fig. 4.2). Recent guidelines suggest this should be a parasternal short axis view.

- Optimize a parasternal long axis view with the septum and posterior wall lying parallel (or a parasternal short axis mid-ventricle view).
- Drop the M-mode cursor through opposing walls so that it intersects both at right angles. In the long axis view the cursor should lie at the level of the mitral valve tips (some guidelines suggest chordal level).
- Look at the M-mode trace and identify the 2 walls. Measure from edge-to-edge where the walls are closest together (peak systole) and furthest apart (end diastole). Report the *left ventricle systolic* and *end-diastolic* diameters.
- The M-mode trace from a parasternal long axis view can also be used to measure septal and posterior wall thickness at end diastole.

2D-imaging

This follows the same principle as M-mode but relies on clear 2D images.

- Record a loop of an optimized parasternal long axis or short axis (mid ventricle) view. Identify the end-diastolic frame (largest ventricle).
- Measure from endocardial border to border at right angles to each wall (Fig. 4.3). In the long axis view the line should pass through the mitral valve tips. Report the *left ventricular end-diastolic diameter*.
- Scroll through the loop to identify the end-systolic frame (smallest ventricle) and using the same technique measure the *left ventricular end-systolic diameter*.

2D vs. 3D volume measurements

- Volumes obtained from 3D measurements are significantly larger than the volumes measured with 2D techniques, contrast enhanced 3D volumes are larger than corresponding volumes in native 3D echo.
- 3D LV ejection fraction are lower than in 2D (lower limit 49%).
- For longitudinal studies, the same imaging software and postprocessing units should ideally be used in order to maintain consistency.

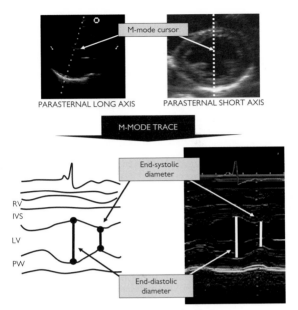

Fig. 4.2 Measurements using M-mode in parasternal views.

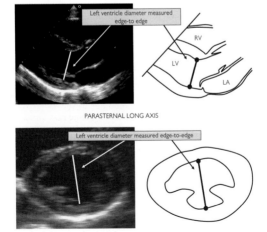

Fig. 4.3 Examples of 2D measures in parasternal views.

2D volumetric measures

Simpson's method

Simpson's method (Fig. 4.4) is based on the principle of slicing the left ventricle from apex down to mitral valve annulus into a series of discs. The volume of each disc is then calculated (using the diameter and thickness of each slice). All the disc volumes are added together to provide the total left ventricular volume. If done in a single plane (based on apical 4-chamber view) it is assumed the left ventricle is circular at each level. Accuracy is improved by using diameters in 2 perpendicular planes (biplane—apical 4- and 2-chamber) so that the disc surface area is more precisely defined. Although this can be done 'by hand' by measuring the diameter at multiple levels, in reality, you trace the outline of the ventricle and the machine or off-line software automatically calculates the volume.

- In the apical 4-chamber view obtain a clear image of the left ventricular cavity with a clear endocardial border.
- Record a loop and scroll through to find the end-diastolic image (usually just before the aortic valve opens or on the R-wave of the ECG). This image should have the largest left ventricular volume.
- Trace around the endocardial border going from one side of the mitral valve annulus to the other and joining the 2 ends with a straight line. Record the *left ventricular end diastolic volume*.
- Measure the length of the left ventricle from apex to middle of mitral valve. Depending on the machine, identification of the apex may be automatic after tracing the border. Record *left ventricular long axis*.
- Scroll through the loop again and find the smallest left ventricular volume at end-systole (usually just before the mitral valve opens or on the T-wave of the ECG). Trace around the endocardial border, as before, and record *left ventricular end systolic volume*.
- The method described will provide single plane measures of left ventricular volumes. For biplane measures repeat the process for diastolic and systolic images using an optimized apical 2-chamber view.

Normal ranges depend on technique, sex and body size

Systematic differences between techniques mean 'normal' ranges vary. For instance, direct 2D measures tend to produce slightly smaller measures than M-mode. Also, normal ranges depend on the sex and size of the person. Always report the method you used and demographic data.

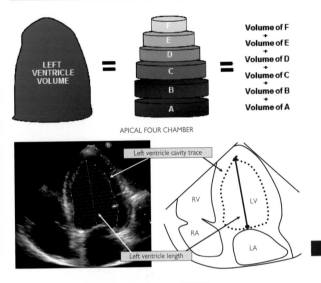

APICAL FOUR CHAMBER

APICAL TWO CHAMBER

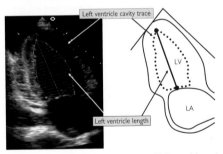

Fig. 4.4 Biplane Simpson's method for measurement of left ventricle cavity size.

Area length equation (Fig. 4.5)

This method can be used if apical definition is poor and it is difficult to trace the border. It is based on an equation that models a 'bullet-shaped' ventricle (and therefore does not take account of regional abnormalities). For the equation you need the length of the ventricle and the cross-sectional area at the mid papillary level.

- Obtain a clear parasternal short axis (mid ventricle level) view with good endocardial border definition and record a loop.
- Trace around the endocardial border in the end diastolic frame to obtain the *end-diastolic cross sectional area*.
- In an apical 4-chamber view record the distance from the middle of the mitral valve annulus to the left ventricle apex at end-diastole and record the *end diastolic left ventricle long axis lengths*.
- Ventricular volume at *end-diastole* is then:

$$(5 \times \text{cross-sectional area in parasternal short axis} \times \text{ventricle length})/6$$

- Ventricular volume at *end-systole* can be measured in exactly the same way but using parasternal and apical images frozen at end-systole.

Avoid foreshortening—ensure a clear endocardial border

- Accurate left ventricular volume measurements require an unforeshortened ventricle. Foreshortening leads to underestimation of volume and changes ventricle shape. Foreshortening can usually be avoided by moving more lateral ± 1 intercostal space further down. 3 pointers to be confident you have identified the true apex:
  - Apex is fixed and does not move towards the base in systole.
  - Apical myocardium is thinner than the rest of the ventricle.
  - The view is the one with the longest ventricle (if apical view).
- If the endocardial border is not clear, volumes will be overestimated. Clear definition is particularly important to see regional wall motion abnormalities. Endocardial definition can be enhanced by machine controls to improve grey levels (such as harmonic imaging, gain, and contrast) or probe position (increased pressure, better contact, slight changes in window). If these factors make no difference, intravascular contrast agents provide excellent border definition.

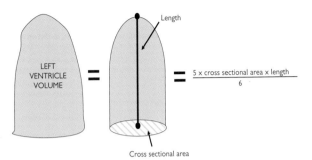

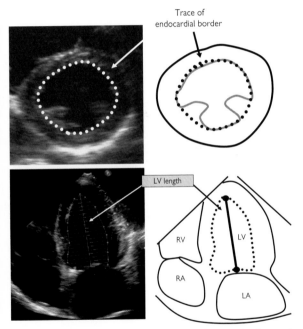

Fig. 4.5 Area length equation based on measurement of cross-sectional area and left ventricle length.

3D volumetric measures

3D echocardiography is an advance on Simpson's method as it allows contouring of the cavity within the 3D space of the echocardiographic volume acquisition. Therefore there is no need to assume that the short axis view of the ventricle follows the shape of a circle (or oval) and sum together a 'stack of discs'. Instead you can contour the actual shape of the ventricle in all dimensions.

- In order to process full volume data sets, a 4D semi-automated contour detection program with manual correction options written specifically for the left ventricle is needed.
- Commercially available scanners contain software tools which allow the assessment of left ventricular volumes and ejection fraction. An alternative is off-line processing with a commercially available software package (4D-LV Function, TomTec, Germany) that is able to process 3D datasets from different scanner systems.
- After acquisition of a 3D dataset, sliced planes are viewed in 4-chamber view, 2-chamber view, and one or more short axis views (C-planes) (Figs. 4.6 and 4.7).
- The left ventricular volumes are calculated by summing the areas for each slice through the complete volume data set (volumetric 3D echo).

How to get optimal 3D volumes

- Good image quality on 2D echocardiography is important when selecting patients to undergo 3D image acquisition.
- If the endocardial definition is poor then a left-sided contrast agent can be used (📖 p.561).
- Full volume datasets are triggered from the ECG trace and so it is important that the patient has a regular heart rhythm.
- To reduce the incidence of stitch artefacts the probe and patient position should be maintained in a stable position.
- Acquisition with the patient holding their breath is advised if the full volume dataset is going to be acquired over several heartbeats.

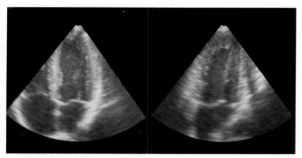

Fig. 4.6 Biplane view during 3D apical LV acquisition showing the 4-chamber view (left) and 2-chamber view (right). See 📹 Video 4.1 and 📹 Video 4.2.

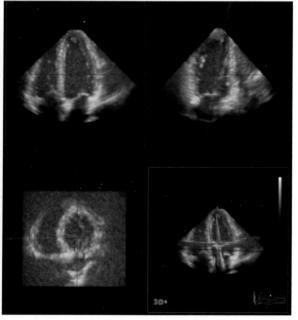

Fig. 4.7 3D full volume LV data presentation on Philips QLAB 7.1. Apical 4-chamber view (top left), biplane apical 2-chamber view (top right), short axis (C plane) view (bottom left), and representation of the 3 displayed planes (bottom right).

Acquisition of 3D volume for assessment of LV

- Position the probe at the apex in the same position as for acquisition of 2D 4-chamber view. Modified windows may be used if selected parts of the left ventricle need to be assessed.
- A biplane preview screen is used so that the 4- and 2-chamber views can be seen simultaneously to help avoid foreshortening, see Fig. 4.6.
- Depth, gain, and TGC are adjusted in 2D imaging in order to achieve the best possible endocardial definition.
- For full volume datasets maximize the number of subvolumes (beats) used to generate the 3D image according to patient breath holding capabilities and the regularity of the heart rhythm. The greater the number of subvolumes that can be acquired and effectively stitched together without artefacts, the greater the temporal and spatial resolution.
- Acquire a 3D dataset and then evaluate it for quality.
- Commercially available 3D scanners allow the acquired image to be viewed on the machine in several short axis planes as well as a rendered 3D volume. This is important in order to identify any stitching artefacts which may have occurred.
- Assess endocardial visualization using the cropping tools of the scanner.
- If not adequate, discard and acquire another. Keep doing this until you are happy that you have a volume you will be able to post-process effectively.

Preparing the dataset

Postprocessing systems will normally automatically display an apical 4-chamber view, 2-chamber view, and C-planes (short axis view). How you then handle the images varies with the different software packages but typically:

- The planes can then be adjusted by the operator to ensure the 4-chamber plane has been accurately identified and is unforeshortened. Similarly the plane used to create the 2-chamber view can also be adjusted.
- Once happy that the long axes of the heart have been identified the ventricular volumes and ejection fraction can then be calculated. To do this typically the operator is asked to:
  - Identify the end-diastolic and end-systolic frame (some software will require you to mark these frames).
  - Identify anatomical points on the 4- and 2-chamber left ventricular views (e.g. left ventricular walls, left ventricular apex, or mitral valve, see Fig. 4.8) so that the semi automated programme can delineate the left ventricular contour. The software then will delineate the contours in the other slices and frames, see Fig. 4.9.

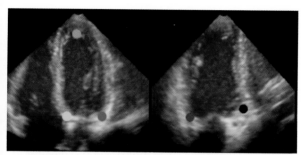

Fig. 4.8 Setting anatomical landmarks for estimation of 3D end-diastolic volume (Phillips QLAB). Once the appropriate frame for end diastole has been selected and the image has been orientated to reduce foreshortening the post processing programme prompts the operator to mark the basal septum (yellow dot), basal lateral wall (red dot), basal anterior wall (purple dot), basal inferior wall (black dot), and the apex (blue dot).

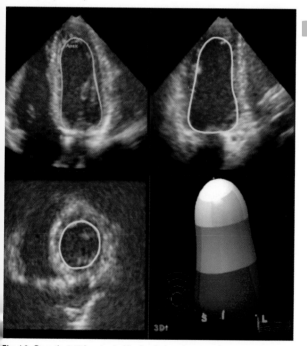

Fig. 4.9 Once the initial anatomical landmarks have been set, the post processing programme will delineate the LV contour for view in the 4 chamber (top right), 2 chamber (top left) and short axis or C-Plane views (bottom left). In doing this a 17 segment model of the LV is created (bottom right). See 📷 Video 4.3.

Review of contouring and calculation of volumes

- Once the postprocessing package has completed contouring the left ventricle (Fig. 4.10), check that it has accurately delineated the true left ventricular border by slicing through the left ventricular cavity in the short axis planes and make corrections if you observe major deviations.
- The end-diastolic, end-systolic volumes, stroke volume, and ejection fraction are judged as in 2D echocardiography.
- Visually assess the regional left ventricular wall motion in the standard apical and serial short axis views to ensure that the calculated ejection fraction is similar to what the operator would expect visually.
- The left ventricular volume can be subdivided into 16 or 17 subvolumes. These create a pyramid volume with the peak in the centre of the left ventricle, which is often coloured in by the software (Fig. 4.11).
- The end-diastolic, end-systolic volumes and ejection fraction can be assessed for each of the subvolumes, but the generally accepted normal values are not yet available. At present the display of the subvolumes helps to visualize regional wall motion abnormalities in conjunction to the findings in the 2D cut planes.
- The timing of peak contraction can be assessed using the subvolume curves (Fig. 4.11).
- The 3D analysis software measures the time from end-diastole until the smallest left ventricular volume is recorded (lowest point of the curve) and calculates the mean and standard deviation.

Left ventricular size: 3D normal ranges

Upper normal values (mean + 2 standard deviations [SD])
- LV end-diastolic volume index (LVEDVI): 82mL/m^2
- LV end-systolic volume index (LVESVI): 38mL/m^2

Lower limit (mean – 2 SD)
- LVEF: 49%

For left ventricular subvolumes no generally approved normal values have been established.

EF, ejection fraction; LVEDVI, LV end-diastolic volume index; LVESVI, LV end-systolic volume index.

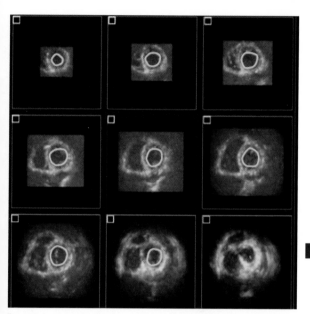

Fig. 4.10 Following initial placement of the required landmarks on the apical 4- and 2-chamber views the post processing programme will contour the volume. The accuracy of this automatic process can be checked by slicing down the short axis planes and checking if the delineated contour (yellow line) tracks the LV endocardial border well. Adjustments can then be made if there are discrepancies. See 📹 Video 4.4.

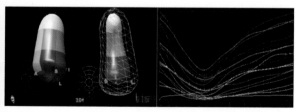

Fig. 4.11 17 segment 3D LV volume shell at end diastole (left) and at end systole (right) with diastolic volume represented as a wire frame. A = anterior, S = septum, L = lateral, I = inferior. 16 segment 3D LV volume curves during a cardiac cycle. See 📹 Video 4.5.

Left ventricular size:
2D normal ranges (Table 4.1)

Table 4.1 Ranges for measurement of left ventricular size. (Adapted from Recommendations for Chamber Quantification: A Report of the American Society of Echocardiography Guidelines and Standards Committee and the Chamber Quantification Writing Group, Developed in Conjunction with the European Association of Echocardiography. *J Am Soc Echocardiogr* 2005; **18**: 1440–1463.)

Part 1, Values for women

	Women			
	Normal	Mild	Moderate	Severe
LV dimension				
LV d diameter, cm	3.9–5.3	5.4–5.7	5.8–6.1	>6.1
LV d diameter/BSA, cm/m²	2.4–3.2	3.3–3.4	3.5–3.7	>3.7
LV d diam/height, cm/m	2.5–3.2	3.3–3.4	3.5–3.6	>3.7
LV volume				
LV d vol, mL	56–104	105–117	118–130	>130
LV d vol/BSA, mL/m²	**35–75**	**76–86**	**87–96**	**>96**
LV s vol, mL	19–49	50–59	60–69	>69
LV s vol/BSA, mL/m²	**12–30**	**31–36**	**37–42**	**>42**
Linear method: fractional shortening				
Endocardial, %	27–45	22–26	17–21	<17
Mid wall, %	15–23	13–14	11–12	<11
2D method				
Ejection fraction, %	**>54**	**45–54**	**30–44**	**<30**

BSA, Body surface area; d, diastolic; s, systolic.
Bold rows identify best validated measures.

Table 4.1 (Contd.)

Part 2, Values for men

	Men			
	Normal	Mild	Moderate	Severe
LV dimension				
LV d diameter, cm	4.2–5.9	6.0–6.3	6.4–6.8	>6.8
LV d diameter/BSA, cm/m^2	2.2–3.1	3.2–3.4	3.5–3.6	>3.6
LV d diameter/height, cm/m	2.4–3.3	3.4–3.5	3.6–3.7	>3.7
LV volume				
LV d vol, mL	67–155	156–178	179–201	>201
LV d vol/BSA, mL/m^2	**35–75**	**76–86**	**87–96**	**>96**
LV s vol, mL	22–58	59–70	71–82	>82
LV s vol/BSA, mL/m^2	**12–30**	**31–36**	**37–42**	**>42**
Linear method: fractional shortening				
Endocardial, %	25–43	20–24	15–19	<15
Mid wall, %	14–22	12–13	10–11	<10
2D method				
Ejection fraction, %	**>54**	**45–54**	**30–44**	**<30**

BSA, Body surface area; d, diastolic; s, systolic.
Bold rows identify best validated measures.

Left ventricular thickness and mass

All measurements of left ventricular mass are based on the principle of estimating the difference between the epicardial and endocardial left ventricular volumes and then calculating the mass of this 'shell' using the known myocardial density (i.e. multiplication of the volume by 1.05). The measurement techniques are the same as for quantification of left ventricular size (📖 p.196). However, they are applied to obtain both a *cavity* volume and a *total* volume. Measurements are done at end-diastole.

Linear measures of wall thickness can be reported directly or used to estimate mass based on simple formulae but do not take account of changes in left ventricular geometry. Volume measures are preferred and 3D echocardiography can also be used to assess mass as long as there is good epicardial border definition.

Linear measures

Interventricular septum and posterior wall thickness

The simplest and most widely used assessments of left ventricular thickness are *interventricular septum* and *posterior wall thickness* from M-mode or 2D images (Fig. 4.12).

- In a parasternal long axis or parasternal short axis (mid papillary level) drop an M-mode cursor through the ventricle perpendicular to the walls at the level of the mitral valve leaflet tips.
- Identify the lines that relate to the septum and posterior wall and measure the thinnest part (end-diastole).
- Report wall thickness and if increased consider further characterization of hypertrophy (📖 p.218).
- Measurements can also be done directly from parasternal 2D images, frozen in end-diastole. Measure with calipers from edge to edge.

Volume measures from linear measures

Teichholz method or prolate ellipse of revolution

Left ventricular mass can be estimated from linear dimensions (see 📖 'Linear Measures', p.210) using a 'prolate ellipse of revolution' formula. Traditionally, this was based on M-mode measures. The equation uses cubed measurements so slightly off-axis views or small errors in diameter are amplified into large differences in volume. The method takes no account of abnormal left ventricular morphology and is rarely used now.

- In parasternal long or short axis (mid papillary level) views obtain measures of *left ventricular end-diastolic diameter* (LVEDD), *interventricular septum thickness* (IVS) and *posterior wall thickness* (PWT).
- In an apical 4-chamber view obtain a measure of *end-diastolic left ventricular length* (from apex to middle of mitral valve annulus).
- Left ventricular mass is automatically calculated using the formula:

$$\left[0.8 \times \left(1.05 \times \left(\left(LVEDD + PWT + IVS \right)^3 - \left(LVEDD \right)^3 \right) \right) \right] + 0.6 \text{ g}$$

(the constants (0.8 and 0.6) improve the accuracy of the basic equation (in bold) in studies based on postmortem hearts).

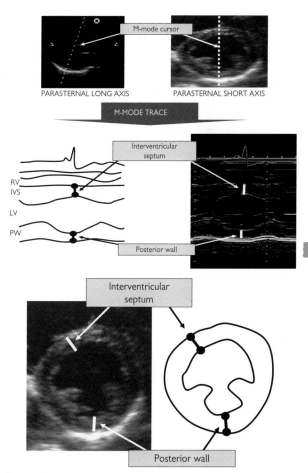

PARASTERNAL LONG AXIS

PARASTERNAL SHORT AXIS

M-MODE TRACE

Interventricular septum

RV
IVS

LV

PW

Posterior wall

Interventricular septum

Posterior wall

Fig. 4.12 Position for linear measures of left ventricle thickness.

2D volume measures (Fig. 4.13)

Area-length and ellipsoid models

There are two validated methods available for estimating left ventricular mass based on the *area–length* formula (📖 p.200) and the *truncated ellipsoid* model. Both methods use the same set of measurements in end-diastole—*total* and *cavity* myocardial area (short axis view, mid-papillary level) and *left ventricle length* (apical 2 chamber view)—and only vary in the equation they use to estimate volumes.

- Obtain a clear parasternal short axis view (mid ventricle level) with good endocardial and epicardial border definition.
- Record a loop and scroll through to the end-diastolic frame.
- Trace around the endocardial border and record the *endocardial* or *left ventricular cavity* cross sectional area. Do not include the papillary muscles in the tracing.
- Trace around the epicardial border and record the *epicardial* or *total* cross sectional area.
- Myocardial area is the difference between the *total* cross-sectional area and the *cavity* cross sectional area.
- In a non-foreshortened apical 2-chamber view record a loop and identify the end-diastolic frame (when the ventricle is largest). Measure the distance from apex to the middle of the mitral valve annulus. Record the *left ventricular length*.
- The machine or off-line software will automatically calculate left ventricular mass from these measurements.
- The truncated ellipsoid equation for a volume is:

$$8 \times (\text{cross-sectional area in parasternal short axis}) 2/3 \times \pi \times \text{ventricle lenght}$$

Biplane Simpson's model

It is possible to use a *biplane Simpson's* method (📖 p.198) to calculate mass from 2D images as long as epicardial border definition is good. The accuracy of the technique is dependent on obtaining a clear epicardial border in both planes but, unlike other methods, will take account of regional wall motion abnormalities or asymmetric variation in wall thickness. The principle behind this technique is also the basis for how mass is measured in 3D echocardiography. To undertake this with 2D:

- Measure total end-diastolic left ventricular volume using Simpson's method by tracing the *epicardial* border in apical 4- and 2-chamber views.
- Subtract *left ventricular end-diastolic volume* assessed with Simpson's method from this total volume. Multiply the difference by 1.05 to obtain a left ventricular mass.

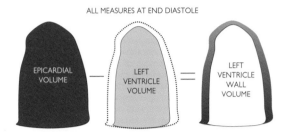

ALL MEASURES AT END DIASTOLE

LEFT VENTRICLE WALL VOLUME × MYOCARDIAL DENSITY (1.05) = LEFT VENTRICLE MASS

Traced endocardial border

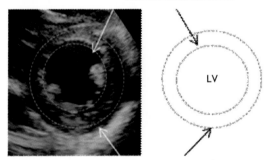

Traced epicardial border

APICAL TWO CHAMBER

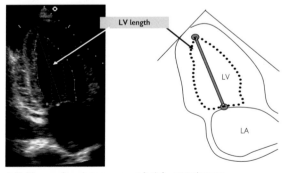

Fig. 4.13 Measures for volume assessment for left ventricular mass.

3D volume measures

3D assessment of mass is an improvement on the 2D biplane Simpson's approach to assessment of mass but instead of just using 2 planes the contours of the epicardial and endocardial 'shells' are identified in 3D by automated software. This technique of measuring the volume in 3D is a key reason why left ventricular mass can be measured so accurately with cardiovascular magnetic resonance. With good image quality, 3D left ventricular mass measures with echocardiography are now as good as gold standard techniques. To measure left ventricular mass with 3D:

- Acquire a 3D apical full volume data set, see 📖 p.202.
- Continue to discard and acquire full volumes until you are happy you have the best quality 3D dataset without artefact and with good border definition.
- Load the dataset into postprocessing software. This will display the left ventricle in the standard views, typically, 4-chamber, 2-chamber, and short axis stack.
- The exact approach to analysis depends on the software package. However, typically (Fig. 4.14).
  - In the 4-chamber view the operator will have to mark the mitral valve hinge points and contour the end diastolic endocardial border.
  - The operator then identifies the contour of the outer ventricular wall.
  - This procedure is repeated for the 2-chamber view.
  - The software package then automatically estimates the end-diastolic volumes and, base to apical length to generate a measure of left ventricular mass.

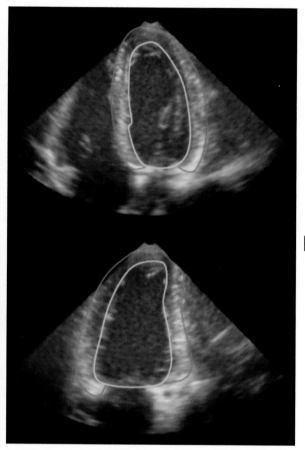

Fig. 4.14 3D estimation of LV mass using Phillips QLAB. End-diastolic frames in the apical 4-chamber and apical 2-chamber views are selected. The mitral valve insertion points and endocardial border is contoured (yellow line). Following this the outer LV wall is contoured (green line). The software will then calculate the end diastolic volume, base to apical length and LV mass.

Left ventricular thickness and mass: normal ranges (Table 4.2)

Table 4.2 Ranges for measurement of left ventricular mass. (Adapted from Recommendations for Chamber Quantification: A Report of the American Society of Echocardiography Guidelines and Standards Committee and the Chamber Quantification Writing Group, Developed in Conjunction with the European Association of Echocardiography. *J Am Soc Echocardiogr* 2005; **18**: 1440–1463.)

Part 1, Values for Women

	Women			
	Normal	**Mild**	**Moderate**	**Severe**
Linear method				
LV mass, g	67–162	163–186	187–210	>210
LV mass/BSA g/m²	**43–95**	**96–108**	**109–121**	**>121**
LV mass/height, g/m	41–99	100–115	116–128	>128
LV mass/height², g/m²	18–44	45–51	52–58	>58
Relative wall thickness, cm	0.22–0.42	0.43–0.47	0.48–0.52	>0.52
Septal thickness, cm	**0.6–0.9**	**1.0–1.2**	**1.3–1.5**	**>1.5**
Posterior wall thickness, cm	**0.6–0.9**	**1.0–1.2**	**1.3–1.5**	**>1.5**
2D method				
LV mass, g	66–150	151–171	172–182	>182
LV mass/BSA, g/m²	**44–s88**	**89–100**	**101–112**	**>112**

BSA, Body surface area.
Bold rows identify best validated measures.

Table 4.2 (Contd.)

Part 2, Values for men

	Men			
	Normal	**Mild**	**Moderate**	**Severe**
Linear method				
LV mass, g	88–224	225–258	259–292	>292
LV mass/BSA g/m²	**49–115**	**116–131**	**132–148**	**>148**
LV mass/height, g/m	52–126	127–144	145–162	>163
LV mass/height², g/m²	20–48	49–55	56–63	>63
Relative wall thickness, cm	0.24–0.42	0.43–0.46	0.47–0.51	>0.51
Septal thickness, cm	**0.6–1.0**	**1.1–1.3**	**1.4–1.6**	**>1.6**
Posterior wall thickness, cm	**0.6–1.0**	**1.1–1.3**	**1.4–1.6**	**>1.6**
2D method				
LV mass, g	96–200	201–227	228–254	>254
LV mass/BSA, g/m²	**50–102**	**103–116**	**117–130**	**>130**

BSA, Body surface area.
Bold rows identify best validated measures.

Left ventricular hypertrophy

General

The clinical importance of left ventricular mass relates to identification of pathological left ventricular hypertrophy. Left ventricular hypertrophy can occur secondary to other pathology (e.g. aortic valve disease or hypertension), or be a primary problem with the myocardium (e.g. hypertrophic cardiomyopathy, infiltrative cardiomyopathy). With hypertrophic cardiomyopathy there may be asymmetric changes with septal or apical changes. Physiological hypertrophy is also found (e.g. athletes or in pregnancy) that is thought to be reversible. In the elderly there is sometimes septal angulation and thickening which creates the impression of septal hypertrophy but left ventricle mass is usually unchanged.

Assessment

If hypertrophy is present base further assessment on: (1) a description of the pattern (global or asymmetric) (Fig. 4.15), (2) a description of severity using overall mass and mass relative to ventricular size, (3) characterization of related pathology (e.g. valve disease or outflow tract obstruction) and unusual appearances (e.g. speckling texture of amyloid, localized hypertrophy of tumour).

Appearance

- Using all views make a qualitative judgement of hypertrophy. Parasternal short axis view is good for seeing concentric hypertrophy. Parasternal long axis and apical 5-chamber views pick up septal hypertrophy. Apical and subcostal views can look for apical hypertrophy. Report the pattern and, if asymmetric, wall thickness measures at different points.
- A common reported abnormal texture is amyloid 'speckling'. This can be influenced by contrast and gain settings. Localized hypertrophy with abnormal echolucency might suggest malignant infiltration.

Grading severity

Left ventricular mass can be clinically graded into 4 categories: (1) normal, (2) increased relative wall thickness with increased mass (concentric left ventricular hypertrophy), (3) increased mass with normal relative wall thickness (eccentric left ventricular hypertrophy) or (4) normal mass with increased relative wall thickness (concentric remodelling). Concentric changes suggest pressure overload (e.g. due to aortic stenosis or hypertension). Eccentric changes suggest volume overload (e.g. due to aortic regurgitation). Grade severity by reporting overall mass and/or wall thickness, and relative wall thickness.

- Overall severity: Fig. 4.15 provides a guide to grading hypertrophy based on mass and wall thickness measures.
- Relative wall thickness: use left ventricular posterior wall thickness (PWT) and left ventricular end diastolic diameter (LVEDD). Relative wall thickness is calculated as: $(2 \times PWT)/LVEDD$.
  - If relative wall thickness is >0.42 report concentric hypertrophy.
  - If relative wall thickness is <0.42 report eccentric hypertrophy.

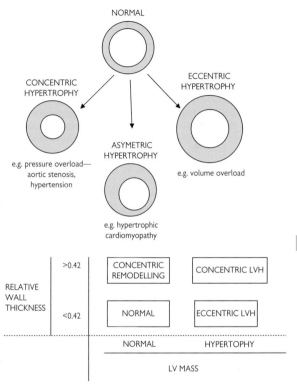

Fig. 4.15 Patterns of hypertrophy.

Hypertrophic cardiomyopathy

General

Hypertrophic cardiomyopathy describes marked left ventricular hypertrophy secondary to specific genetic abnormalities. There are multiple gene defects that lead to hypertrophy and more are being identified. The responsible genes commonly control muscle fibre function. The hypertrophy can be of many different patterns and towards the end of the disease process left ventricular failure can develop (in 10% of cases). The classic pattern is of marked septal hypertrophy (Fig. 4.16) associated with significant outflow obstruction. LVOT obstruction occurs in about a quarter of patients. Symptoms of breathlessness may be due to any or a combination of: reduced diastolic or systolic left ventricular function, mitral regurgitation, left LVOT obstruction or microvascular dysfunction.

Assessment

- If hypertrophic cardiomyopathy is suspected report the pattern and measures of *wall thickness*, *relative wall thickness* and *mass*.
- Assess the LVOT at rest and consider exercise-induced gradients.
- Report left ventricular systolic and diastolic function and look at mitral valve function and regurgitation.
- Assessment of strain or myocardial velocities using TDI or speckle tracking may help identify impaired cardiac function prior to cardiac hypertrophy.

Left ventricular outflow

Historically, *M-mode* has been used to demonstrate outflow obstruction.

- Systolic anterior motion of mitral valve is seen with M-mode placed through the mitral leaflets. It is considered severe (i.e. obstructive) if the leaflet touches the ventricular septum or the outflow tract is narrowed by the anterior mitral valve leaflet for >40% of systole.
- Obstruction tends to be in mid to late systole leading to a drop in flow through the aortic valve towards the end of systole. Therefore, an M-mode trace through the aortic leaflets can demonstrate early closure of the valve and the valve may appear to flutter as flow drops.

Doppler should be used as the main method to quantify obstruction.

- In an apical 5- or 3-chamber view place colour flow mapping over the outflow tract. This may demonstrate turbulent, high velocity, flow (an irregular scattering) in the outflow tract.
- In the apical 5-chamber view align the CW Doppler through the outflow tract, aortic valve, and aorta. Record a spectral trace to obtain peak and mean velocities. The trace may appear as a scimitar shape demonstrating the classic, late, dynamic obstruction (Fig. 4.17).
- Place PW Doppler at the bottom of the outflow tract and move it towards the valve. If the gradient is due to hypertrophy the peak velocities will be present in the outflow tract below the valve and the trace will start aliasing due to the high velocities.
- In a symptomatic patient—particularly if symptomatic on exercise—without obstruction, an exercise stress protocol can be used and outflow tract gradient measured at peak exercise.

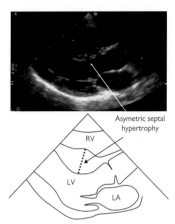

Fig. 4.16 Parasternal long axis view demonstrates septal hypertrophy.
See 📹 Video 4.6.

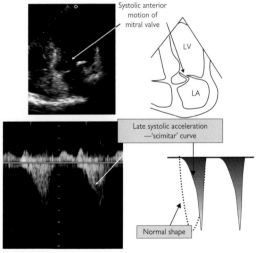

Fig. 4.17 Top: apical 4-chamber view demonstrates systolic anterior motion of
mitral valve. Bottom: scimitar-shaped spectral trace characteristic of late systolic
acceleration.

Left ventricular non-compaction

- Left ventricular non-compaction is an inherited condition characterized by marked left ventricular trabeculation (Fig. 4.18) within the left ventricular apex and if more pronounced extending towards the midventricular or even basal segments.
- The inferior and lateral segments are more commonly affected than the septum.
- Left ventricular non-compaction may lead to impaired ventricular function and can be a substrate for left-sided thrombi and arrhythmias. To identify non-compaction left-sided contrast agents are helpful. In apical views the trabeculation is seen as a partially contrast-filled layer. Report the thickness of the trabeculation relative to the myocardium.
- A ratio of >2:1 of the non-compacted (trabeculations) myocardium to compacted (normal) myocardium at end-systole suggests left ventricular non-compaction. Colour Doppler often demonstrates flow between the trabeculations. Cardiovascular magnetic resonance imaging aids diagnosis.

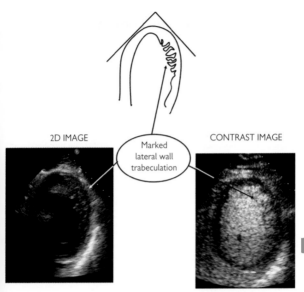

Fig. 4.18 An apical 4-chamber view demonstrating lateral wall trabeculation. The abnormal trabeculations of left ventricular non-compaction can be highlighted with contrast (note improved image quality between native and contrast images) or colour flow mapping. See ☷ Video 4.7 and ☷ Video 4.8.

Restrictive cardiomyopathy

True restrictive cardiomyopathy is rare and tends to occur due to infiltrative disease such as amyloidosis. Symptoms develop due to myocardial thickening and stiffening leading to diastolic dysfunction. Late in the disease systolic dysfunction can develop as contractile function diminishes.

- A full assessment of the left ventricle (size and mass, systolic and diastolic function; 📖 p.246) is needed for diagnosis. Classic appearance is normal systolic function and cavity dimensions but abnormal diastolic function with varying increases in wall thickness.
- The usual diagnostic conundrum is differentiation from constrictive pericarditis. Techniques such as tissue Doppler imaging and mitral inflow are useful and described in the pericardium section on 📖 p.302.

Dilated cardiomyopathy

Dilated cardiomyopathy describes left ventricular dilatation and impaired function and can be accompanied by right ventricular dilatation. There can be many underlying causes, such as ischaemic heart disease, tachycardia-induced, metabolic conditions (e.g. hyperthyroidism, phaeochromocytomas), postpartum, or post-myocarditis. The term idiopathic dilated cardiomyopathy is used if no underlying cause is identified. Echocardiography should provide information on ventricle size and function and, be used for follow-up to gauge recovery or deterioration.

Myocarditis

Myocarditis occurs due to a viral infection either acutely or as a post-viral phenomenon. It can affect left ventricular global systolic function with or without left ventricular dilatation and can range from mild to severe. A pericardial effusion may also develop. LV dysfunction can resolve, stabilize, or deteriorate and myocarditis is a common cause for dilated cardiomyopathy. Recovery is assessed by repeated echocardiography to determine changes in left ventricular function. Cardiovascular magnetic resonance imaging may be useful to determine the degree of myocardial damage.

3D echocardiography in cardiomyopathies?

Real-time 3D echocardiography has advantages over 2D echocardiography which may be helpful in the assessment of patients with cardiomyopathies:

• It permits more accurate assessment of ventricular volumes.
• 3D imaging allows detection of early changes in myocardial mechanics prior to changes in conventional measures of ventricular function with the use of 3D speckle tracking. This has been shown to provide results similar to that for 2D speckle tracking although as real-time 3D uses only one apical view rather than multiple views, post-processing is less time consuming.
• For the assessment of cardiomyopathies with poor ventricular function, real-time 3D has been used to quantify left ventricular mechanical dyssynchrony to identify patients who may be suitable for cardiac resynchronization therapy.
• In patients with hypertrophic cardiomyopathy, 3D echocardiography has been shown to provide important insights into the mechanics and deformational geometry of the left ventricular outflow tract. 3D echocardiography has helped to show that in patients with hypertrophic cardiomyopathy and systolic anterior motion of the mitral valve the anterior segment of the anterior mitral valve leaflet causes the development of the left ventricular outflow tract gradient.
• In patients with apical hypertrophic cardiomyopathy, 3D echocardiography allows cropping to visualize the left ventricular apex in multiple directions planes to help assess for hypertrophy.
• The use of 3D echocardiography in the diagnosis of left ventricular non-compaction has also been reported. By rotating and cropping the dataset it allows the extent of non compaction to be determined in a segmental approach.

Left ventricular function

Assessment of left ventricular function is one of the most frequently requested echocardiography studies, with ejection fraction the most sought after parameter. This is driven by several issues:

- The number of patients presenting with dyspnoea and possible congestive heart failure is increasing, there is clear prognostic significance to the parameter of ejection fraction.
- To help guide therapy (especially decisions for device therapy in heart failure and surgery for valve disease). Remember that congestive heart failure is a clinical diagnosis and even before clinical signs are evident abnormalities of left ventricle function may be apparent. Early detection is critical to prevent progression of heart failure.

Assessment

An assessment of left ventricle function should be comprehensive. Box 4.1 outlines the techniques for a complete examination. Not all will be felt necessary for all patients and selection should be based on the clinical indication for the study. However, the minimal requirements are an assessment of:

- Left ventricle size and shape.
- Systolic function, including regional differences.
- Diastolic function.

Box 4.1 Assessment of left ventricular function

- *Global systolic function:*
  - Subjective evaluation of size, shape, regional and global function.
  - Measurement of left ventricle volumes/dimensions, ejection fraction (Simpson's or 3D).
  - Doppler: volumetric measurements, dP/dt in patients with mitral regurgitation.
  - New techniques for myocardial function (strain, strain rate).
  - LV response to exercise stress.
- *Left ventricle shape and wall stress.*
- *Regional systolic function:*
  - Subjective evaluation of segmental function, wall motion score.
  - Myocardial contrast enhancement.
- *Diastolic function:*
  - Transmitral flow categorization.
  - Strategies for recognition of pseudonormal filling.
  - LA size (area or volume).
  - Annular tissue Doppler (E/E').
  - Response to Valsalva manoeuvre.
  - Others (pulmonary vein flow, mitral flow propagation).
- *Synchrony:*
  - M-mode intraventricular delay.
  - Doppler assessment of interventricular delay.
  - Tissue Doppler imaging.

Global systolic function

Left ventricular systolic evaluation is commonly performed by eye. Although the eyeball of an experienced reader is equivalent to the trackball, the desirability of visual assessment is dependent on the circumstances. Visual assessment alone is appropriate in an emergency but inappropriate in most circumstances when elective decisions are being made. Global systolic function should be quantified. The standard approaches are detailed here and the most accurate (and therefore the preferred methods) are based on volumetric measures ($\square$ p.198).

2D measures

Ejection fraction

This represents the fraction of blood within the left ventricle which is ejected in 1 cardiac cycle (Fig. 4.19). To calculate, use the end-diastolic (LVEDV) and end-systolic (LVESV) volumes ($\square$ p.198). The ejection fraction is:

$$\frac{LVEDV - LVESV}{LVEDV} \times 100\%$$

EF can be calculated from linear measures ($\square$ p.196) using Teicholz' equation, but this is notoriously inaccurate, especially if regional function is reduced. If apical images are suboptimal, use of LV opacification may permit measurement using Simpson's rule, and 3D imaging may be performed from the parasternal window. Teicholtz equation:

$$\frac{LVEDD^3 - LVESD^3}{LVEDD^3} \times 100\%$$

Fractional shortening (fractional area change)

Fractional shortening and *fractional area change* represent summary measures of changes in left ventricle size in mid cavity. Fractional shortening is based on the standard linear measures (Fig. 4.20 and $\square$ p.196):

$$\frac{LVEDD - LVESD}{LVEDD} \times 100\%$$

Fractional area change (Fig. 4.21) uses end-diastolic (LVEDA) and end-systolic (LVESA) cavity cross-sectional area traced in parasternal short axis (mid-ventricle level) view (to measure area see $\square$ p.199):

$$\frac{LVEDA - LVESA}{LVEDA} \times 100\%$$

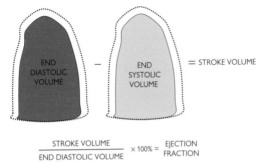

$$\frac{\text{STROKE VOLUME}}{\text{END DIASTOLIC VOLUME}} \times 100\% = \text{EJECTION FRACTION}$$

Fig. 4.19 Principle of ejection fraction. This can also be estimated from linear measures.

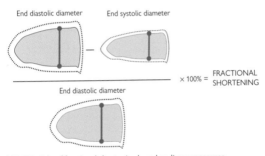

Fig. 4.20 Principle of fractional shortening based on linear measures.

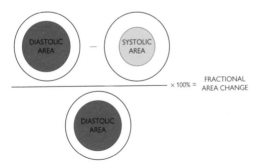

Fig. 4.21 Principle of fractional area change.

3D measures

- Inaccuracy of the earlier described measurements is inherent in the projection of the 3D structure of the heart in 1D or 2D, which necessitates both geometric assumptions and appropriate plane location.
- These considerations are especially important for repeat imaging, for which exact plane duplication is almost impossible. A wealth of evidence supports 3D to be a more accurate means of obtaining LV volumes than standard imaging—although the benefit is less marked for EF.
- Patients most likely to benefit are those with ischaemic cardiomyopathy and those having repeat studies. There remains some underestimation of LV volumes due to suboptimal resolution of trabeculations.
- Further technical developments are needed to improve imaging quality and frame rate, but the technique is ready for routine use.

Doppler evaluation

Stroke volume and cardiac output

- Doppler measurements of stroke volume are more commonly written about than performed.
- The volume of blood that forms the ejection fraction (LVEDV − LVESV) represents the *stroke volume*. Normally this is around 75–100mL. These measures vary with body size and should be divided by body surface area (body surface area = sq root(height (m) × weight (kg)/36)) to give a *stroke volume index* (normally 40–70mL/m^2) and *cardiac index* (normally 2.5–4L/min/m^2) respectively.
- If the mitral valve is competent then this can be multiplied by heart rate to calculate *cardiac output*. Normally this is around 4–8L/min.
- Stroke volume may be derived from EDV and ESV measures, but this depends on good image orientation.
- Doppler may be useful for stroke volume assessment (Fig. 4.22), but depends on accurate outflow tract measures (errors of which are squared to calculate area).
- Measurement of dP/dt can be a useful extra measure in patients with severe mitral regurgitation.

Calculating stroke volume

- In apical 5-chamber view record a PW Doppler in the outflow tract and trace the shape. Record the velocity time integral (vti).
- In a parasternal long axis view, zoom the LVOT and measure the width (edge to edge, just below aortic valve).
- Stroke volume is the area of the outflow tract ($\pi \times$ [LVOT diameter/2]^2) multiplied by the outflow tract vti.
- Cardiac output is stroke volume multiplied by heart rate.

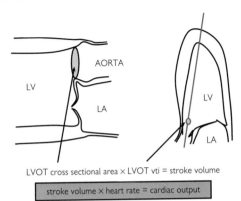

LVOT cross sectional area × LVOT vti = stroke volume

stroke volume × heart rate = cardiac output

Fig. 4.22 Stroke volume can be used as a Doppler-based assessment of left ventricle function.

dP/dt

dP/dt describes the rise in intraventricular pressure during early systole (Fig. 4.23). The change in pressure is determined by systolic contraction so the faster the rise the better the left ventricular systolic function. Theoretically this should be less dependent than ejection fraction on the loading condition of the heart. It can only be measured if there is significant mitral regurgitation.

- In an apical 4-chamber view align the CW Doppler through the mitral valve and the associated regurgitant jet.
- Record a spectral trace at a sweep speed of 100mm/s to broaden the tracing. Set the scale to focus on the 0 to 4m/s range.
- Measure the time taken for the velocity of the regurgitant jet to rise from 1 to 3m/s (the measure has been standardized for this pressure rise from 4 to 36mmHg). The machine or software will normally automatically calculate dP/dt if the 1m/s and 3m/s points are marked although it can be calculated by hand.
- dP/dt >1200mmHg/s (roughly <27ms between points) relates to normal function and <800mmHg/s (roughly >40ms) is severely depressed function.

Left ventricular outflow vti

To gain an impression of whether cardiac output is *normal*, *low*, or *high* measure vti in the left ventricular outflow tract using PW Doppler from an apical 5-chamber view. In the general population if the heart rate is between 60–100 then normal range is 18–22. This technique can also be applied to assess right ventricular output using PW Doppler in the right ventricular outflow tract in a parasternal short axis view. Normal values should be 76% (or three-quarters) of left ventricle outflow vti.

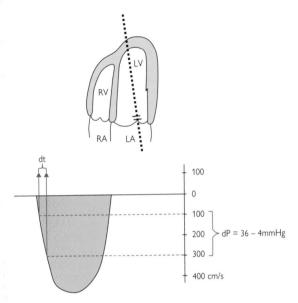

dt < 27ms = normal function
dt > 40ms = severely impaired function

Fig. 4.23 dP/dt measures the rise in intraventricular pressure. A mitral regurgitant jet has been assessed with continuous wave Doppler in an apical 4-chamber view.

Regional systolic function

Although regional changes can occur in cardiomyopathies, the most common cause of regional left ventricle dysfunction is coronary artery disease. Regional abnormalities are usually assessed by eye and are dependent on operator experience. Basic assessment is of wall movement in coronary artery territories. This should be refined to gauge movement of wall segments and can then be semi-quantified with wall motion scores. There are fully quantitative methods although not yet in routine clinical practice.

Qualitative assessment

The key to reporting regional dysfunction is to use a standard system to segment the heart. The standard 16-segment model of the American Society of Echocardiography (septal, lateral, anterior, and inferior at the apex, as well as anteroseptal and posterior segments at the base and mid-papillary muscle level) is still widely used, although the American Heart Association has moved to a 17-segment model (which includes a true apical segment) to encourage similar segment models between imaging techniques (Fig. 4.25).

Wall motion

- Record parasternal long and short axis and, apical 4-, 3-, and 2-chamber views. Avoid foreshortening and ensure a clear endocardial border. Enhance the border with left-sided contrast agents if needed (see ☐ p.561).
- Generally: anterior wall, apex, and septum are supplied by the left anterior descending artery; lateral and posterior (inferolateral) walls by the circumflex artery; and inferior wall by the right coronary artery. However, basal septum in an apical 4-chamber view is right coronary artery territory and supply of the apex and posterior wall varies slightly depending on which coronary system is dominant (left or right) (Fig. 4.24).
- In each loop look at each segment and score as normal, hypokinetic (endocardial excursion <5mm), akinetic (endocardial excursion <2mm), or dyskinetic (endocardium moves out in systole).
- As movement may be passive, look for thickening in segments you are unsure about. Normal segments will thicken by >50% between diastole and systole. If present, report as normal or hypokinetic.
- Present the findings as a diagram.

Wall motion scores

Wall motion scoring permits semi-quantitative evaluation of the regional function assessment.

- Score normal regions as 1; hypokinetic as 2; akinetic as 3; and dyskinetic as 4. Score aneurysms as 5; and thinning with akinesis as 6; or thinning with dyskinesis as 7.
- Calculate (or let the software calculate) a *wall motion score index* by averaging scores of all individual segments. This is a semi-quantitative index of global systolic function analogous to ejection fraction.

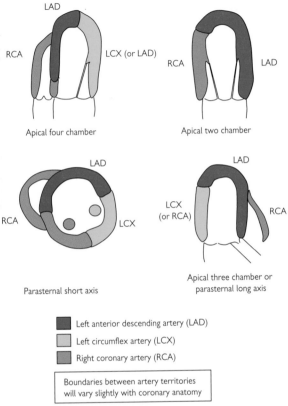

Fig. 4.24 Coronary artery supply to walls of left and right ventricle.

Quantitative assessment

Concordance of wall motion assessment between centres may be improved with the use of standard reading criteria, but remains imperfect. The benefit of a suitable objective measure would be to supplement wall motion scoring and help less expert readers.

Quantitation of regional function has been performed with a number of echocardiographic and Doppler modalities (Table 4.3). Although some are encouraging, none have entered mainstream practice.

Table 4.3 Assessment techniques for regional function

	Radial	Longitudinal
Displacement and thickening	Centre-line (from 2D)	Annular M-mode
	Color kinesis	Tissue tracking
	Anatomical M-mode	
	Speckle	Speckle or TDI
Velocity	Speckle	TDI or speckle
Deformation	Speckle	TDI or speckle
Timing	TDI (time to peak systole or onset of diastole)	TDI (time to peak systole or onset of diastole)

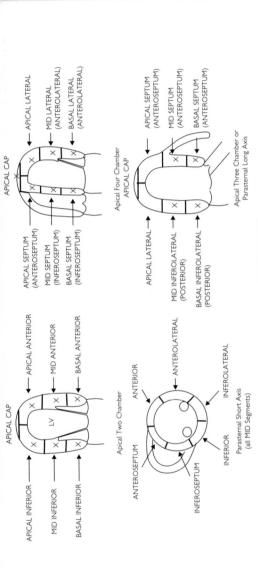

Fig. 4.25 17-segment model (16-segment is the same without the apical cap). Note that some segments are seen in multiple views. The posterior wall can also be referred to as the inferolateral wall. 'X's mark the 17 different segments of the ventricle, some of which are seen in the other views (unmarked segments).

APICAL CAP

APICAL LATERAL

MID LATERAL
(ANTEROLATERAL)

BASAL LATERAL
(ANTEROLATERAL)

APICAL SEPTUM
(ANTEROSEPTUM)

MID SEPTUM
(INFEROSEPTUM)

BASAL SEPTUM
(INFEROSEPTUM)

Apical Four Chamber
APICAL CAP

APICAL SEPTUM
(ANTEROSEPTUM)

MID SEPTUM
(ANTEROSEPTUM)

BASAL SEPTUM
(ANTEROSEPTUM)

Apical Three Chamber or
Parasternal Long Axis

APICAL LATERAL

MID INFEROLATERAL
(POSTERIOR)

BASAL INFEROLATERAL
(POSTERIOR)

APICAL CAP

APICAL ANTERIOR

MID ANTERIOR

BASAL ANTERIOR

APICAL INFERIOR

MID INFERIOR

BASAL INFERIOR

LV

Apical Two Chamber

ANTERIOR

ANTEROLATERAL

ANTEROSEPTUM

INFEROSEPTUM

INFERIOR

INFEROLATERAL

Parasternal Short Axis
(all MID Segments)

X marks the distinct seventeen segments (some are seen in multiple views)

Left ventricular strain

Background

Strain is a fundamental physical property of myocardium that reflects its deformation under an applied force. Two methods are used: (1) tissue Doppler—which derives strain from strain rate, a gradient of adjacent velocities over a sampling distance, and (2) speckle tracking—which derives strain from excursion of the speckles.

Complete assessment of strain—radial, longitudinal, circumferential, and the shear stress—may be achievable but is likely to be too much information for routine clinical use. The most robust and reproducible measure is longitudinal strain, for which there is the most clinical data. Circumferential strain (Figs. 4.26 and 4.27) can be assessed with speckle tracking but radial strain is difficult to measure by any method.

Which technique?

- Speckle strain is simpler and provides strain in multiple dimensions—potentially in 3D. Speckle strain is the preferred option apart from when high frame-rate is needed (e.g. for strain rate or stress imaging), in which case tissue velocity is likely superior.
- Neither tissue velocity nor speckle techniques are perfect and require further development—for example, studies suggest strain values in the same myocardium differ depending on the machine.

Global strain

- Although ejection fraction is simple and intuitive, as well as being supported by a wealth of prognostic information, it has important limitations including image quality dependence, geometric assumptions, load dependence, and insensitivity to early disease (which is characterized by disturbances of longitudinal function).
- Global strain avoids inaccuracy due to inaccurate border tracing, but is dependent on both loading conditions and image quality.
- Global strain is an analogue of ejection fraction, and can be measured as either longitudinal (GLS) or circumferential strain (GCS), derived as the mean of interpretable regional strains. These parameters have predicted outcome in two studies.
- Global strain is likely to be of value for sequential studies (e.g. left ventricular response to therapy), and the detection of early disease (e.g. infiltration, cardiotoxicity).
- Global strain is the average of the strain measurements in all 16 or 17 myocardial segments (or the segments where strain measurements are available).

Normal values for strain measurements

By convention, shortening is described by a negative value and lengthening by positive strain. If the myocardium did not contract then strain would be 0. Longitudinal strain is the most robust clinically and normal regional peak systolic strain in the longitudinal direction is approximately −18%. Longitudinal strain values of −14% or even closer to 0 are probably abnormal and a global longitudinal strain of −12% corresponds to an EF <35%. So far there is only very limited data available on normal ranges for all the parameters but the values given here have been published as normal ranges (mean ± SD) for the different types of strain (modified from Saito K et al.[1]). Note longitudinal and circumferential strain are negatives as the left ventricle reduces in size during systole, whereas, because radial strain describes thickening of the myocardium in systole, it is positive.

	3D speckle tracking*	2D speckle tracking
Longitudinal, %	−17.0±5.5	−19.9±5.3
Circumferential, %	−31.6±8.0	−27.8±6.9
Radial, %	34.4±11.4	35.1±11.8

3DT=3D speckle tracking; 2DT=2D speckle tracking, *Artida (Toshiba)

Reference

1 Saito K et al. Comprehensive evaluation of left ventricular strain using speckle tracking echocardiography in normal adults: comparison of three dimensional and two dimensional approaches. Am Soc Echocardiogr 2009; 22(9): 1025–30.

Regional strain

- The most important application of regional strain is to the recognition of ischaemic heart disease. The recognition of scar (resting imaging), viability (low-dose response), and ischaemia (peak dose imaging) is subjective and depends on image quality and observer expertise. Strain may offer a sensitive and reproducible alternative.
- The use of strain to recognize resting wall motion abnormalities may improve the detection of coronary disease in the ICU, operating room, and Chest Pain Unit (cut-offs of $-0.83/s$ for strain rate and -17.4% for strain have been proposed).
- Diastolic strain disturbance may persist for hours and represent a potential 'ischaemic memory' signal. Strain has also been used to anticipate the transmural extent of scar.
- The augmentation of viable segments in response to dobutamine may also be quantified with strain. Speckle strain appears to be inferior to Doppler-based strain, especially in the basal segments, possibly due to image quality.
- The assessment of strain during ischaemia remains extremely difficult. A human study has shown an increment of both sensitivity and specificity by combination of strain rate with wall motion. However, Doppler-based strain rate is onerous and subject to artefact, and speckle-based imaging is limited by image quality and frame-rate.
- The application of strain to the timing of regional contraction (mechanical dispersion) has potential applications in cardiac resynchronization therapy and possibly in the prediction of ventricular arrhythmias.
- Other strain applications that will likely assume importance are RV and atrial strain.

Advantages and disadvantages of strain imaging

The advantages of strain include:
- A sensitive and automated marker of regional and global function.
- It is relatively homogeneous in different LV segments.
- It is a marker of contractility.
- It is independent of tethering.

The disadvantages of strain include:
- Methods are time-consuming, complex, and require a knowledgeable user to avoid misleading results due to artefact.
- Speckle strain is dependent on good image quality.
- Tissue velocity requires imaging of the structure as close as possible to the ultrasound beam.

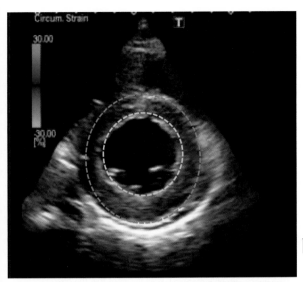

Fig. 4.26 2D circumferential strain. Postprocessing to delineate endocardial and epicardial borders (Toshiba Artida 2D wall motion tracking software).

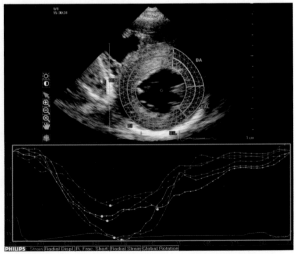

Fig. 4.27 2D circumferential strain with post processing on QLAB demonstrating regional circumferential strain at basal LV short axis level (Phillips QLAB 8.1). See Video 4.9.

Strain assessment by 2D speckle tracking

Image acquisition

- Good 2D image quality is necessary to ensure clear visualization of the endocardium.
- For complete 2D strain analysis all of the standard views for assessment of left ventricular regional wall motion will need to be acquired: left ventricular parasternal view; left ventricular short axis view (basal, mid and apical level) and left ventricular apical 4-, 3-, and 2-chamber views.
- Optimize the 2D image, adjusting the sector size, and depth to focus on the left ventricle.
- Ensure the frame rate is between 50–90 frames/s.
- Acquire images at end expiration.

Postprocessing

- A number of postprocessing software packages exist.
- After loading the appropriate view of the left ventricle the software package will ask the operator to confirm which view it is.
- Some software packages allow the gain of the image to be altered again if necessary.
- The operator will be prompted to identify specific points on the image to mark (usually up to 3 points). From this the software automatically will delineate the endocardial and epicardial borders (Fig. 4.26).
- The image can then be played. It is important that the operator visually assesses how well the automated borders are tracking the true endocardium/epicardium through the cardiac cycle.
- If the tracking is poor it will be necessary to adjust the automated border as required.
- When happy, the operator can then select which type of strain is to be analysed (Fig. 4.27).
- A colour overlay which corresponds to the colour bar on the left of the screen will be seen (see Fig. 4.28).

Each image of the left ventricle which is being assessed will be displayed segmentally and also displayed on a segmental strain graph.

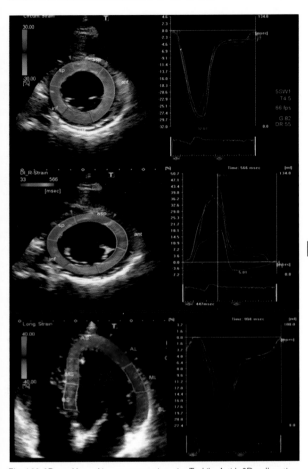

Fig. 4.28 2D speckle tracking post processing using Toshiba Artida 2D wall motion tracking. The LV in each view is segmented and has a colour overlay which corresponds to the strain value on the colour bar (far left of each image). Segmental strain curves also shown (right). Top: normal circumferential strain basal LV level. Middle: normal radial strain basal LV level. Bottom: normal longitudinal strain apical LV 4-chamber view. See 📹 Video 4.10 and 📹 Video 4.11.

Strain assessment by 3D speckle tracking

Image acquisition

- For adequate 3D speckle tracking analysis it is important that the 2D windows are good so that the endocardial border can be seen.
- Once the optimal 2D left ventricular apical 4-chamber view has been obtained, select 3D view.
- 3D full volume acquisition mode should be used.
- In the biplane view, adjust the depth and sector width to ensure you focus on the left ventricle.
- For 3D speckle tracking the image resolution should be optimized so that an adequate frame rate is achieved. Adjust the line density and use the maximal number of subvolumes (beats) possible depending on patient breath-holding capabilities.
- Acquire a full volume at end expiration.
- Check for the presence of stitching artefacts in the 4-chamber view and also by slicing the left ventricle to view in several short axis planes.
- If adequate, accept the image or else delete and start acquisition again.

Postprocessing

- Several different postprocessing software packages exist and whilst there may be some variation in individual algorithms, the general principles of estimating 3D strain are similar.
- Select the 3D full volume left ventricular acquisition to be used.
- The left ventricle will then be displayed in a number of planes—usually an apical 4-chamber view, apical 2-chamber view, and 3 short axis slices (Fig. 4.29).
- The left ventricular orientation in the biplane view can be adjusted to correct for foreshortening.
- The level of the 3 short axis planes can also be adjusted to ensure that the left ventricular apex, mid left ventricle (papillary muscle view), and basal left ventricle are being displayed.
- The software package will then prompt the operator to identify and mark anatomical landmarks (usually between 3–5) on the left ventricular biplane view. The automated software will then delineate the endocardium and epicardium in all of the on-screen left ventricular views.
- The operator can then play the loop of the cardiac cycle to see whether the epicardial and endocardial borders are being tracked appropriately.
- In addition to end-diastolic volume, end-systolic volume, and ejection fraction, the software calculates left ventricular mass. The left ventricular mass is measured during the cardiac cycle and a flat curve is an indicator for good tracking of the endocardium and epicardium as it is consistent with mass being constant. The following values are available within 30 seconds after initiating the analysis:
  - Global and segmental displacement.
  - Global and segmental strain strain rate, displacement.
  - A special feature is 3D strain which probably comes closest to the real movement of speckles.
  - Rotation and twist.

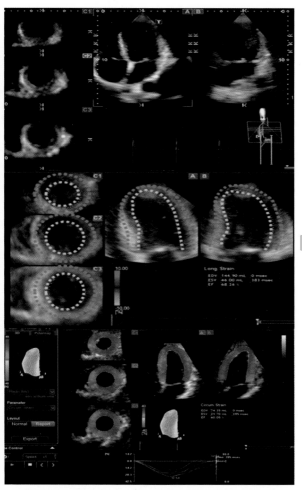

Fig. 4.29 3D strain acquisition and postprocessing on Toshiba Artida system. Top: from the apical LV window, the LV is displayed in two apical views and three short axis views. Middle: contouring of the epicardial and endocardial border. Bottom: normal LV 3D circumferential strain analysis. See 📹 Video 4.12.

Diastolic function

Diastolic dysfunction is increasingly recognized as an important influence on symptoms and haemodynamic status. Diastole extends from aortic valve closure to mitral valve closure and has 4 distinct phases:
• Isovolumetric relaxation—before the mitral valve opens.
• Early filling—accounting for up to 80% of ventricular filling.
• Diastasis—as left atria and left ventricle pressures equalize.
• Atrial systole—accounting for the remainder of ventricular filling.

Diastolic dysfunction during the early phases is due to problems with active myocardial relaxation. This is usually present early in disease development (e.g. ischaemia, aortic stenosis, hypertension, hypertrophy) and is termed *abnormal relaxation*. With disease progression, fibrosis develops and chamber compliance reduces (also seen with infiltrative disease). These changes affect later diastole and lead to *restrictive filling*. During the transition there is a period of apparently *pseudonormal filling* on some echocardiographic parameters at the mitral valve although diastolic function remains impaired.

Assessment

Measurement of *transmitral flow* (left ventricular filling) is the cornerstone of diastolic function evaluation (i.e. E/A ratio). This measure is refined with: (1) *pulmonary vein flow* and *left atrial size* (to understand left atrial pressure) and (2) *tissue Doppler imaging* of the mitral annulus (to study changes in myocardial movement) (see Fig. 4.16). *Colour M-mode propagation* has also been used. The report should comment on the presence and pattern of diastolic dysfunction (*abnormal relaxation*, *pseudonormal filling* or *restrictive filling*). Also comment on likely underlying pathology, if identified, during the examination.

Mitral valve inflow

• In the apical 4-chamber view position the PW Doppler sample volume at the mitral leaflet tips (Fig. 4.30). Use colour Doppler if necessary to optimize beam alignment with mitral inflow. Record a tracing.
• E/A ratio: measure peak E-wave velocity and peak A-wave velocity. Normal filling is generally characterized by an E/A ratio of 0.75–1.5.
• Other measures:
  • *Deceleration time*: measure the distance from start to end of the E-wave. If the end is obscured by the A-wave extrapolate the slope to the baseline. A deceleration time of 160–260ms is normal.
  • *Isovolumetric relaxation time*: measure the time from the end of the aortic outflow trace to the start of the mitral inflow trace. This normally requires two different Doppler recordings (one of aortic outflow and one of the mitral inflow) with timings taken relative to a fixed point on the ECG. Normal range for 21–40yrs is 67 ± 8ms; 41–60yrs is 74 ± 7ms; over 60yrs is 87 ± 7ms.
  • *Valsalva manoeuvre*: the mitral inflow pattern can be recorded again with the patient performing a Valsalva. If there is *pseudonormal* or *reversible restrictive filling* the trace will revert to an *abnormal relaxation* pattern.

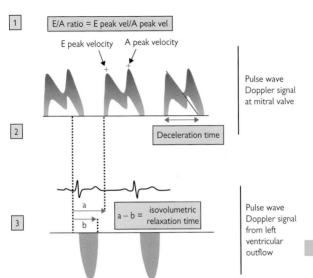

Fig. 4.30 Doppler measures of diastolic function. E/A ratio uses peak of E and A wave velocities from PW Doppler at mitral valve tips. Deceleration time is time from peak of E wave to baseline. Isovolumetric relaxation time: a = time from R wave on ECG to start of mitral valve inflow, b = time from R wave to end of aortic outflow.

Left atrial size
- Determine left atrial size by standard methods (p.280). Increased left atrial size implies raised left atrial pressure.

Pulmonary vein flow
- In the apical 4-chamber view ensure there is enough depth to see the pulmonary vein inflow. The easiest vein to see (and best aligned for Doppler) is the right upper pulmonary vein near the atrial septum. Placement can be optimized with colour flow mapping to demonstrate the pulmonary vein flow.
- Place the PW Doppler sample volume just inside the pulmonary vein and record a spectral tracing. A good tracing confirms a satisfactory position.
- The tracing will consist of 2 forward flow phases, systolic and diastolic, followed by an atrial reversal (due to atrial systole). Normally the systolic wave is dominant or equal to the diastolic wave.
- A prominent atrial reversal (>30cm/s peak velocity of the atrial wave and >20–30ms longer duration of the atrial wave compared to the duration of the A wave on the mitral inflow) is a specific but not very sensitive marker of raised filling pressure. Blunting of the systolic flow wave is a reliable marker of raised filling pressure in patients with systolic dysfunction, but not normal function.

Tissue Doppler imaging
- In apical 4-chamber views place the PW tissue Doppler on the septal or lateral annulus of the mitral valve (there is no clear consensus about which is optimal). The tissue Doppler spectrum can be optimized by decreasing the sample volume and optimizing gain settings (excessive gain causes spectral broadening). Ensure it is aligned with the long axis of the ventricle.
- The Doppler pattern should be the same as the mitral valve inflow with an E wave and A wave (but below the baseline away from the probe). Measure the peak velocity of both. They are usually referred to as E' and A' (see Tables 4.4 and 4.5).
- E/E' can also be calculated and relates to left atrial pressure. E/E' <8 suggests normal left atrial pressure and E/E' >15 suggests elevated left atrial pressure.
- E/E' is central to recent recommendations for the diagnosis of heart failure with a normal ejection fraction (HFNEF) (see Fig. 4.32).

Diastolic function: tips and measures

Transmitral flow categorization (see Figs. 4.16 and 4.31)

1. Impaired relaxation This is characterized by reduction of the peak transmitral pressure gradient (hence lower E velocity and E/A ratio [<1 in young, <0.5 in elderly]) and prolongation of the E deceleration slope (>220ms in young, >280ms in elderly). Cardiac pacing, left bundle branch block, and RV overload may provoke the same changes.

2. Pseudonormal filling As left atrial pressure increases with progressive left ventricle disease, E velocity and deceleration time return to normal. With exception of patients with more marked elevations of filling pressure and low heart rate, who may show a mid-diastolic ('L') wave, transmitral flow patterns cannot be distinguished from normal without the performance of other steps. The first step is to suspect the condition—'normal' transmitral flow in the setting of left ventricle enlargement, hypertrophy, or systolic dysfunction is likely to be pseudonormal. The second step is to assess left atrial size, followed by estimation of filling pressure (as E/E') and tissue Doppler of the mitral annulus. Note that when left ventricle ejection fraction is preserved, E deceleration time, the Valsalva response, blunting of the pulmonary venous S wave (and S/D ratio), and flow propagation velocity may be unreliable indicators of diastolic dysfunction.

3. Restrictive filling Continued elevation of filling pressure leads to increased E velocity (increase in E/A ratio >2) and shorter E deceleration time (<150ms). This finding is unusual with normal ejection fraction (indicating a restrictive cardiomyopathy, e.g. amyloidosis), and is more commonly associated with left ventricle dilatation and severe systolic dysfunction. The presence of reversibility (i.e. normalization with Valsalva or after diuresis) is prognostically very important.

Table 4.4 Age-adjusted normal cut-offs for selected diastolic parameters

	<40 years	40–60 years	>60 years
E deceleration time (ms)	<220	140–250	140–275
Septal E' velocity (cm/s)	>9	>7	>6
Lateral E' velocity (cm/s)	>11	>10	>7

Table 4.5 Useful criteria for differentiating normal from pseudonormal filling in adult subjects with normal left ventricular systolic function

	Normal	Pseudo-normal
Lateral E' velocity (depending on age)	>7–11	<7–11
Lateral E/E'	<10	>10
PV A velocity (cm/s)	<35	>35
PV A duration – transmitral	<30	>30
A duration (ms)		
Valsalva manoeuvre	No significant change in E/A ratio	E/A <1 or E/A decrease by >50%

PV = pulmonary venous.

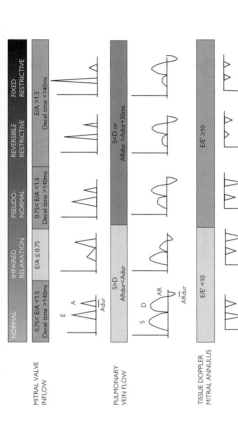

Fig. 4.31 Doppler patterns for mitral valve, pulmonary vein, and mitral annulus to characterize diastolic function. The mitral inflow can be repeated with a Valsalva manoeuvre and if there is pseudonormal filling the mitral inflow will change to an impaired relaxation pattern. Reversible restrictive describes a restrictive pattern in which the mitral valve inflow also changes to an impaired relaxation pattern on Valsalva. Mitral: E = peak E wave velocity, A = peak A wave velocity, Adur = duration of A wave. Tissue Doppler mitral annulus: E' = peak velocity; A' = peak velocity. Pulmonary vein flow: S = peak systolic wave; D = peak diastolic flow; AR = peak atrial reversal flow; ARdur = duration of atrial reversal wave.

HFNEF

Clinically, it is increasingly recognized that there is a group of patients who require treatment for symptoms of heart failure (shortness of breath etc.) but who have normal systolic cardiac function. These symptoms appear to relate to underlying diastolic dysfunction and they are increasingly referred to as patients with heart failure with a normal ejection fraction (HFNEF). HFNEF could be a precursor of heart failure with reduced ejection fraction. Guidelines have been established to help guide diagnosis and treatment of this group of patients.

The diagnosis of HFNEF requires the following conditions to be fulfilled:
- Signs or symptoms of heart failure.
- Normal or mildly reduced LV systolic function (LVEF >50% and LV end diastolic volume index <97mL/m^2.
- Evidence of diastolic dysfunction.

Assessment for a diagnosis of HFNEF (Fig. 4.32)
- Left ventricular end-systolic and end-diastolic volumes should be calculated from standard views to obtain a Simpson's biplane or 3D evaluation (📖 p.228).
- If left ventricular ejection fraction is >50% and the left ventricle is not dilated (<97mL/m^2) then proceed on to obtain an assessment of diastolic function based on both tissue Doppler imaging of the mitral annulus and transmitral inflow velocities by PW Doppler (Fig. 4.30).
- Using these Doppler measures calculate the ratio of E/E'. This correlates closely with left ventricular filling pressure and if E/E' is >15 then this is considered diagnostic for HFNEF. If E/E' <8 then, conversely, HFNEF is excluded.
- If E/E' is between 8 and 15 then further echocardiographic evaluation is required. Any of the following are considered to support a diagnosis of HFNEF:
  - E/A <0.5 and deceleration time >280ms (age >50 years).
  - LA indexed volume >40mL/m^2.
  - LV mass index >122g/m^2 (female) or >149g/m^2 (male).
  - Duration of reverse pulmonary vein atrial flow—duration of mitral valve atrial wave flow >30ms.

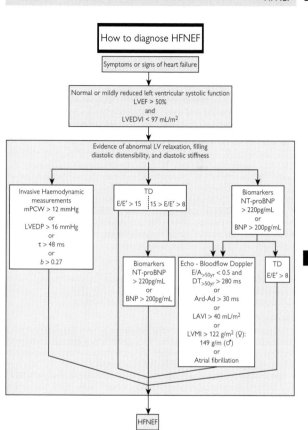

Fig. 4.32 Diagnostic flowchart on 'How to diagnose HFNEF' in a patient suspected of HFNEF. LVEDVI, left ventricular end-diastolic volume index; mPCW, mean pulmonary capillary wedge pressure; LVEDP, left ventricular end-diastolic pressure; t, time constant of left ventricular relaxation; b, constant of left ventricular chamber stiffness; TD, tissue Doppler; E, early mitral valve flow velocity; E0, early TD lengthening velocity; NT-proBNP, N-terminal-pro brain natriuretic peptide; BNP, brain natriuretic peptide; E/A, ratio of early (E) to late (A) mitral valve flow velocity; DT, deceleration time; LVMI, left ventricular mass index; LAVI, left atrial volume index; Ard, duration of reverse pulmonary vein atrial systole flow; Ad, duration of mitral valve atrial wave flow. Paulus WJ et al. Eur Heart J 2007. **28**(20):2359–550.

Left ventricular synchrony

The current selection criteria for cardiac resynchronization therapy include NYHA class III or IV heart failure symptoms and left ventricle ejection fraction <35% on maximal medical therapy, in the setting of a widened QRS (the relevant QRS width varies between trials, but usually is >120ms (usually left bundle branch block)). Despite using these criteria 20–30% do not respond and it may be that others with heart failure would benefit.

Markers of dyssynchrony (Fig. 4.33)

Echocardiographic assessment of synchrony can be used for patient selection, pacing site selection, or both. Synchrony can be assessed between right ventricle and left ventricle (interventricular dyssynchrony—electromechanical delay in right ventricular outflow tract and left ventricular outflow tract) or within the left ventricle (intraventricular dyssynchrony—M-mode, tissue Doppler, strain, 3D). There are few comparisons between the markers and centres often offer a 'menu' of measurements. A list follows, with findings that would suggest dyssynchrony:

- M-mode septum to posterior delay >130ms.
- Inter-ventricular delay >40ms.
- Systolic strain (% delayed contraction >30).
- Septal to posterior wall delay >65ms by tissue Doppler imaging.
- Dyssynchrony index >32.6ms.
- Parametric markers: tissue strain index, tissue tracking.

Interventricular dyssynchrony

Interventricular dyssynchrony is the difference in time between onset of pulmonary flow and onset of aortic flow (≥40ms suggests dyssynchrony). Because separate measurements are needed for each measurement the onset of flow in each view is timed relative to the ECG trace.

- Obtain a parasternal short axis view (aortic valve level). Record a PW Doppler tracing through the pulmonary valve. Ensure there is a surface ECG recording.
- In an apical 4-chamber view place a PW Doppler in the outflow tract and record a tracing. Ensure there is a surface ECG trace.
- Measure the distance from the start of the QRS to the start of the pulmonary valve flow on the first view then measure the distance from the start of the QRS to the start of the aortic valve flow on the second view. The difference is the interventricular delay.

Intraventricular dyssynchrony (septal vs. lateral wall)

Intraventricular dyssynchrony is the delay between the septal and posterior wall peak contraction (≥130ms suggests dyssynchrony), i.e. the delay between the opposite walls of the left ventricle being fully contracted.

- In a parasternal long axis view drop the M-mode cursor perpendicular to the septal and posterior wall. On the tracing identify the peak of septal and posterior wall systolic motion. Measure the time difference between the 2 walls and this is the intraventricular delay.

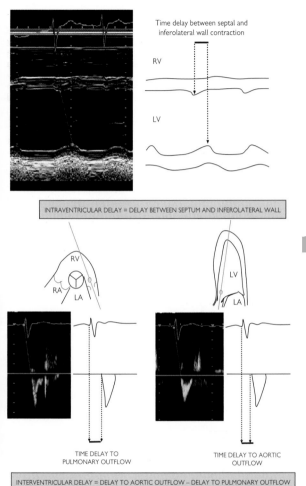

Time delay between septal and
inferolateral wall contraction

RV

LV

INTRAVENTRICULAR DELAY = DELAY BETWEEN SEPTUM AND INFEROLATERAL WALL

RV

RA   LA

LV

LA

TIME DELAY TO
PULMONARY OUTFLOW

TIME DELAY TO AORTIC
OUTFLOW

INTERVENTRICULAR DELAY = DELAY TO AORTIC OUTFLOW – DELAY TO PULMONARY OUTFLOW

Fig. 4.33 Measurement of inter- and intraventricular dyssynchrony.

Tissue Doppler measures

Differences in movement of the mid and basal segments of each wall of the left ventricle can be assessed by tissue Doppler imaging to provide some impression of the coordination of the ventricle. The assessment can be based on 8 measures from apical 4- and 2-chamber views, or 12 measures, which include measures in the apical 3-chamber view (Fig. 4.34).

- In apical 4-chamber place the tissue Doppler sample volume on each side of the mitral valve annulus and in the mid segments of the septum and lateral wall. Record tracings in each position.
- Repeat the process in the apical 2-chamber view on each side of the annulus and the mid segments of the inferior and anterior walls.
- This can then be repeated in the apical 3-chamber view in all 4 basal and mid segments.
- Measure the time from the start of the QRS to the systolic phase of motion on each tracing.
- The standard deviation of the 8 (or 12) measures provides a global index of dyssynchrony (>33ms suggests dyssynchrony).
- An alternative measure is the delay between the basal septum and basal lateral wall in the apical 4-chamber view (>60ms suggests dyssynchrony).
- Finally if any of the 8 (or 12) measures are >100ms different then this suggests dyssynchrony.

Use in follow-up: how to define success?

The most widely used markers include clinical improvement (formalized as improvement in heart failure class or quality of life score) and improved exercise capacity (e.g. lengthening of a 6-minute walk). Echocardiographic markers include ≥15% decrease in left ventricle volumes, ≥5% increase in ejection fraction, any decrease in left ventricle mass, or a decrease in mitral regurgitation severity.

Unresolved issues

Current guidelines for CRT therapy do not include dyssynchrony measurements. There are controversial studies on the value of routine synchrony studies for decision on CRT treatment. A number of potential contributions from echocardiography remain unresolved:

- What is the optimal synchrony marker to predict recovery?
- Predicting response to CRT using 2D echocardiography has been seen with varying degrees of success.
- Should echocardiography be used to assess ischaemia/viability?
- Is guidance regarding optimal pacing site useful?
- Should echocardiography be used to make adjustments to pacing parameters over time as cardiac function varies?

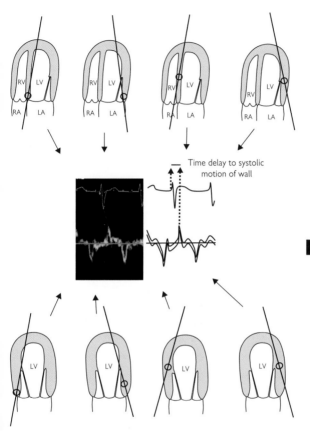

Fig. 4.34 Tissue Doppler imaging in basal and mid segments of left ventricle walls from apical 4- and 2-chamber views. For a 12-segment model the apical 3-chamber view is used as well.

3D for assessment of dyssynchrony? (Fig. 4.35)

- Real-time 3D echocardiography has been used to quantify global LV mechanical dyssynchrony in patients with and without prolonged QRS duration.
- Using real-time 3D echocardiography, data sets for global and segmental LV volumes can be processed to analyse the time–volume relationship during the cardiac cycle.
- From 3D LV acquisition, a series of volume curves can be obtained to show the variation of segmental volume during the cardiac cycle. In a synchronous ventricle, the individual segmental volume curves should reach their minimum volumes at a similar time at end systole. With a dyssynchronous LV, the segmental volume traces vary with respect to time.
- A systolic dyssynchrony index (SDI) has been proposed which can be used to identify chronic heart failure patients who may not otherwise be considered for CRT. Here, the SDI is defined as the standard deviation of the time taken to reach minimal regional volume using a 16-segment model and expressed as a percentage of the cardiac cycle. It has been shown that clinical responders to CRT had larger SDI at baseline versus non-responders and that an SDI >6.4% had a sensitivity of 88% and a specificity of 86% to predict acute volumetric response to CRT.

Advantages and disadvantages of 3D for dyssynchrony

The use of real-time 3D imaging has advantages over 2D echocardiography:
- There is simultaneous acquisition of all LV segments during the same cardiac cycles.
- All LV segments are recorded simultaneously and thus avoid problems with heart rate variability which may be seen in 2D echocardiography.

The use of real-time 3D imaging has the disadvantages:
- The image quality of real time 3D echocardiography is lower than that for 2D echocardiography with lower temporal resolution than 2D tissue Doppler imaging.
- Stitching artefacts may be more prevalent in the population of patients being assessed due to breath-holding problems and also rhythm disturbances.

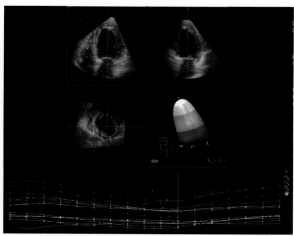

Fig. 4.35 Example of segmental volume traces in a patient with LV dyssynchrony. Bottom: segmental volume curves varying with time during the cardiac cycle. In each curve, the red triangle is a marker of the minimum systolic volume.

Optimization

Optimization procedures often do not lead to clinical improvement but two pacing parameters can be altered to test for benefit. Delay between pacing atrium and ventricle (AV delay) and delay between pacing left and right ventricle (VV delay).

Assessment

Start

Ensure you have the appropriate pacemaker programmer and a technician. Start by collecting the standard baseline dyssynchrony measures (🕮 p.254) and record the current programmed AV and VV delay.

AV delay (Fig. 4.36)

The aim is to choose the shortest AV delay that still allows complete ventricular filling. There are 2 approaches. Both use apical 4-chamber view with a PW Doppler profile of mitral valve inflow.

Iterative method

- Program a short AV delay (e.g. 50ms) on the pacemaker. Look at the A-wave and decrease the delay in 20ms steps until the A-wave starts to be truncated. Then gradually extend the delay by 10ms steps until the A-wave is just complete (Fig. 4.36).

Ritter method

- Program a short AV delay (e.g. *short delay* = 50ms) and measure distance from start of QRS to end of A wave (*QAshort*).
- Program a long AV delay (e.g. *long delay* = 150ms) and measure distance from start of QRS to end of A wave (*QA long*).
- Calculate optimal delay as = long delay + QAlong – QAshort.

VV delay (Fig. 4.37)

In an apical 5-chamber view place PW Doppler in left ventricular outflow tract. Keep it in the same position throughout the study.

- Start the VV delay with left ventricle paced 80ms before the right.
- Record a spectral profile and annotate with the VV delay.
- Calculate the vti by tracing the spectral profile.
- Reduce the delay by 20ms to 60ms and record another vti.
- Repeat, reducing delay by 20ms until there is no delay (0ms). Then start pacing right ventricle first, increasing in 20ms increments up to 80ms.
- Also, try left and right ventricle pacing alone.
- Look at results and identify parameter with maximal vti. There should be a graded pattern away from the optimal delay. Choose this as the new VV delay.
- If decision is to pace right ventricle first AV delay should be reset.

new optimal AV delay = previous optimal AV delay − VV delay.

Finish

Program new AV and VV delay. Finish study with full re-evaluation of synchrony to ensure improvement following reprogramming.

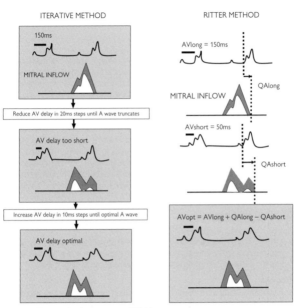

Fig. 4.36 Two methods to measure AV delay.

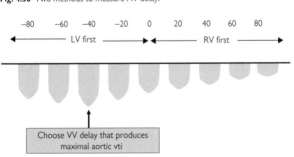

Fig. 4.37 VV delay assessed from recordings of aortic vti at different programmed delays. The VV delay with maximal aortic vti is selected.

Right ventricle

Normal anatomy

The right ventricle is made up of inflow (sinus), apical trabecular, and outflow (conus) regions though there is no clear demarcation between each. Towards the apex a muscular *moderator band* connects the free wall and septum. The combination of a thin free wall and thick septum leads to an irregular crescent shape when viewed in short axis with asymmetric contraction. The right ventricle maintains blood flow from the venous system to the pulmonary vasculature and from there to the left atrium and left ventricle. Size and function can therefore be affected by pulmonary problems (e.g. pulmonary hypertension, embolism), left-sided heart disease (e.g. left ventricle failure, mitral valve disease), and right ventricular disorders (e.g. infarction, dysplasia). Septal defects have important effects on right ventricular function because the right heart is exposed to systemic pressures.

Normal findings

Views

- Key views are: parasternal long axis; parasternal right ventricular inflow and outflow; parasternal short axis (aortic valve, mitral valve and mid-papillary levels); apical 4- and 3-chamber; subcostal (Fig. 4.38).

Findings

- Parasternal long axis: right ventricle nearest probe. View can be used for M-mode measures of the proximal RVOT.
- Parasternal right ventricular inflow and outflow: these give excellent views of tricuspid and pulmonary valves. TR jet velocity can be measured if there is good alignment.
- Parasternal short axis (aortic valve, mitral valve, and mid-papillary levels): right ventricle wraps around the left ventricle and therefore can be scanned through at multiple levels (as for the left ventricle). At the aortic valve it can be seen with both tricuspid and pulmonary valves and Doppler measures can be performed. As the plane moves towards the apex, the right ventricle is seen as a crescent to the left of the left ventricle. These views can give an impression of size and, in combination with septal appearance, of right ventricular pressure.
- Apical views: this can be used to assess function based on tricuspid annulus movement. Cranial tilt of probe may demonstrate right ventricular outflow. Visualization of TR jet is improved by medial and cranial displacement of the probe.
- Subcostal view: right ventricle nearest probe with ventricular septum horizontal. Best view for septal defects (colour flow) as well as measuring wall thickness. A short axis view of basal right ventricle can be achieved in certain patients, particularly if thin. Doppler interrogation of outflow and main pulmonary artery can be undertaken.

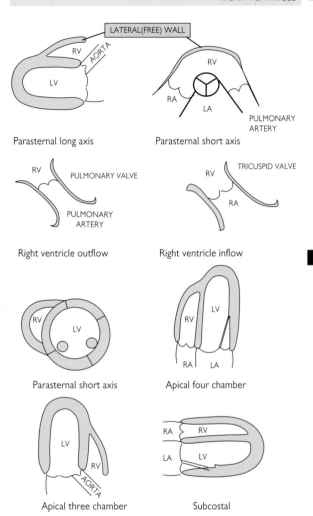

Fig. 4.38 Key views to assess the right ventricle.

Right ventricular size

The right ventricle has a complex shape so assessment of size is often performed qualitatively. However, the right ventricle has significant clinical relevance and a more thorough quantitative assessment is now warranted. This task has been aided by recent guidelines which have provided guidance on quantification and normal values.

Assessment

Assess the right ventricle in several views. If it does not appear normal comment on cavity size, as well as wall thickness, outflow tract size, and right atrial area.

2D measures of size

Right ventricular cavity size

- The apical 4-chamber view should be focused to maximize the size of the RV such that it transects the acute margin of the RV while keeping the LV apex in view. The latter is key since it is easy artificially to make the RV form the apex and be bigger than the LV.
- A useful rule of thumb is that the normal RV should be two-thirds the size of the LV. However this relies on the LV being normal sized itself. Appearances of the cardiac apex can be instructive: with moderate amounts of dilatation, the acute angle formed by the RV free wall and septum increases. In severe RV dilatation, the RV apex can dominate over the left.
- Overall, it is more helpful to assess RV size quantitatively using the *diameter at the tricuspid annulus and mid cavity diameter* which should be less than 4.2cm and 3.5cm respectively.
- If so this can be reported as *apex forming*.
- The RVOT can be measured in the left parasternal (and subcostal views if necessary). The proximal RVOT is seen in the PLAX and PSAX at the level of the aortic valve (RVOT1) where a value >33mm is abnormal, but it is preferred to take the distal RVOT (RVOT2) where the PV and infundibulum meet. The RVOT is dilated here if >27mm. (See Fig. 4.39 and Table 4.6.)

Right atrial area can be measured from planimetry in the apical 4-chamber view and a value >18 cm^2 considered to reflect RA enlargement.

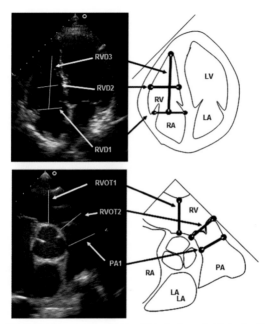

Fig. 4.39 Six standard measures of right ventricle size from apical 4-chamber (top) and parasternal short axis (bottom) views.

Table 4.6 2D parameters to assess right ventricle size and function (ASE guidelines)

Measure	Abnormal
Chamber dimensions	
RV basal diameter (RVD1)	>4.2cm
RV subcostal wall thickness	>0.5cm
RVOT PSAX distal diameter (RVOT2)	>2.7cm
RVOT PSAX proximal diameter (RVOT1)	>3.3cm
Systolic function	
TAPSE	<1.6cm
Tissue Doppler peak velocity at the annulus	<10cm/s
Pulsed Doppler myocardial performance index	>0.40
Tissue Doppler myocardial performance index	>0.55
Fractional area change (%)	>35%

3D measures of size

Analysis of 3D right ventricular views is currently possible with a commercially available software package (4D-RV Function, TomTec, Germany). Only patients with very good image quality should be considered for 3D echocardiography of the right heart. Also, for accurate assessment there should be no arrhythmia, and breath-holding capacity should be good. Following initial acquisition of the 3D dataset, cut planes are reviewed in the short axis view (in order to outline the tricuspid valve in the optimal position), apical 4-chamber plane (to outline the apex) and the coronal plane (to outline the RVOT). The right ventricular volumes are calculated by summing the areas for each slice through the complete volume data set (Table 4.7).

Acquisition of 3D volume for assessment of RV and RA volumes

- Position the probe at the apex in the same position as for acquisition of 2D 4 chamber views.
- The biplane preview (Fig. 4.40) screen is used so that the 4- and 2- chamber views can be seen simultaneously to help avoid foreshortening.
- Sometimes the probe will need to be tilted anteriorly towards the RVOT.
- Depth, gain, and TGC are adjusted in 2D imaging in order to achieve the best possible endocardial definition.
- For full volume datasets maximize the number of subvolumes (beats) used to generate the 3D image according to patient breath-holding capabilities. The greater the number of subvolumes, the greater the temporal resolution.
- Acquire 2D or more 3D datasets as artefacts are common and then inspect the dataset.
- Use short axis planes to make sure there are no stitching artefacts. Use the cropping tool to ensure there is good endocardial delineation and that the right ventricular outflow tract is included in the dataset.
- If the listed criteria are not adequate delete and reacquire.

Table 4.7 Normal values for 3D RV volumes and ejection fraction

	LRV (95% CI)	Mean (95% CI)	URV (95% CI)
3D RV EF (%)	44 (39–49)	57 (53–61)	69 (65–74)
3D RV EDV indexed (mL/m²)	40 (28–52)	65 (54–76)	89 (77–101)
3D RV ESV indexed (mL/m²)	12 (1–23)	28 (18–38)	45 (34–56)

CI, confidence interval; EF, ejection fraction; EDV, end-diastolic volume; ESV, end-systolic volume; LRV, lower reference value; URV, upper reference value.

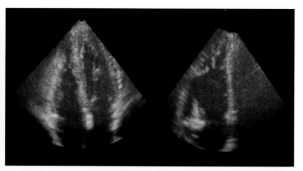

Fig. 4.40 Acquisition of full volume RV 3D dataset showing initial biplane view used to optimize the RV and to avoid foreshortening. 4-chamber view (left) and 2-chamber view (right).

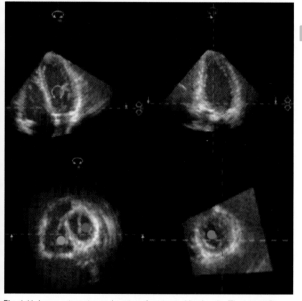

Fig. 4.41 Image orientation and setting of anatomical landmarks. The initial 3D dataset is displayed as three 2D images: 4-chamber (top left), 2-chamber (top right), and 2 short axis (sagittal) views (bottom). Moving the blue dashed cursor up and down the ventricle will allow the coronal view to be altered accordingly. The program prompts the operator to mark the centre of the tricuspid valve (blue dot), centre of the mitral valve (red dot) and centre of the LV apex (green dot). Once this has been completed, then RV contouring can be performed. See 🎥 Video 4.13.

Processing the dataset

Image orientation and setting of anatomical landmarks

- TomTec (Germany) allows post processing of full volume 3D right ventricular datasets. Initially the operator is prompted to select the orientation from which the image was acquired (apical-lateral, apical-medial or subcostal).
- Play the dataset initially and confirm that the chosen end-systolic and end-diastolic frames are correct or adjust if needed.
- The initial display shows the 3D volume as a sequence of three 2D slices: the apical window, the 2-chamber window (coronal view), and the short axis window (sagittal view).
- When the cropping mode is activated these views usually are displayed but often have to be adjusted in order to obtain the right ventricle in full length, to include RVOT and to get the sagittal mid right ventricle view around 90° angulated to the apical 4-chamber view.
- The postprocessing system will prompt you to identify certain anatomical landmarks on the sagittal (e.g. centre of tricuspid valve, centre of mitral valve, and the left ventricular apex), Fig. 4.41. The landmarks are obtained by slicing the apical view using the slice prompt (see Fig. 4.42 blue dashed line). When the centre of the tricuspid valve is located the position is marked on the sagittal view (see Fig. 4.41, blue dot). The centre of the mitral valve is then marked (see Fig. 4.41, red dot). Finally the horizontal cutting plane (yellow dashed line) is moved so that the sagittal view is cutting the left ventricular apex and again this is marked on the sagittal view (see Fig. 4.41, green dot).

RV contouring

- The initial contours are then set in the apical 4-chamber view; sagittal and coronal cut planes in end-systole and end-diastole, see Fig. 4.42.
- During contouring of the sagittal and coronal planes, the program helps the operator to delineate the endocardial border by showing circular targets which the contour should pass through (see Fig. 4.42).
- Trabeculations are included in the endocardial rim, but the apical component of the RV moderator band is excluded from the cavity. The software then will calculate the contours in the other slices and frames.
- After the 3 planes have been contoured, check the calculated contours with reference to the true anatomical structure of the right ventricle by slicing through the right ventricular cavity and making corrections if major deviations are observed.
- The TomTec programme will then estimate the right ventricular end-diastolic, end-systolic, and stroke volumes as well as calculating the right ventricular ejection fraction.
- The right ventricular motion can be reviewed in a 3D model and rotated to be seen from different angles (Fig. 4.43).
- The right ventricular motion can also be viewed, for instance with a static wire frame, see Fig. 4.43.

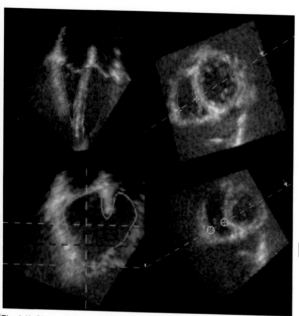

Fig. 4.42 RV contouring (green line) in the 3 cut planes: apical (top left), sagittal (top right), coronal (bottom left). Circular yellow targets created by the program to help the operator contour the RV (bottom right). See 📹 Video 4.14, 📹 Video 4.15, 📹 Video 4.16.

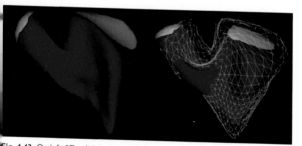

Fig. 4.43 On left, 3D solid display of RV. This is described as a Beutel display. On right, Beutel display with a static wire frame representing the end-diastolic Beutel overlaps a dynamic 3D surface model (green). See 📹 Video 4.17.

Right ventricular wall thickness

This can be assessed at end-diastole using M-mode imaging in the parasternal long axis view, or more consistently from the subcostal view (Fig. 4.44) Normal is <0.5 cm.

- In the subcostal view use a clear 2D image frozen in end-diastole (or perpendicular M-mode trace). Measure from edge-to-edge of the free wall at the level of the of the tip of the anterior tricuspid valve leaflet.
- In the parasternal view use a 2D image or M-mode trace with cursor perpendicular to the ventricle wall at the mitral valve tip level.
- In either view take care not to include epicardial fat, coarse trabeculations, or papillary muscles in the measurement.

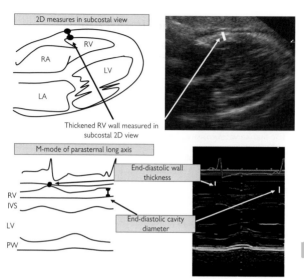

Fig. 4.44 Measurement of RV wall thickness from a 2D subcostal view (top) and M-mode in parasternal long axis view (bottom).

Right ventricular function

- Although it can be evaluated qualitatively by studying the movement of the right ventricle free wall and assigning a label of normal or impaired to right ventricular systolic function, quantitation of right ventricular systolic function is now recommended.
- A number of measures of right ventricular systolic function have evolved whose purpose is to sidestep the difficulties of using volumetric techniques established in the left ventricle for the geometrically complex right ventricle.
- The number of surrogates for right ventricular systolic function is a reminder that no single index predominates. More recently, quantifying right ventricular systolic function using volumetric techniques has been simplified by advances in 3D imaging acquisition and analysis.

Assessment

- Assess right ventricular function from the apical 4-chamber view.
- Confirm your impression in parasternal and subcostal views.
- Concentrate on movement of the tricuspid annulus to get an overall impression of function.
- Support this by looking at regional wall motion abnormalities and thickening along the free wall to the apex, note whether areas are *normal*, *akinetic* or *dyskinetic* (use same criteria as left ventricle regional assessment, ☐ p.234).

When assessing regional wall motion abnormalities, bear in mind that the right ventricular free wall is predominantly supplied by the right coronary artery and that the septum, apex, and, in some patients, the distal free wall is supplied by the left anterior descending artery. Where possible, use the 4 methods described in this section to quantify right ventricular systolic function:

Myocardial Performance Index (MPI) or TEI index

- Considered a cumulative measure of right ventricular systolic and diastolic dysfunction.
- It is calculated by dividing the *isolvulumic time* by *ejection time*.
- These measures can be derived using pulsed Doppler. The *ejection time* is derived from the spectral trace in the RVOT and the *isovolumic time* from the pulsed Doppler of inflow across the tricuspid valve. Ensure heart rates are similar when each pulsed Doppler measure is recorded as variation in cardiac cycle length will make the measures inaccurate. This means it is particularly unreliable in atrial fibrillation.
- Alternatively, both indices can be derived at the same time from the TDI trace of the tricuspid annulus (Fig. 4.45).
- A value >0.40 for the pulsed Doppler method and 0.55 for the TDI are abnormal.

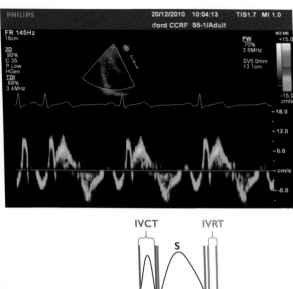

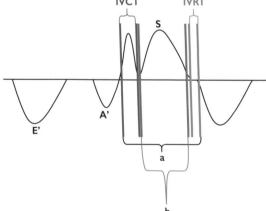

Fig. 4.45 Tei index. A' = myocardial lengthening velocity during atrial contraction; E' = myocardial velocity during early diastole; a = time interval from the end of the A' wave to the beginning of the E' wave; S = myocardial shortening velocity during ventricular systole; b = time interval from beginning to the end of the S wave; IVCT = isovolumic contraction time; IVRT = isovolumic relaxation time. Myocardial performance index (TEI) index: (a—b)/b.

Tricuspid annular plane systolic excursion (TAPSE)

In the normal right ventricle, the lateral side of the tricuspid annulus moves towards the apex during systole reflecting right ventricular longitudinal function. TAPSE is a way of measuring how much it moves.

- Obtain an apical 4-chamber view.
- Place the M-mode cursor through the lateral annulus of the tricuspid valve and record a trace (Fig. 4.46).
- Measure the maximum excursion.
- A value <16mm indicates right ventricular systolic dysfunction.

Although a simple, reproducible measure it relies on the assumption that longitudinal motion is a surrogate for right ventricular systolic function as a whole.

Peak systolic velocity of right ventricular basal free wall TDI (Fig. 4.45)

Similar to TAPSE this measure assesses movement of the right ventricular free wall. However, instead of looking at the distance the tricuspid annulus moves it uses tissue Doppler imaging to measure how quickly the annulus moves.

- Obtain an apical 4-chamber view.
- Place the pulse wave TDI cursor either on the lateral edge of the tricuspid annulus or basal segment of the right ventricular free wall close to the annulus (normally well seen with transthoracic echo).
- Obtain a tissue Doppler trace and measure the maximal systolic velocity of the basal right ventricular free wall. This is referred to as S'.
- S' velocity <10cm/s reflects right ventricular systolic dysfunction.

Ejection fraction and fractional area change (FAC)

Right ventricular ejection fraction is difficult to measure on 2D because of complex geometry but, if available, 3D volume acquisitions can be post-processed using dedicated software to calculate volumes over the cardiac cycle and derive an ejection fraction.

On 2D imaging fractional area change can be assessed from an apical 4-chamber view (Fig. 4.47). To perform this measure

- Obtain a clear apical 4-chamber view.
- Identify the end-diastolic frame (largest ventricle). Trace around the endocardial border being careful to exclude right ventricular trabeculae and obtain an area.
- Identify the end-systolic frame and repeat the process to obtain the end-systolic area.
- The difference between the 2 measures can be reported as a percentage relative to the end-diastolic area.
- A 2D fractional area change of <35% indicates right ventricular systolic dysfunction.

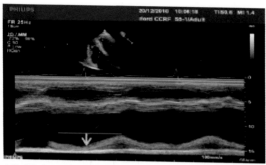

Fig. 4.46 Calculation of TAPSE: M-mode cursor is aligned with the tricuspid valve annulus in the 4 chamber view and the systolic excursion measured (yellow arrow).

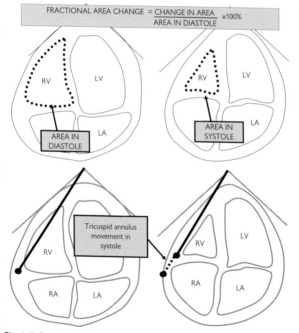

Fig. 4.47 Right ventricle function assessed by fractional area change or (more commonly) movement of tricuspid annulus.

Right ventricular overload

Identifying volume or pressure overload in the right ventricle can aid clinical assessment of right heart function. Although often considered together they usually represent 2 different initial pathologies. Right *volume overload* suggests a left-to-right shunt or right-sided valvular regurgitation. *Pressure overload* suggests pulmonary hypertension or pulmonary stenosis. *Pressure overload* can develop from *volume overload*, and occasionally vice versa, in which cases features of both will be present.

Assessment

The key points to look at when evaluating the 2 situations are:
- What happens to right ventricle size and thickness (📖 pp.264–71)?
  - *Volume overload* leads to increased cavity size and *pressure overload* leads to increased wall thickness. However, one can lead to the other and the two findings will coexist.
- How does the interventricular septum behave during the cardiac cycle?
  - Simply, *volume overload* is related to a flattened septum in *diastole* whereas *pressure overload* is associated with a flattened septum in both *diastole* and *systole*.

Assess *right ventricular systolic pressure* (📖 p.162) to help support your impression of right ventricle pressure or volume overload.

Volume overload (Fig. 4.48)

- Obtain a clear parasternal short axis (mid papillary level) view.
- *Ventricle size and wall thickness*: in volume overload the right ventricle should be *dilated* (the same size or bigger than the left ventricle) so comment on size. In chronic overload the right ventricle may start to hypertrophy but this will be *eccentric* as there will still be dilatation.
- *Septum*: the septum will flatten in *diastole* due to the large right ventricular volume and create a D-shaped ventricle (as volume overload worsens it will start to bow into the left ventricle). But then in *systole* the left ventricle reverts to a circular shape. This creates abnormal septal motion towards the left ventricle in diastole and towards the right ventricle in systole.

Pressure overload

- Use the same parasternal short axis (mid papillary level) view.
- *Ventricle size and wall thickness*: in chronic pressure overload the right ventricle free wall thickens (normally half left ventricle thickness) but the cavity will remain the same until the right ventricle starts to fail.
- *Septum*: as pressure increases the septum will flatten out towards the left ventricle through both *diastole* and *systole*. With chronic pressure overload and increase in wall thickness the right ventricle will start to behave more like a left ventricle, the septum will bow into the left ventricle and contract towards the right ventricle during systole. This also creates *paradoxical septal motion* (but for a different reason from volume overload).

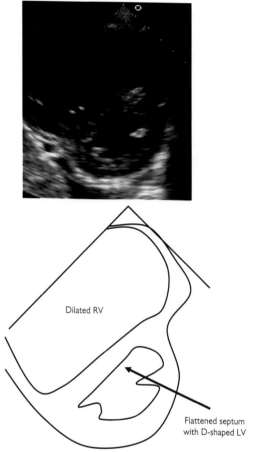

Fig. 4.48 Example of right ventricle volume overload in a parasternal short axis view. Note dilated right ventricle and flattened septum in diastole. See 🖥 Video 4.18.

Left atrium

Normal anatomy
The left atrium receives blood from the 4 pulmonary veins. It acts as a reservoir and as a conduit to transport blood to the left ventricle. It has contractile function and atrial systole contributes approximately 25% of left ventricle filling. Morphologically the atrium can be considered as having a body and an appendage. The common anatomical variations related to the atrium are those associated with the atrial septum, such as aneurysm, patent foramen ovale, atrial septal defect, or lipomatous hypertrophy. Rare anatomic variants can occur within the atrium such as cor triatum, in which the left atrium is separated into a superior and an inferior chamber.

Normal findings
Views
- The key views for the left atrium are: parasternal long axis, and apical 4- and 2-chamber (Fig. 4.49). The apical views are the most useful to assess left atrial volume and left atrial haemodynamics.
- The parasternal short axis (aortic valve level) includes the left atrium and can be useful to look at the septum. The subcostal view aligns the left and right atrium perpendicular to the probe so can be useful for Doppler assessment of the septum.

Findings
- Parasternal long axis: the left atrium lies below the aortic root and the view is used for simple linear measures of left atrial size.
- Parasternal short axis (aortic valve level): the left atrium lies below the aortic valve. The interatrial septum is seen on the left and the left atrial appendage can occasionally be seen on the right.
- Apical 4- and 2-chamber: the left atrium lies at the bottom of the images and the views allow assessment of left atrial volume. The septum can also be studied. However, it lies vertically in the image and it is difficult to identify defects or do Doppler measures. Pulmonary veins are seen at the back of the atrium in the apical 4-chamber (particularly the right upper vein that lies by the septum). In the apical 2-chamber the left atrial appendage can sometimes be seen pointing out to the right. Generally, the left atrial appendage is only rarely visualized by transthoracic imaging.
- Subcostal view: the septum lies horizontal in the image and this is the best view to look for septal defects with colour flow and Doppler.

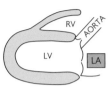

Parasternal long axis

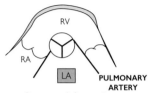

Parasternal short axis

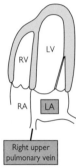

Apical four chamber

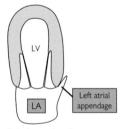

Apical two chamber

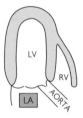

Apical three chamber

Fig. 4.49 Key views to assess left atrium.

Left atrial size

Left atrial enlargement is of clinical importance as it is associated with adverse cardiovascular outcome from a range of pathologies including myocardial infarction, stroke, dilated cardiomyopathy, and diastolic left ventricular failure with increased filling pressure. Atrial enlargement is also associated with atrial fibrillation.

Assessment

Preferred assessment is with volumes measured in apical views. Historically linear measures are quoted in parasternal views. This is the anteroposterior diameter. If the atrium has enlarged along the long axis of the heart this may be missed with single anteroposterior linear measures.

Volumetric measures

Volume measures use the same principles and equations as for left ventricle volume assessment (📖 p.196). The left atrium can be modelled with the area–length formula, Simpson's method (that cuts the atrium into a series of disks and adds up the volumes of each disk), and the ellipsoid method. All calculations are usually done automatically by the machine software but require measurement of atrial length and diameters or planimetry of cross-sectional area. If measures are done in the 4-chamber view it is assumed that the atrium is spherical. Use of both 4- and 2-chamber views allow 3D assessment.

- Obtain a clear apical 4-chamber view with enough depth to include the whole of the left atrium.
- Record a loop and scroll through to identify end-systole.
- Planimeter around left atrium excluding the junction of the pulmonary veins and left atrial appendage (if visible). Record the area.
- Measure the length from back of the left atrium to the midpoint of a line across the mitral annulus (Fig. 4.51).
- Repeat the process in the apical 2-chamber view.
- Use the shorter of the 2 lengths as the measure of atrial length.
- The machine will calculate volumes by *Simpson's* method.
- The *area length formula* for left atrial volume is calculated as:

$$\frac{8 \times \text{area in 4-chamber} \times \text{area in 2-chamber}}{3 \times \pi \times \text{atrial length}}$$

- The *ellipsoid formula* is:

$$\frac{4\pi \times (\text{length}/2) \times (\text{anteroposterior diameter}/2) \times (\text{apical view diameter}/2)}{3}$$

Linear measures

- In a parasternal long axis view, record a 2D loop and identify end-systole. Measure perpendicularly across the atrium from edge-to-edge.
- Alternatively, drop the M-mode cursor across the atrium at the level of the aortic valve tips, perpendicular to the walls. Measure left atrial size at end-systole (maximal size) (Fig 4.50).

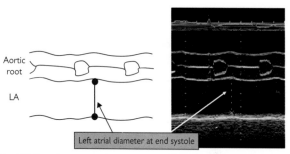

Fig. 4.50 M-mode measures of anteroposterior left atrial size in parasternal long axis view.

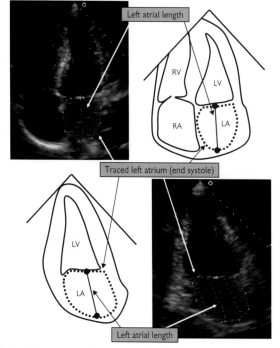

Fig. 4.51 Area tracing of left atrium in apical views to provide a more accurate assessment of left atrial size.

Left atrial function

Indices of left atrial function, that incorporate left atrial ejection fraction corrected for cardiac output and body surface area have been reported in the literature, but are not in clinical use.

Indirect measures of atrial function include the presence of P waves on the ECG, a transmitral A wave on pulse wave Doppler (the best way to demonstrate normal atrial contraction) and the presence of an atrial reversal wave on PW Doppler of the pulmonary vein. The presence of a P-wave on ECG but absent A-wave on mitral inflow suggests atrial dysfunction. This can occur, for example, early after cardioversion from atrial fibrillation.

Left and right atria: normal ranges (Table 4.8)

Table 4.8 Parameters to assess left and right atria

	WOMEN			
	NORMAL	MILD	MODERATE	SEVERE
Atrial dimension				
LA diameter, cm	2.7–3.8	3.9–4.2	4.3–4.6	>4.6
LA diameter, BSA, cm/m²	1.5–2.3	2.4–2.6	2.7–2.9	>2.9
RA minor axis, cm	2.9–4.5	4.6–4.9	5.0–5.4	>5.4
RA minor axis/BSA, cm/m²	1.7–2.5	2.6–2.8	2.9–3.1	>3.1
Atrial area				
LA area, cm²	<20	20–30	31–40	>40
Atrial volume				
LA volume, mL	22–52	53–62	63–72	>72
LA volume/BSA, mL/m²	**<29**	**29–33**	**34–39**	**>39**
	MEN			
	NORMAL	MILD	MODERATE	SEVERE
Atrial dimension				
LA diameter, cm	3.0–4.0	4.1–4.6	4.7–5.2	>5.2
LA diameter, BSA, cm/m²	1.5–2.3	2.4–2.6	2.7–2.9	>2.9
RA minor axis, cm	2.9–4.5	4.6–4.9	5.0–5.4	>5.4
RA minor axis/BSA, cm/m²	1.7–2.5	2.6–2.8	2.9–3.1	>3.1
Atrial area				
LA area, cm²	<20	20–30	31–40	>40
Atrial volume				
LA volume, mL	18–58	59–68	69–78	>78
LA volume/BSA, mL/m²	**<29**	**29–33**	**34–39**	**>39**

BSA, Body surface area.
Bold rows identify best validated measures.

Right atrium

The right atrium acts as reservoir for blood from the coronary sinus, and inferior and superior vena cava. It has some unique anatomical features that can be mistaken for pathology. These include the Eustachian valve, which *in utero* directs blood from the inferior vena cava through the foramen ovale but becomes redundant after birth. If it does not regress it is seen attached to the right atrial wall between the inferior vena cava and border of the fossa ovalis. A Chiari network is a remnant from the embryological stage before the Eustachian valve forms and is a thin membrane, typically fenestrated, near the orifice of the inferior vena cava and extending further across the right atrium than the Eustachian valve.

Normal views and findings
- The right atrium can be seen in a modified right ventricle inflow view and parasternal short axis view (aortic valve level) (Fig. 4.52).
- The apical 4-chamber view is useful for volume measurements and Doppler interrogation of tricuspid valve inflow.
- The subcostal view often provides excellent views of the right atrium and right atrial inflow from the inferior vena cava.

Right atrial size

Techniques to measure right atrial size are borrowed from those for the left atrium but assessment is less clinically relevant. Right atrial size measurements are most often used in assessment of right ventricular systolic pressure (p.264). There is little research or clinical data so normal ranges are fairly simplistic without reference to sex or body size.

Qualitative measures
- The simplest assessment is to compare the left and right atria in an apical 4-chamber view (Fig. 4.53). If the right atrium appears larger than the left it is dilated.

Quantitative measures
- *Minor axis* is a simple linear measure. On an apical 4-chamber view measure across the middle of the atrium from lateral wall to septum. Ranges are in Table 4.8.
- Area can be reported. Trace around the right atrium joining the lateral and septal sides of the tricuspid annulus with a straight line.
- A volume can be calculated using the area length equation (p.196) with measures from an apical 4-chamber view. Right atrial length is required and can be measured from the back of the atrium to the middle of the annulus.

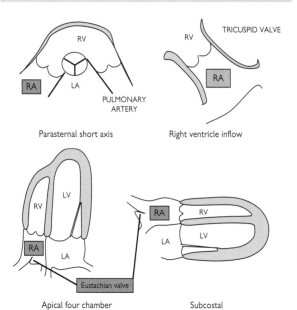

Fig. 4.52 Key views to assess right atrium.

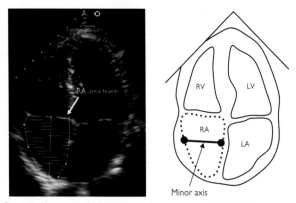

Fig. 4.53 Assessment of right atrial size from area measures in apical views.

Interatrial septum

Normal anatomy

The atrial septum divides the left and right atrium. Embryologically it develops as two distinct sheets, the *primum* and *secundum* septum. *In utero* the septum, specifically the foramen ovale, acts as a portal for blood to pass from the inferior vena cava, directed by the Eustachian valve, to the left side of the heart, bypassing the lungs. After birth the foramen closes. In around 80% of people it seals but remains evident as a depression in the septum called the *fossa ovalis*. In 20% it remains as a potential communication between right and left heart.

Normal findings

Views

The atrial septum is best assessed in a subcostal view (Fig. 4.54). This is the only view that has the septum perpendicular to the probe and therefore aligns the septum for Doppler or colour flow assessment. The atrium can also be assessed in the parasternal short axis (aortic valve level) and apical 4-chamber view. Agitated saline contrast can be used to investigate the possibility of a *patent foramen ovale*.

Findings

- Parasternal short axis (aortic valve level): the septum lies in the far field extending from the aortic ring (usually at the bottom left) with the left atrium on the right and right atrium on the left.
- Apical 4-chamber: the septum can be seen lying between the atria in the far field. Because it is in line with the probe there may be areas of ultrasound dropout that can be confused for defects. Colour flow mapping in this view can be tried.
- Subcostal view: the right atrium lies nearest the probe and the septum lies across the screen. This view can be used for colour flow mapping and Doppler alignment through the septum.

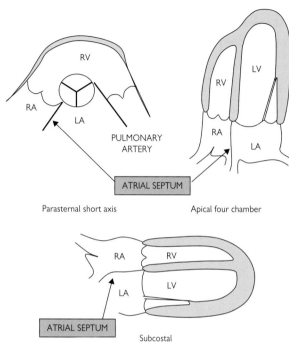

Parasternal short axis

Apical four chamber

Subcostal

Fig. 4.54 Key views to assess the atrial septum.

Atrial septal defects

Atrial septal defects are the commonest congenital heart defect. Although they can occur on their own they are frequently associated with other defects and a full echocardiographic assessment should be performed. They can also be iatrogenic (e.g. after cardiac surgery and transseptal puncture) or accidental (e.g. after pacing). There are 4 types of congenital defect:
- Secundum atrial septal defect (65%)—fossa ovalis/central septum.
- Primum atrial septal defect (15%)—more muscular septum by valves.
- Sinus venosus defect (10%)—near the superior vena cava/posterior and superior septum.
- Coronary sinus defects are much rarer.

Assessment

Initial assessment should be with 2D imaging, followed by colour flow mapping to study direction of flow (Fig. 4.55) and then Doppler to quantify the size of the shunt. Where suspicion of a defect remains high, a contrast study can be performed with Valsalva to identify a left-to-right shunt (📖 p.572). Full assessment may require a transoesophageal study (see Chapters 5 and 7).

2D and colour flow mapping

Study the septum in all the standard views and look for gaps in the septum. To avoid overcalling septal dropout the defect should be apparent in different planes. There may be indirect evidence of a problem that prompts more careful study, in particular: right atrial and right ventricular enlargement without other cause; an abnormally directed colour flow jet in the right atrium on colour flow mapping; abnormal septal motion or an aneurysmal septum. Comment on:
- The position of the defect and, therefore, likely classification.
- Any associated defects (particularly relevant for primum defects).
- The size of the defect in two directions if possible (this can be done in subcostal views with long axis and sagittal planes through the defect).
- Direction and timing of flow from colour flow mapping. Usually predominantly left to right during systole but with chronic right ventricle overload flow starts to occur right to left.
- RV size and function.
- RV systolic pressure.

Doppler quantification of shunt

The principle of shunt quantification is comparison of right and left ventricle stroke volumes. Their ratio (called Qp/Qs) should be 1 but with shunting to the right the ratio increases and to the left the ratio declines. Accuracy depends on accurate measures of outflow tract diameter.
- Obtain LVOT PW Doppler vti from apical 5-chamber view and diameter from parasternal long axis.

$$Qs = \pi \times (\text{LVOT diameter}/2)^2 \times \text{aortic vti}$$

- Measure RVOT PW Doppler vti and diameter from a parasternal short axis (aortic valve level) view.

$$Qp = \pi \times (\text{RVOT diameter}/2)^2 \times \text{pulmonary vti}$$

- Report the ratio Qp/Qs.

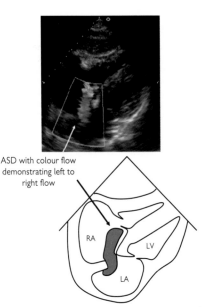

ASD with colour flow
demonstrating left to
right flow

RA   LV

LA

Fig. 4.55 Colour flow mapping of atrial septum in subcostal view. See 📱 Video 4.19, 📱 Video 4.20, 📱 Video 4.21, 📱 Video 4.22.

Primum atrial septal defects and associated defects

Primum defects occur when there is failed development of the primum septum. To make the diagnosis there must be no atrial septal tissue extending from the base of the atrio-ventricular valves.

The atrial septal defect on its own is a *partial atrio-ventricular canal* defect. If extending to involve the ventricular septum and atrio-ventriular valves it forms a *complete atrio-ventricular canal* or *endocardial cushion defect*. The valves often have abnormal atrio-ventricular valve rings and lie in the same plane in apical views (instead of the usual apical displacement of the tricuspid valve i.e. loss of off-setting).

If there is a primum septal defect look for and comment on:
- Inlet ventricular septal defect.
- Cleft mitral valve leaflet—generally involving the anterior mitral valve leaflet at around '12 o'clock' in the parasternal short axis (mitral valve level) view. Invariably associated with regurgitation, often eccentric.
- Mitral and tricuspid regurgitation.
- Partial attachment of the anterior mitral valve leaflet to the ventricular septum—best seen from the parasternal long axis view after forward and backward displacement of the probe.

Patent foramen ovale

If the foramen ovale fails to seal after birth (~20–30% of the population) it remains possible for pressure changes in the left and right atria to reopen the hole. This is of clinical interest because patent foramen ovale are amenable to percutaneous closure and their presence raise the possibility that emboli, e.g. clots or fat, could pass from the right heart to the systemic circulation and cause strokes. Furthermore foramen ovale are associated with decompression illness and, possibly, migraines.

To identify a patent foramen ovale right-to-left flow needs to be identified for a short period during the cardiac cycle (flow throughout the cardiac cycle identifies a septal defect). Sometimes this can be done with colour flow but usually means contrast is needed (see Chapter 9).

Atrial septal aneurysm

Atrial septal aneurysms are an area of excessive mobility of the atrial septum and in 75% of cases are associated with patent foramen ovale. The technical definition is movement of the septum (at least 10mm in width) away from the normal plane of the septum (to left or right) by ≥10mm (Fig. 4.56). Usually the septum will move back and forth as the relative pressure gradient between atria varies, but may be fixed. Comment on presence and look for underlying reasons.

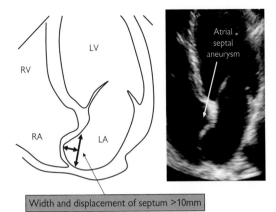

Fig. 4.56 Demonstration of septal aneurysm. At least 10mm wide with at least 10mm movement. See ⚎ Video 4.23.

Ventricular septum

Normal anatomy

The ventricular septum divides the left and right ventricle. The ventricular septum can be divided simply into: (1) a small membranous portion below the aortic valve and forming part of the left ventricular outflow tract, and (2) a muscular septum, spreading inferiorly, anteriorly and apically. These have separate embryological origins.

The muscular septum can be subdivided into 3 areas: the *inlet* septum between the mitral and tricuspid valves; the *trabecular* septum extending to the apex and forming the bulk of the septum on echocardiographic views; and the *outlet* septum close to the aortic and pulmonary valves. These subdivisions are used to classify ventricular septal defects.

Normal findings

Views

Any view that studies the ventricles can also be used to study the ventricular septum. Therefore, parasternal long and short axis views, apical 4-, 5-, and 3-chamber and subcostal are all useful (Fig. 4.57).

Findings

- Parasternal long axis: the membranous septum (or sometimes part of the muscular outlet septum) is seen in the LVOT, with the mid segments of the trabecular (muscular) septum lying to the left.
- Parasternal short axis (aortic valve level): the membranous and outlet septum are seen around the aortic ring.
- Parasternal short axis (midpapillary muscle level): the septum lies between the right and left ventricle and mainly consists of the muscular (trabecular) septum. The muscular inlet septum may be seen at the bottom of the septum.
- Apical 4- and 5-chamber: the trabeculated (muscular) septum can be viewed right up to the apex. In a 4-chamber view the muscular inlet septum is seen between mitral and tricuspid valves. In the 5-chamber view the membranous septum by the aortic valve comes into view.
- Subcostal view: the septum lies perpendicular to the probe and this view provides an opportunity for aligning colour flow mapping and Doppler through the septum.

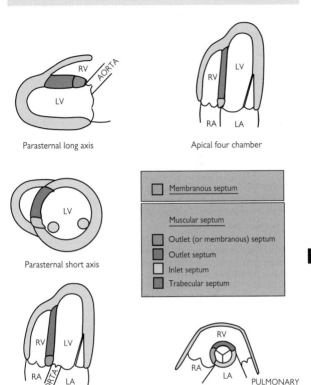

Parasternal long axis

Apical four chamber

Parasternal short axis

Membranous septum

Muscular septum

Outlet (or membranous) septum
Outlet septum
Inlet septum
Trabecular septum

Apical five chamber

Parasternal short axis

Fig. 4.57 Key views to assess the ventricular septum and areas of septum.

Ventricular septal defects

Ventricular septal defects are one of the common congenital heart defects. They can occur anywhere within the septum and are named according to their location—*membranous* or *muscular* (inlet, outlet, or trabeculated) (Fig. 4.58). If they involve both the membranous and muscular septum they are called *peri-membranous*. *Gerbode defects* are a specific type from left ventricle to right atrium. As well as being congenital they can occur due to ischaemia (post infarction, often quite apical in trabecular septum with multiple holes) or be iatrogenic following cardiac surgery or pacing. Membranous (and peri-membranous) are easiest to identify, with muscular defects the most often missed because the defect is small or altered in shape by ventricular contraction.

Assessment

Initial assessment should be with 2D imaging, followed by colour flow. Doppler can quantify the size of any shunt.

2D and colour flow imaging

- Study the septum in all views and look for gaps. To avoid overcalling septal drop-out the defect should be apparent in different planes.
- Colour flow imaging over the septum, particularly in the subcostal and parasternal views, is essential to scan for abnormal colour flow jets appearing in the right ventricle and originating from the septum.
- The septum is curved and can not be seen entirely in one plane. Peri-membranous defects are easiest to see in parasternal long axis and short axis (aortic valve level) views with tilting to scan through the septum. These views also identify outlet defects, which can be differentiated from peri-membranous defects because they lie nearer the pulmonary valve. The inlet and trabecular defects are better seen in apical and subcostal views but may need probe tilting to scan the septum.

Comment on

- Position of the defect and, therefore, likely classification.
- Characteristics of the defect, e.g. multiple small defects.
- Size of the defect (in 2 directions if possible, e.g. subcostal views with long axis and sagittal planes through the defect). Measure size from 2D images or colour flow jet.
- Direction and timing of flow from colour flow mapping. With large chronic defects right ventricular pressure will increase and the left-to-right flow will reduce. Colour flow may be less evident.
- If possible, use PW or CW Doppler aligned across the defect to measure the pressure gradient between ventricles using the Bernouli equation ($= 4 \times$ velocity^2). Right ventricular pressure can be measured from the pressure gradient. If the aortic valve is normal then systolic blood pressure will equal left ventricular systolic pressure. Right ventricular systolic pressure = systolic blood pressure—gradient across the defect.
- Left and right ventricle size and function, as well as evidence of right ventricle pressure or volume overload (📖 p.276).
- Associated problems, e.g. aortic valve dysfunction and regurgitation.

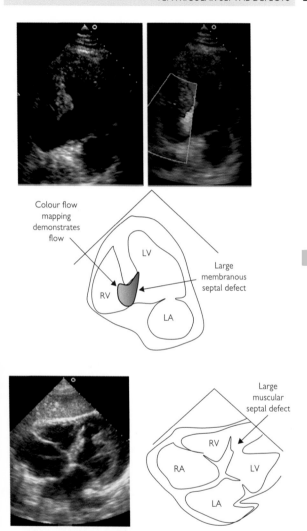

Fig. 4.58 Examples of ventricular septal defects. The top figure shows a large congenital peri-membranous defect in an apical view. The lower figure demonstrates a trabecular muscular defect secondary to ischaemia seen in a subcostal view. See 📹 Video 4.24, 📹 Video 4.25, 📹 Video 4.26, 📹 Video 4.27.

Pericardium

Normal anatomy

The pericardium surrounds the heart. An outer, supportive, *fibrous pericardium* blends superiorly into the aorta and pulmonary arteries and inferiorly attaches by ligaments to the diaphragm, sternum and vertebrae. On the inside of the fibrous layer and the outer surface of the heart are two *serous membranes* which allow the heart to move. There are two irregular holes through the membranes; one around the aorta and pulmonary arteries, and the other around the pulmonary veins and vena cavae. The membranes join around the edges of the holes to create an enclosed, 'deflated' sac which can fill with fluid. Because they wrap round the blood vessels two pockets (or sinuses) are created; the *transverse sinus* between aorta and pulmonary artery, and the *oblique sinus* between the pulmonary veins on the back of the left atrium. These are important because localized collections can form in the pockets.

Normal findings

Views
- Part of the pericardium can be seen in all views and should be studied in all scan planes—only part of the pericardium may be affected in disease or there may be a localized collection.
- The best views are: parasternal long and short axis, apical 4-chamber, and subcostal (Fig. 4.59).

Pericardium
- The *pericardial surfaces* are difficult to see because they adhere to surrounding structures but may appear as a thin, slightly brighter line around the heart.
- Measures of pericardial thickness do not correlate well with pathology specimens but the pericardium is normally 1–2mm thick. CT or magnetic resonance imaging should be used to measure thickness.

Pericardial space
- The *pericardial space* is seen as a black line around the heart. It is normal to have a few millimetres of fluid.

Distinguishing pericardial from pleural fluid

In the parasternal long axis view use the descending aorta as a landmark. The pericardial sac tucks in between the aorta and left atrium, so pericardial fluid will extend up to the gap and lie in front of the aorta. Pleural fluid will track behind the aorta and over the left atrium.

If both pericardial and pleural fluid are suspected look for the pericardium lying as a continuous dividing line within the fluid in an apical view.

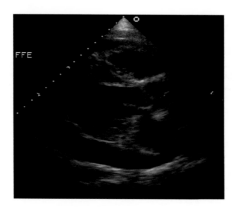

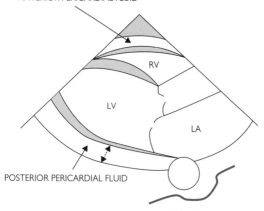

ANTERIOR PERICARDIAL FLUID

RV

LV

LA

POSTERIOR PERICARDIAL FLUID

PLEURAL FLUID WOULD LIE
BEHIND AORTA

Fig. 4.59 Parasternal long axis view showing heart lying in global pericardial effusion. Measure depth on 2D (double ended arrow) or M-mode and report measurement site. See 📹 Video 4.28 and 📹 Video 4.29.

Pericardial effusion

Amount of pericardial fluid
- Measure fluid thickness using 2D or M-mode in several places and views. Report the depth and where the measurement was made.
- For global effusions, grade as *mild*, *moderate*, or *large* based on depth (depth also approximates to volume of fluid).
  - <0.5cm   Minimal   50–100mL
  - 0.5–1cm   Mild   100–250mL
  - 1–2cm   Moderate   250–500mL
  - >2cm   Large   >500mL
- More accurate volume measures can be made with planimetry from traced pericardial and heart borders in apical views. It is possible to produce even more accurate measures with 3D echocardiography, although there is not usually any clinical indication.

Thickness does not relate to clinical severity

Rapid accumulation of a small quantity can have as severe a haemodynamic effect as slow accumulation of a large quantity. Look for features of tamponade.

Appearance of pericardial space
- *Fluid* is the black echolucent area and will be serous, blood, or pus. It is difficult to differentiate with echocardiography.
- *Strands* (fibrin) can occur in any condition which causes inflammation (infection, haemorrhage, or uraemia) (Fig. 4.60).
- *Masses* are more unusual and could be haematoma, tumour, cyst, or related to infection, e.g. fungus. Comment on size, shape, appearance, movement, attachments to surfaces, e.g. pericardium, ventricle. Haematoma is usually the same echocardiographic density as myocardium—so may be difficult to see—but suggests a haemopericardium.

Localization Look at effusion in all views and comment whether global (most common) or localized. Specify where the effusion is localized.

Problems with localized effusions

- Suspect localized effusions after cardiac surgery (blood) or infections (loculation). Localized effusions may only be evident because of restricted pulmonary vein flow (oblique sinus) or unusual compression of a cardiac chamber. Consider transoesophageal echocardiography in patients with haemodynamic problems after cardiac surgery to look for localized effusions.
- Apparent posterior localization may be because a small effusion has shifted posteriorly due to gravity in a supine patient.
- A localized anterior space in parasternal views may actually be mediastinal (e.g. fat, fibrosis, thymus).

Evidence of cardiac tamponade see 📖 p.300.

Best site for pericardiocentesis

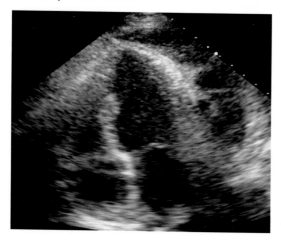

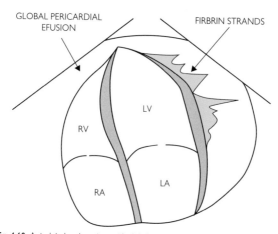

Fig. 4.60 Apical 4-chamber view with global pericardial effusion and fibrin strands. Comment on strands and attachment to ventricle.

Cardiac tamponade

Cardiac tamponade is a clinical diagnosis based on tachycardia (>100bpm), hypotension (<100mmHg systolic), pulsus paradoxus (>10mmHg drop in blood pressure on inspiration), raised JVP with prominent x descent. Echocardiography provides supporting evidence.

2D findings suggestive of tamponade (Fig. 4.61)

As intrapericardial pressure rises and begins to exceed right heart pressure, parts of the cardiac chambers collapse during the cardiac cycle. Clinical signs usually appear before the left heart is affected.

- Right atrium appears to collapse faster than usual in atrial systole.
- Parts of right ventricle start to collapse during ventricular diastole. First the right ventricular outflow during early diastole (at lowest pressure) then as intrapericardial pressure increases collapse extends to involve whole of right ventricle and whole of diastole.
- Combination of rapid atrial collapse in atrial systole followed by rapid ventricular collapse in ventricular diastole creates the appearance of a 'swinging right atrium and ventricle'.

Doppler findings suggestive of tamponade

Doppler findings in tamponade are the echocardiographic demonstration of the exaggerated variation in right and left ventricle inflow during respiration—clinically demonstrated as pulsus paradoxus.

- In an apical 4-chamber view place PW Doppler at tricuspid valve inflow. Switch on physiological respiration trace (if available) and slow sweep speed to 25cm/s.
- Acquire a tracing and measure maximum and minimum E-wave velocities (these correspond with respiration: maximum in inspiration).
- Do the same at the mitral valve (E-wave maximum in expiration).
- Normal variation is <15% at mitral valve and <25% at tricuspid valve. Greater than this supports tamponade but clinical signs are usually associated with ~40% variation at the mitral valve.

Exaggerated flow changes through the heart during respiration can also be demonstrated in the left and right ventricle outflow tracts (increased flow in inspiration on the right and in expiration on the left).

- Use PW Doppler in RVOT in parasternal short axis. Record vti and peak velocity in inspiration and expiration.
- Do the same at the LVOT in apical 5-chamber.
- Normally vti and peak velocity vary <10% during respiration.

Problems with assessment of tamponade

2D and Doppler measures are only accurate with 'normal' relations between intrapericardial, intrathoracic, and intraventricular pressures. Increased ventricular 'stiffness' (ventricular hypertrophy, intraventricular haematoma) or increased right ventricular pressure (pulmonary hypertension) makes the ventricle less likely to collapse. Low volume states mean the change in ventricular inflow on Doppler is less pronounced. Doppler indices are not validated in ventilated patients.

Pulsus paradoxus

There is normally a swing of 5mmH$_2$O in intrathoracic pressure with respiration. Inspiration leads to an increase in blood flow into the lungs and therefore an increase in flow into the right heart and reduced flow into the left heart. Expiration forces blood out of the lungs and increases flow into the left heart and reduces flow into the right heart. This accounts for the normal variation in blood pressure ('left-sided pressures') with respiration. Increased pericardial fluid increases intrapericardial pressure. Left and right ventricular filling is impaired and this filling is exacerbated on the left on inspiration leading to an exaggerated drop in blood pressure on inspiration.

Changes in 2D and Doppler with increasing tamponade

1. Tricuspid valve inflow pattern.
2. Mitral valve inflow pattern.
3. Abnormal right atrial collapse in atrial systole.
4. Right ventricular outflow collapse in ventricular diastole.
5. Left ventricular outflow collapse in ventricular diastole.

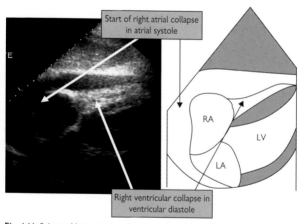

Start of right atrial collapse in atrial systole

Right ventricular collapse in ventricular diastole

RA

LV

LA

Fig. 4.61 Subcostal long axis view showing early atrial systolic collapse and ventricular diastolic collapse.

Constrictive pericarditis

Constrictive pericarditis is uncommon and often has vague signs and symptoms with a long history. It can be due to chronic inflammation as a result of infection (classically tuberculosis), cardiothoracic surgery, radiation, or connective tissue disease. It can be transient with pericardial inflammation. Diagnosis is clinical. Echocardiography can be supportive and differentiate from restrictive cardiomyopathy. Magnetic resonance imaging or CT are also usually required to assess the pericardium.

2D findings suggestive of constriction

- Look for the pericardium: may appear normal thickness (1–2mm) or thickened (up to 10mm) (measurements are inaccurate so use other modalities for actual measures). May appear bright or there may be shadowing from calcium (a marker of chronic inflammation).
- Assess the left ventricle: usually normal systolic function—consider other causes if not. Assess septal motion in parasternal views with 2D and M-mode. Classically, septum appears to 'flutter' as left and right ventricles fill during diastole. Probably due to waves of competitive filling of the 2 ventricles. Seen as early diastolic notching on M-mode, or paradoxical and then normal motion on 2D.

Differentiation from restrictive cardiomyopathy (Table 4.9)

Table 4.9 Clinical features of constrictive pericarditis and restrictive cardiomyopathy are similar. Echocardiography is useful to differentiate

	Restrictive cardiomyopathy	Constrictive pericarditis
Similarities between conditions:		
E/A ratio	Increased	Increased
Deceleration time	Decreased	Decreased
Differences between conditions:		
LV function	May be abnormal	Usually normal
Pericardium	Normal	May be bright or thick
Septal motion	Usually normal	May be abnormal
Atria	Biatrial enlargement	Usually normal size
Mitral annulus velocity	Decreased	Normal
Ventricular inflow	Normal variation	Increased variation on respiration

Doppler findings suggestive of constriction

- Assess mitral and tricuspid inflow during respiration just as for tamponade (Fig. 4.62). Constrictive pericarditis causes the same changes as tamponade (>25% variation at tricuspid and >15% at mitral). As the ventricles are supported by 'stiff' pericardium no ventricular collapse.
- Look for features of diastolic dysfunction (□ p.246). Exaggerated E/A ratio on mitral inflow and shortened deceleration time (time from peak to end of E-wave: normal >160ms).
- Use tissue Doppler (if available). In apical 4-chamber place cursor on lateral mitral annulus. In constrictive pericarditis myocardial function is normal and peak mitral annulus velocity is therefore normal (>10mm/s). If reduced, consider restrictive cardiomyopathy (Fig. 4.63).

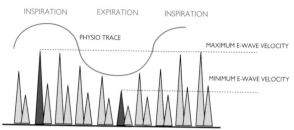

Fig. 4.62 Diagram representing pulsed wave Doppler trace at tricuspid valve. There is significant variation in tricuspid valve inflow (>25%) consistent with cardiac tamponade or constrictive pericarditis. The same recording can be done at mitral valve but maximum E-wave velocity will be in expiration and normal variation is <15%.

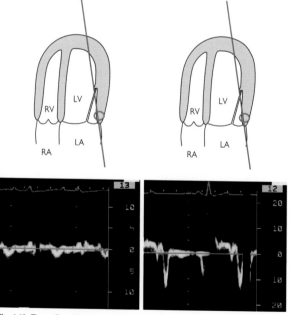

Fig. 4.63 Tissue Doppler imaging of lateral mitral annulus showing reduced movement in restrictive cardiomyopathy (left) compared to normal myocardial function (right). Normal motion is >10cm/s.

Congenital pericardial disease

Congenital absence of pericardium is rare. Usually suspected in 2D because of an obvious gap or herniation of part of the heart (often left or right atrial appendage or parts of ventricle). The heart may be abnormally positioned with right atrial or ventricular dilatation and paradoxical septal motion. Record where the pericardium is missing and any functional effects of herniation.

Congenital pericardial cysts are more common. Usually benign. Comment on size, mobility, position, attachment, appearance (fluid, masses).

Pericardial tumours

Primary cardiac tumours or *metastatic tumours* can involve the pericardium. Comment on any masses, reporting the position, size, appearance, attachments, and functional effects on cardiac function.

Acute pericarditis

There are no echocardiographic features diagnostic of acute pericarditis. Echocardiography should be used in suspected pericarditis to look for:
• Complications (e.g. effusions).
• Left ventricular function (e.g. abnormal function may suggest myocarditis).
• Underlying causes (e.g. tumour or regional wall motion abnormalities suggestive of myocardial infarction).
• Other causes for clinical signs (e.g. endocarditis, pericardial effusion).

Pericardiocentesis

Echocardiography is very useful during pericardiocentesis. Pericardio-centesis is usually done from subcostal or apical positions so assess pericardial fluid in both views (Fig. 4.64).

Before the procedure record:
• Depth of fluid in each position.
• Depth from skin to the outer boundary of fluid (a guide as to how far to introduce the needle).

During the procedure:
• Angle of the echo probe to achieve images can be a guide to the angle to be used for the needle.
• The needle can sometimes be seen advancing into pericardial space.
• If unclear whether needle is in pericardial space, inject agitated saline contrast down needle. Contrast should be seen clearly filling the pericardial space if needle is correctly positioned . . . or filling another cardiac chamber if not!

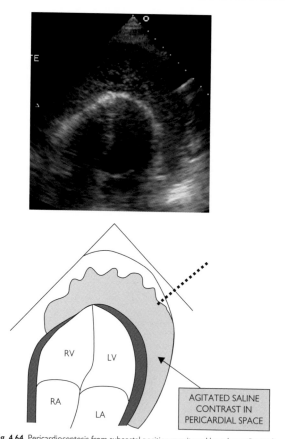

Fig. 4.64 Pericardiocentesis from subcostal position monitored by echocardiography from apex. Agitated saline contrast has been injected down the pericardiocentesis needle and is seen circulating in the pericardial space. This confirms the correct location of the needle.

Aorta

Normal anatomy

The aorta is the main conductance artery of the body, carrying blood from the heart to all major branch vessels. It has a functional role, distending during systole and recoiling in diastole, to propel blood. The aortic wall has 3 layers: tunica intima, a thin inner layer, lined by endothelium; tunica media, a thicker middle layer of elastic tissue for tensile strength and elasticity; tunica adventitia, a thin outer layer, predominantly collagen, housing the vasa vasorum and lymphatics.

There are 4 major sections: (1) ascending aorta from aortic valve annulus including sinuses of Valsalva, sinotubular junction (the narrowest point) and up to right brachiocephalic artery; (2) aortic arch from brachiocephalic to aortic isthmus (just distal to left subclavian artery); (3) descending aorta from isthmus to diaphragm; (4) abdominal aorta from diaphragm to aortic bifurcation and origin of iliac arteries.

Normal findings

Views

Parts of the aorta can be seen in all windows (Fig. 4.65). Full evaluation requires a combination of views and additional, non-standard transducer positions.

Proximal ascending aorta

- Proximal ascending aorta is best seen in the parasternal long axis view. Additional views include, particularly if dilated, the right parasternal views or left parasternal views from higher intercostal spaces for ascending aorta, (particularly with patient in extreme left lateral position to bring aorta more anterior). Doppler interrogation is limited to qualitative assessment of flow and aortic regurgitation severity.
- Apical views: the ascending aorta can also be visualized in apical 5- and 3-chamber views. 2D image quality is limited at this depth but orientation is optimal for Doppler to assess aortic regurgitation.

Aortic arch

- Suprasternal views (and supraclavicular views) allow assessment of aortic arch and brachiocephalic vessels. Both transverse and longitudinal views are possible but the latter is most useful to identify head and neck vessels. Descending aorta is only partially in plane and, artefactually, appears to taper. Descending aorta blood flow can be used to assess aortic regurgitation severity and aortic coarctation.

Descending thoracic aorta

- Descending thoracic aorta is seen in cross-section posterior to the left atrium in the parasternal views. The proximal segment of descending aorta is seen in the suprasternal view. Additional views of the longitudinal section of the descending thoracic aorta can normally be visualized from an apical 2-chamber view with lateral angulation and clockwise rotation of probe. The distal thoracic aorta and proximal abdominal aorta can be visualized from the subcostal view.

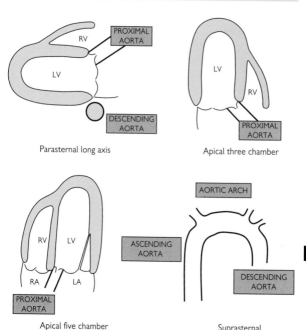

Parasternal long axis

Apical three chamber

Apical five chamber

Suprasternal

Fig. 4.65 Key views to assess the aorta.

The pathological significance of the aortic isthmus

The isthmus is the point where the relatively mobile ascending aorta and arch become fixed to the thorax and thus the aorta is vulnerable to trauma at this point. Coarctations also commonly develop here. The isthmus is just distal to the left subclavian.

Aortic size

The terms *proximal aorta* or *aortic root* refer to the aortic annulus, sinuses of Valsalva, sinotubular junction, and proximal ascending aorta. Measurement of the aortic root is of crucial importance in the diagnosis of Marfan syndrome, and in the serial monitoring of patients with, or at risk of, progressive dilation of the ascending aorta. While a single measurement of the proximal aorta may suffice in the normal examination, when monitoring aortic root dilatation a minimum of 4 measurements should be routinely made and recorded from the parasternal long axis view.

Different methods for assessing aortic root dilation are quoted in the literature (e.g. systolic versus diastolic measurement; inner to inner or leading edge to leading edge dimensions). Normative data in adults were calculated using leading edge methodology in diastole. However, to try and achieve consistency with both other chamber measurements and other imaging methods it is now more common to measure inner edge to inner edge at the widest diameter, i.e. in systole. Differences are likely to be small but it is important that the method used is stated and consistent methodology used in follow-up.

Assessment (Fig. 4.66)

- Make measurements from a parasternal long axis view in systole (with valve leaflet tips open to their maximum).
- 2D measurement at the sinuses gives higher values than M-mode measurements and are preferred. Make measurements parallel to aortic annular plane from inner edge to inner edge.
- A complete assessment includes measurement of:
  - Annulus (normal 2.3 ± 0.3cm).
  - Sinus of Valsalva, at aortic leaflet tip level (normal 3.4 ± 0.3cm; <2.1cm/m^2).
  - Sinotubular junction.
  - Proximal ascending aorta (normal 2.6 ± 0.3cm).
- Comment on how the measurements were made and use the appropriate normal values. In a normal study a single aortic diameter may be sufficient. When possible, report size relative to body surface area.
- Where needed, continue the assessment by providing measurements of the arch from suprasternal views, descending aorta from parasternal views and, for completeness, abdominal aorta from subcostal views.
  - Aortic arch.
  - Descending thoracic aorta (normal <1.6 cm/m^2).
  - Abdominal aorta (normal <3 cm; <1.6 cm/m^2).

Serial measurements and identification of dilatation

- In serial measurements the annulus is not prone to dilation. Any significant change should raise suspicion of methodological error and caution over interpreting measurements elsewhere. In effect, the annulus acts as a control for serial studies.
- Measurements at the sinus of Valsalva are the key. They tend to be the site of initial ectasia when the aortic root does dilate in Marfan syndrome. In the normal adult it measures <3.7cm but can vary with body surface area (Fig. 4.67). Normograms that adjust for body surface area maximize sensitivity for the detection of aortic dilation in adults, but for practical purposes the upper normal limit in the adult is 2.1cm/m^2 and anything below this can be reported as normal.

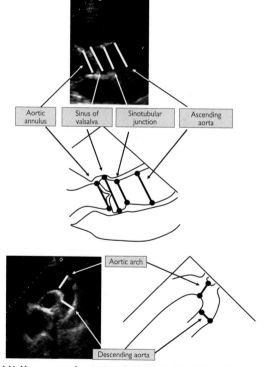

Fig. 4.66 Measurement of aortic size at key locations from parasternal long axis (top) and suprasternal (bottom) views.

Calculating a z-score: Cornell data-based formulae for children and adults in different ranges of age

Z-scores for aortic root size are used extensively in the new Ghent criteria for Marfan syndrome. Therefore it is important to know what they are.

A z-score is a way to take account of expected variability in a measure so that you can assess how abnormal the value you have obtained really is. The z-score represents the proportion of a standard deviation that the value you have measured lies away from the expected mean for that measure, given the level of another factor. For example, the distribution of aortic root size varies with age. Therefore, you can not know if the aortic root size you measure is abnormal unless you know what the normal range is for the age group of patient you are studying. For aortic root size this is further complicated by the fact that aortic root size also varies with body surface area so this also needs to be taken into account in the z-score. The formulae listed here allow you to calculate an 'aortic root size' z-score for different age groups based on what the predicated aortic root size would be for the patient body surface area. To use these formulae you need to know for your patient their: *1) age, 2) body surface area 3) measured aortic root diameter* (originally measured in diastole—leading edge to leading edge; inner edge measurements in systole now recommended). Then, choose the formulae below that suit the age of the patient and calculate their predicted aortic root size using the patient's body surface area. Then, calculate the z-score using the measured root diameter and the predicted root diameter. This number tells you how many standard deviations the patient lies away from the mean.

Age up to 15:
Mean predicted aortic root (cm) = 1.02 + 0.98 × BSA

Z = (Measured root diameter − predicted aortic root diameter)/0.18

Age 20 to 40:
Mean predicted aortic root (cm) = 0.97 + 1.12 × BSA

Z = (Measured root diameter − predicted aortic root diameter)/0.24

Age >40
Mean predicted aortic root (cm) = 1.92 + 0.74 × BSA

Z = (Measured root diameter − predicted aortic root diameter)/0.37.

Mean predicted aortic root size is based on Dubois formula.

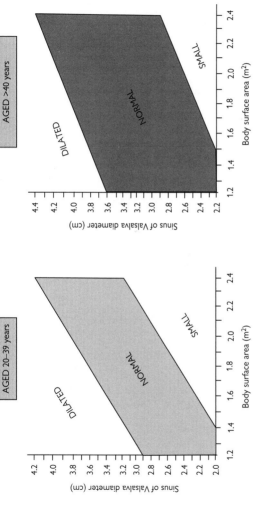

Fig. 4.67 Ranges of normal sinus of Valsalva size according to age.

Aortic dilatation

General (Fig. 4.68)

Dilatation of the aorta is an increase in diameter more than expected for age and body size and is the most commonly identified aortic abnormality. When localized to the sinus of Valsalva the risk of complications is significantly lower than when there is generalized aortic dilatation but still higher than no dilatation! Causes include: degenerative disease (hypertension, atherosclerosis, cystic medical necrosis, post-stenotic); collagen vascular disease (Marfan syndrome, Ehlers–Danlos, Loeys–Dietz, familial aortic aneurysm); inflammatory disorders (rheumatoid, systemic lupus erythematosus, ankylosing spondylitis, Reiter syndrome, syphilis, aortic arteritis); trauma (blunt or penetrating).

Assessment

Measure the degree of dilatation at multiple positions and report where and how the measurements were made.

Differentiation of degenerative dilatation from Marfan

When the aorta dilates due to degenerative disease, the contours of the sinuses of Valsalva and the normal slight narrowing at the sinotubular junction are maintained. In contrast, dilatation of the aorta in Marfan syndrome is characterized by enlargement of the sinuses of Valsalva, resulting in loss of narrowing at the sinotubular junction.

Indications for considering elective aortic root replacement

- Aortic diameter ≥45mm in adults with connective tissue disease, especially if a family history of aortic dissection.
- Aortic diameter ≥50mm in patients with bicuspid aortic valve disease.
- Aortic diameter ≥55mm in adults without connective tissue (atherosclerotic aneurysm).
- Rapid change in the aortic root size: >5mm per year.

If there is an indication for aortic valve replacement, lower thresholds can be used: concomitant root replacement should be considered if aortic diameter ≥40 mm.

There is an increased risk in pregnancy. If the aortic diameter is ≥40 mm, monitoring with echocardiography and clinical examination should be considered monthly. Progressive root dilatation to ≥45 mm should lead to consideration of surgery prior to, or contemporaneous with, delivery of the child. Special precautions would also be required at the time of delivery which should take place under the care of a specialist team managing complex pregnancy with cardiac disease.

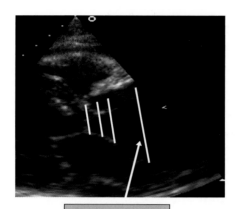

Ascending aorta aneurysm

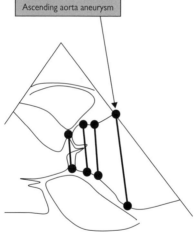

Fig. 4.68 Example of dilatation of the proximal ascending aorta seen in a parasternal long axis view.

Marfan syndrome

Marfan syndrome is an autosomal dominant connective tissue disorder due to mutation in the *Fibrillin 1* gene. It is a multisystem disorder that affects both locomotor and cardiovascular systems, and the eyes. The incidence is approximately 1 in 10,000 births of whom approximately 26% are a spontaneous mutation, i.e. have no family history. Many individuals have some of the skeletal features of Marfan syndrome without the actual condition and the diagnosis is dependent on diagnostic criteria (Ghent criteria).

Assessment

Echocardiography is key for the criteria and should concentrate on aortic root dimensions (Fig. 4.69). To correct for body size, either a Z-score should be calculated using a validated formula, with the Cornell formula the most commonly used, or aortic root dimensions plotted on a validated nomogram against body surface area. An aortic Z-score of ≥2 supports diagnosis of Marfan syndrome. Previous or newly diagnosed aortic root dissection carries the same weight.

The presence of mitral valve prolapse, diagnosed as per standard practice (see 📖 p.128), scores 1 in the systemic score (which has replaced minor criteria) and its presence and severity should therefore also be reported.

2010 Revised Ghent Nosology for Marfan syndrome

Marfan syndrome should be diagnosed if any 1 of these 7 rules is fulfilled:

If no family history of Marfan syndrome:
1. Aortic Z ≥2 and Ectopia lentis
2. Aortic Z ≥2 and *Fibrillin 1* gene mutation
3. Aortic Z ≥2 and Systemic score ≥7
4. Ectopia lentis and *Fibrillin 1* gene mutation with known aortic aneurysm

If positive family history of Marfan syndrome:
5. Ectopia Lentis and confirmed family history
6. Systemic score ≥7 and confirmed family history
7. Aortic Z score ≥2 if over 20 years, ≥3 if below 20 years, and confirmed family history.

For explanation of Z-score see 📖 p.312.

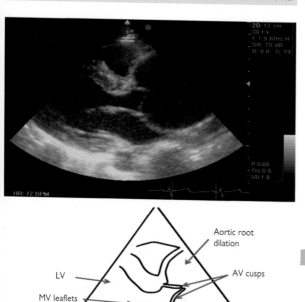

Fig. 4.69 Parasternal long axis view of dilation of the aortic root in a patient with Marfan syndrome. See 📹 Video 4.30.

Aortic dissection

General

Aortic dissection originates from an intimal tear, leading to subintimal haemorrhage which can extend within a false lumen back to the aortic valve or forwards, throughout the aorta. Aortic dissection is life threatening with an early mortality of 1% per hour. Presentation is usually with severe chest pain. The differential includes other causes of chest pain such as acute myocardial infarction or chest wall pain, and aortic intramural haemorrhage or expanding thoracic aneurysm. Risk factors for dissection include: Marfan syndrome, aortic dilatation/aneurysm, hypertension, aortic valve disease—particularly bicuspid valve (risk 5× normal).

The Stanford classification is the simplest and most pragmatic.
- Type A: involvement of the ascending aorta irrespective of involvement elsewhere.
- Type B: limited to the arch and/or descending thoracic aorta.

Assessment

Prompt diagnosis is crucial and transthoracic echocardiography is of value in initial management. Examine for diagnostic features and for secondary complications. A negative transthoracic study does not exclude aortic dissection and where there is a high index of suspicion further imaging with TOE, CT, or magnetic resonance imaging will be required.

Diagnostic features
- Look for the presence or absence of any possible *dissection flap* in *all* aortic views (parasternal, suprasternal, subcostal) (Fig. 4.70). A flap will appear as a linear mobile structure with motion independent of the aortic wall.
- 3D echocardiography can confirm presence of dissection flap—which will appear as sheet-like structure—and extent, helping to exclude or confirm involvement of coronary ostia.
- Look for a *false lumen* using colour flow Doppler placed over the aorta in all aortic views. There will be different patterns of flow in the true and false lumen.

Beam-width artefact and reverberation
- Beam-width artefact and reverberation can mimic a dissection flap.
- M-mode of aortic wall motion and a suspected flap will demonstrate flap motion which is different from aortic wall movement, whereas a reverberation artefact will move with the wall.

Secondary complications
- Measure aortic root size from parasternal views, size of arch and descending aorta from suprasternal views, and size of descending thoracic and abdominal aorta from subcostal views.
- Comment on and quantify aortic regurgitation.

- Comment on pericardial fluid and perform Doppler analysis of transmitral and transtricuspid blood flow to diagnose tamponade. A small acute collection can cause tamponade without obvious pericardial fluid.
- Assess left ventricular systolic function, and comment on any regional wall motion abnormalities which might suggest coronary artery involvement.

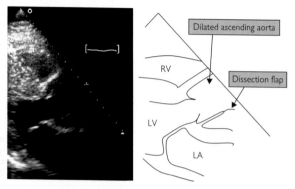

Dilated ascending aorta

RV

Dissection flap

LV

LA

PARASTERNAL LONG AXIS VIEW

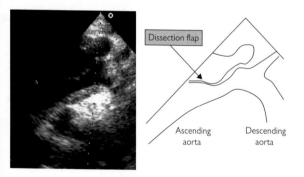

Dissection flap

Ascending aorta   Descending aorta

SUPRASTERNAL VIEW

Fig. 4.70 Examples of aortic dissection flap seen in parasternal long axis and suprasternal views. See 📹 Video 4.31, 📹 Video 4.32, 📹 Video 4.33.

Aortic coarctation

General

Aortic coarctation is a congenital narrowing in the proximal descending thoracic aorta, usually located immediately proximal to the entry site of the *ductus arteriosus*. It may be suspected in a patient with hypertension and a weak femoral pulse, radiofemoral delay or systolic murmur. Aortic coarctation first diagnosed in adulthood is usually asymptomatic as the stenosis is not usually severe and collaterals are present. 50–80% will have a bicuspid aortic valve and other cardiac abnormalities (e.g. subaortic membrane, supravalvular aortic stenosis).

Assessment

Echocardiography is required in diagnosis and follow-up. Aortic coarctation can be relatively complex and further imaging (usually magnetic resonance imaging) is performed if intervention is being considered.

Diagnosis

The suprasternal view is the most useful.

- Identify the brachiocephalic vessels—coarctation usually occurs just distal to the left subclavian with post-stenotic dilatation common.
- Use colour flow mapping of the descending aorta to identify a high-velocity narrowed flow stream with turbulence (even if 2D poor).
- Place CW Doppler through the point of maximum colour flow turbulence to measure a typical systolic velocity gradient. The gradient will typically persist to end diastole ('diastolic tail') (Fig. 4.71).
- CW Doppler tends to overestimate the gradient and better correlation with catheter gradients can be obtained if the proximal velocity is measured with PW Doppler and the modified Bernoulli equation used to calculate flow.
- If coarctation is suspected but difficult to image, CW Doppler using a pencil probe in the suprasternal position will often allow measurement of a gradient in the descending aorta.

Follow-up

All patients with previous repair of coarctation of the aorta should be followed up throughout adult life. Echocardiography should be repeated annually. Where visualization is inadequate alternative imaging such as CT or magnetic resonance imaging may be needed.

- Examine and report the residual gradient.
- Look for abnormalities in the aorta and comment on development of any aneurysm at the site of previous repair.
- Reassess the aortic valve annually: early degenerative disease is common (sometimes in previously unrecognized bicuspid valve).

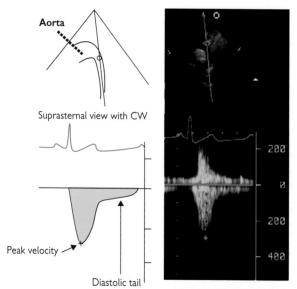

Fig. 4.71 Doppler profile in coarctation of the aorta from a suprasternal view. Note the increased peak velocity and prolonged flow throughout diastole ('diastolic tail').

Sinus of Valsalva aneurysm

Sinus of Valsalva aneurysms can be congenital resulting from incomplete fusion of the distal bulbar septum that divides the aorta and pulmonary arteries. They tend to have a long sac of mobile tissue projecting into adjacent structures, forming a 'wind sock' appearance. Acquired aneurysms, usually due to endocarditis, lead to more symmetrical dilation, with no excess tissue. If rupture occurs, a fistula develops between aorta and adjacent chamber, with left-to-right shunting and clinical features that can vary in severity from acute haemodynamic compromise to a new continuous murmur. 85% affect right coronary sinus and project/rupture into the right ventricle; 10% affect non-coronary sinus and project/rupture into the right atrium; 5% affect left coronary sinus and project/rupture into the left atrium.

Assessment

- Use parasternal long and short axis views to diagnose and measure (Fig. 4.72).
- If rupture suspected, use parasternal short axis view at and above the aortic valve. Colour flow mapping will usually confirm site of communication and continuous flow. If possible the coronary artery should be visualized to exclude coronary artery fistulae.
- CW Doppler will show a high velocity systolic and diastolic signal.
- Comment on the size of the right atrium (which reflects acute right atrial overload) and left atrial and left ventricular size (which will reflect the extent of chronic volume overload).
- 3D echocardiography may be helpful in planning particular surgical or percutaneous approach to repair. Image the aortic valve in parasternal long axis view before acquiring a full 3D volume set.

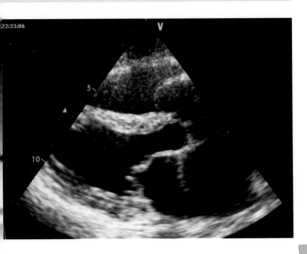

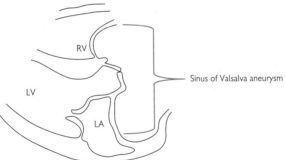

Fig. 4.72 Parasternal long axis left ventricle (LV) showing sinus of Valsalva aneurysm. RV right ventricle, LA left atrium. See 📹 Video 4.34.

Aortic atherosclerosis

General

Atherosclerosis of the aorta can result in dilatation, aneurysm, or dissection and is a risk factor for coexisting coronary artery disease and cerebrovascular disease.

Assessment

Aortic atheroma can be visualized with transthoracic echocardiography (although transoesophageal is more appropriate) in either the proximal ascending aorta or, more commonly, in the descending abdominal aorta.

Atherosclerotic thoracic aortic aneurysm may also be detected by transthoracic imaging, either at the aortic root or behind the left atrium in the descending thoracic aorta (parasternal long axis view). More rarely, descending abdominal aortic aneurysm may be picked up in subcostal views (Fig. 4.73). The extent of the aneurysm cannot usually be accurately quantified, but the extent of dilatation and presence or absence of laminar thrombus can be commented upon. Further imaging will frequently be required.

Modified subcostal view

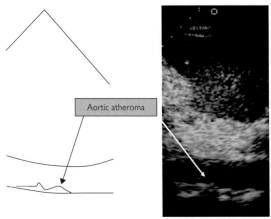

Aortic atheroma

Fig. 4.73 A subcostal view aligned to view the abdominal aorta. Note the thickening of the wall and irregular appearance consistent with an atherosclerotic plaque.

Cardiac tumours

One of the most 'exciting' things to see in echocardiography is a cardiac mass that should not be there. Once seen it is easy to forget about continuing with the systematic collection of information but this is essential in order to understand what effect any mass may be having. Masses will be vegetations, cysts, tumours (benign and malignant), or thrombus (Figs. 4.74 and 4.75).

Primary tumours—benign (80%)

Myxoma

Myxoma is the most common primary tumour (30% of tumours: 74% left atrium, 18% right atrium, 4% left ventricle free wall). 10% are familial so family counselling should be considered if other familial cases.

Appearances and assessment

Globular, finely speckled mass with well-defined edges. May prolapse into left ventricle. Usually attached to interatrial septum (fossa ovalis 90%). Attachment best visualized in apical and subcostal 4-chamber views. Tumour calcification may be seen infrequently. Determine length and diameter of myxoma. Quantify severity of coexisting mitral regurgitation or effective stenosis caused by myxoma.

Myxoma or thrombus?

No specific finding differentiates the two but thrombus is more often irregular, layered, immobile, broad-based (myxoma typically has a stalk) and located near the posterior wall of the left atrium. The left atrium is more likely to be dilated with an abnormal mitral valve.

Papillary fibroelastoma

10% of primary tumours. Found attached most commonly to mitral and aortic valves with small pedicles. Rarely attach to LVOT or papillary muscles.

Appearances and assessment

Small (rarely >1cm in diameter), mobile, pedunculated, echocardiographically-dense mass. May mimic vegetation or Lambl's excrescences. Usually no other valve abnormalities. Comment on size, location, and functional effects.

Other tumours

Lipoma (10%), fibroma (4%), rhabdomyoma (9%—children more common).

Primary tumours—malignant (20%)

Typical tumours are sarcomas, angiosarcomas and rhabdomyosarcomas. Primary lymphomas also reported. Final diagnosis often requires biopsy.

Appearances and assessment

Often irregular and invade into myocardium. Can be recognized as unusual, localized myocardial thickening. Report location, extent, and functional effects (valve or ventricle dysfunction, restrictive or constrictive physiology, pericardial fluid). Comment on concerns about cause.

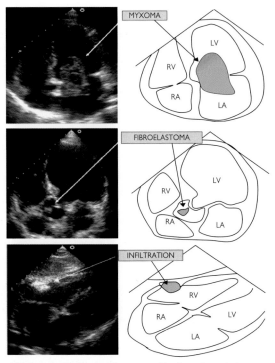

Fig. 4.74 Examples of primary cardiac tumours. Top figure demonstrates a myxoma prolapsing through the mitral valve. The middle figure is an apical 5-chamber view that demonstrates a fibroelastoma on the aortic valve. The bottom figure is a subcostal view of an infiltrative mass, probably malignant tumour. See 📹 Video 4.35.

Secondary tumours—metastases

40 times more common than primary malignant tumours. Cardiac metastases occur in 5% of patients who die of malignant tumours. Most common tumours to metastasize to heart are: melanoma, bronchogenic carcinoma, breast cancer, lymphoma, gastrointestinal adenocarcinoma, laryngeal carcinoma, pancreatic cancer, mucinous adenocarcinoma of cervix/ovary. Often clinical presentation is with tachycardia, arrhythmias, or heart failure and most common finding is a pericardial effusion.

Appearances and assessment

Usually seen as wall thickening and there may be an associated pericardial effusion. Tumour mass may protrude into a cardiac chamber. Comment on size, location, and functional effects.

Valve cysts

Fluid-filled cysts can be found on valves often due to myxomatous degeneration. They appear as round structures, often with a pedicle attachment. The cyst has a fluid-filled appearance and there may be floating structures inside. Comment on location, size, and functional effects.

Pericardial cyst

Cysts can form in pleura or pericardium. Most commonly cysts are seen around the right costophrenic location (70%), then left costophrenic angle (30%) and rarely in upper mediastinum, hila, or left cardiac border.

Appearances and assessment

Pericardial cysts appear as an ovoid space adjacent to a cardiac chamber. The differential is between cyst and loculated pericardial effusion, dilated coronary sinus or ventricular pseudo-aneurysm.

Extra-cardiac tumours

Tumours within the thorax, but separate from the heart, can be incidentally picked up during echocardiography. Parasternal views identify mediastinal cysts or thymomas. Other extra-cardiac tumours include haematoma, teratoma, diaphragmatic hernia, and pancreatic cysts.

Appearances and assessment

Comment on location, suspected cause, and functional effects. Key effects are displacement of the heart, compression of cardiac chambers, evidence of superior vena cava obstruction, cardiac tamponade, constrictive pericarditis, pulmonary or tricuspid stenosis.

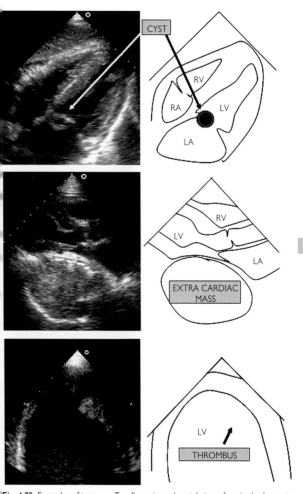

Fig. 4.75 Examples of tumours. Top figure is a subcostal view of a mitral valve cyst. The middle figure demonstrates a large extra-cardiac mass causing chamber compression. The bottom figure shows an apical left ventricle thrombus. See 📷 Video 4.36 and 📷 Video 4.37.

Congenital heart disease

Background

Common congenital heart defects, such as atrial and ventricular septal defects (📖 pp.288, 292) and coarctation of the aorta (📖 p.320) have distinct methods of assessment using standard techniques. More complex congenital disease is dealt with in specialist texts. Imaging of any congenital heart disease, simple or complex, relies on the same basic echocardiographic principles and should not be alarming. All images must be acquired and assessed. If complex, liaise closely with a specialist congenital centre. It is also worth remembering that echocardiography complements other imaging tools and a range of imaging modalities are required in the management of patients with congenital heart disease.

Assessment

Try to obtain as much patient detail as possible prior to scanning such as operation notes, previous procedures and results of previous imaging investigations. This will immediately tell you what you might expect to be seeing and what views may be most useful or required. When starting to image remember:

- Do not be scared: apply basic principles of transthoracic echocardiography—assessment of ventricular function, valvular function, and presence of a pericardial effusion is usually possible in all patients (Fig. 4.76).
- However, experience is essential for imaging of patients with complex congenital heart disease and, in particular, interpretation of imaging can be operator dependent. Therefore, if you are not experienced do not hesitate to ask for advice or support from seniors or a specialist Adult Congenital Heart Disease Centre.
- Beware of endocarditis in the congenital patient.

Particular advantages of echocardiography in congenital heart disease

- Non-invasive detailed anatomical information with serial assessment.
- Doppler assessment of valves, aortic arch (coarctation), shunt calculation (rarely used), baffle obstruction (atrial switch TGA patients).
- Contrast bubble echo for the identification of shunts, e.g. PFOs (see p.572).
- Assisting with percutaneous interventional procedures.
- Dobutamine stress echo for arterial switch TGA patients (ischaemia).
- Advanced techniques: tissue Doppler for ventricular function, 3D for detailed anatomical information (e.g. Ebstein's, AVSD), speckle tracking and dyssynchrony assessment.

Key views and findings

A standard dataset acquisition can be undertaken. However, additionally, abdominal views from the subcostal window can be very helpful and therefore 9 key views are recommended to ensure a systematic approach. It should also be remembered that because of the unusual features of congenital heart disease it is also important to be opportunistic if good images appear in unusual positions. The key 9 views are:

1. Abdominal transverse
- Subcostal window with probe marker at ~3 o'clock: provides information on abdominal situs (liver/stomach) and relationship of aorta and IVC (right) to the spine.

2. Abdominal longitudinal
- Subcostal window with the probe marker towards head ~12 o'clock: used to identify the pulsatile aorta and coeliac axis. If the probe is angled towards the liver it will be possible to identify hepatic veins and inferior vena cava draining to a right-sided atrium.

3. Parasternal long axis including the inflow and outflow views
- Useful for assessment of right ventricular outflow tract and right ventricular inflow.

4. Parasternal short axis
- Especially looking for a perimembranous VSD (at 10 o'clock), LPA/RPA, origins of coronary arteries, mitral valve and LV/RV.

5. Apical 4/3/2 chamber:
- Look for normal off-setting of atrio-ventricular valves (tricuspid should be more apical). Identify the moderator band at apex of right ventricle to establish a morphological right ventricle. Assess for any associated lesions.

6. Apical 5 chamber:
- Detailed assessment of the aorta and valve.

7. Subcostal (epigastric):
- Scan systematically the liver, right atrium, atrial septum, left atrium, and pulmonary veins entering left atrium.

8. Arch view/suprasternal:
- Neck extension may optimize views. Identify ascending aorta, neck vessels and PA. Look for any coarctation or PDA.

9. Right parasternal long axis:
May provide further information on aortic valves.

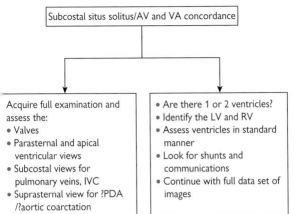

ig. 4.76 Basic questions to ask during transthoracic examination.

Sequential segmental analysis

There is some key information that needs to be established in order t
evaluate a patient with congenital heart disease. This information relates t
how the heart and blood vessels connect together. The sequence given her
can be used to gather all this key information (see also Table 4.10).

Establish arrangement of atrial chambers (situs)

The atria are defined by the appendages (right-broad, left-narrow) an
by the systemic and pulmonary connections. Normal is situs solitus an
abnormal situs inversus (morphological left atrium on right). Abdomina
organs usually match atria (liver on left suggests inversus). Use subcosta
views and look for the features:

- Left atrium has long, thin atrial appendage and rounded shape.
- Right atrium has broad, short appendage, and Eustachian valve.
- Identify where inferior vena cava and pulmonary vein connect (vein
  inflow does not identify atria as connections vary).

Determine ventricular morphology and arrangement: atrioventricular (AV) connections

Normally the heart tube folds to the right and heart lies in left chest wit
right ventricle anteriorly. If the tube folds to the left the right ventricl
lies on the other side of left ventricle. Atrio-ventricular valves stay wit
ventricles. Use the following features to identify the ventricles:

- Identify right ventricle from trabeculations, 3 papillary muscles,
  tri-leaflet valve, moderator band, and triangular cavity.
- Left ventricle has smooth surface, 2 papillary muscles, bileaflet valve,
  and bullet-shape.
- Establish right ventricle from moderator band and tricuspid valve. Left
  ventricle is bullet-shaped and associated with mitral valve.

Determine morphology of great arteries

This identifies arterial transposition and can occur if valves are in 'right'
position but folding rotates ventricles, or if ventricles are right but arterie
are switched.

- Use parasternal short axis and modified long axis views to identify
  pulmonary artery from orientation (heading posteriorly) and
  bifurcation. Ascending aorta heads superiorly.
- Use suprasternal views to see if the arch goes to left (normal) or right.

Ventriculoarterial (VA) connections

- Morphology of arterial valves, arterial relations, and infundibular
  morphology can be established from parasternal and apical windows.

Assess for any associated intracardiac lesions

- Patients may have >1 lesion. A full data set is required looking for flow
  abnormalities and shunts.

Establish cardiac position in the chest and orientation of cardiac apex

- Use subcostal view. The usual arrangement of the heart and body
  organs is situs solitus (left-sided heart, left-sided stomach and spleen
  and a right-sided liver).

Table 4.10 Sequential segmental analysis used in congenital heart disease

Abdominal situs	Solitus (liver on right, stomach on Left)
	Inversus (liver on left/transverse, stomach on right)
Atrial anatomy and systemic venous connections	Solitus (RA on right)
	Inversus (RA on left)
	Ambiguous/indeterminate
Atrioventricular connections	2 AV valves
	Common AV valve
	AV valve atresia
	Straddling or overriding AV valve
Morphology of Ventricles	Right ventricle on right
	Right ventricle on left
	Univentricular heart
Morphology of great arteries	Concordant (normal)
	Discordant (transposition)
	Double outlet (left or right ventricle)
	Common outlet (truncus arteriosus)
	Single artery atresia

Congenital defects

Some of the disorders that may be seen during routine echocardiography include:

Patent ductus arteriosus

Patent ductus arteriosus connects aorta to pulmonary artery and can be identified as follows:

- Identify the aortic end in descending aorta using a suprasternal view focusing just distal to left subclavian.
- The pulmonary end empties into left pulmonary artery just to left of pulmonary trunk and can usually be seen from a modified parasternal short axis views.
- Colour flow will demonstrate a jet directed the wrong way in the pulmonary trunk (towards the pulmonary valve).
- Report functional effects of the left-to-right shunt.

Persistent left superior vena cava

A persistent left superior vena cava drains into the coronary sinus. Usually the right superior vena cava is also present although it is possible only to have a left superior vena cava. To identify these abnormalities:

- Use an apical 4-chamber view adjusted to cut below the mitral valve. This will demonstrate the coronary sinus. It is usually dilated.
- Agitated saline contrast injected into a vein in the left arm will opacify the coronary sinus before the right atrium.
- Then inject agitated saline into a vein in the right arm. If the right superior vena cava is still present contrast will appear in the right atrium first, as normal. If the right superior vena cava is absent the saline will appear in the coronary sinus first.
- There is usually no significant haemodynamic effects but it complicates pacemaker placement.

Anomalous pulmonary drainage

This describes drainage of pulmonary veins into right atrium. Total drainage requires a septal defect for oxygenated blood to reach systemic circulation. In partial drainage 1 or 2 pulmonary veins still drain to left.

- Most easily assessed with TOE.
- Right upper pulmonary vein may drain to right atrium or superior vena cava.
- Right lower pulmonary vein may connect to inferior vena cava.
- Left pulmonary veins may connect to innominate vein.

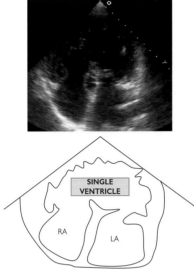

Fig. 4.77 Apical 4 chamber view of a single ventricle.

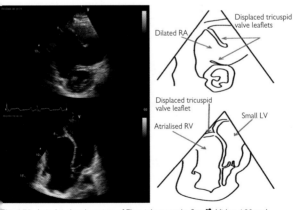

Fig. 4.78 Apical 4-chamber view of Ebstein's anomaly. See 📹 Video 4.38 and 📹 Video 4.39.

Tetralogy of Fallot

Combination of right ventricle outflow obstruction, ventricular septal defect, right ventricular hypertrophy, and aorta overriding the septum. Assessment preoperatively should focus on, and quantify, each aspect.

Double outlet right ventricle

Both aorta and pulmonary artery arise from right ventricle. Ventricular septal defect allows oxygenated blood to reach systemic circulation.

Persistent truncus arteriosus

Single trunk divides into systemic and pulmonary arteries. Associated with ventricular septal defect and single valve in trunk.

Hypoplastic left ventricle

Usually involves whole of left heart with disordered valve development and small left atrium and ventricle.

Single ventricle

Single ventricle with mitral, tricuspid, aortic and pulmonary valves connected. Chamber can be of left or right origin with remnants of other ventricle seen (Fig. 4.77).

Obstructive congenital disorders

Many congenital defects can be organized, and assessed, according to their restriction or obstruction to blood flow. They can be demonstrated using standard 2D imaging and Doppler quantifications.

Right ventricular inflow:
• Ebstein's anomaly and tricuspid atresia (Fig. 4.78 and 📖 p.122).

Right ventricular outflow:
• Subvalvular—outflow tract (use short axis views).
• Pulmonary valve—pulmonary stenosis (📖 p.156).
• Supravalvular—pulmonary artery (use short axis views).

Left ventricular inflow:
• Pulmonary veins—stenosis or obstruction. Usually requires transoesophageal echocardiography to document.
• Atrium—atrial membranes (either across the middle of atrium—cor triatum or supravalvular).
• Mitral valve—congenital stenosis (📖 p.101), double inlet valve.

Left ventricular outflow:
• Subvalvular—fibromuscular (wall thickening) or membranous (discrete membrane present) (use parasternal and apical views).
• Aortic valve—bicuspid valve (📖 p.134).
• Supravalvular level—membranous or fibromuscular thickening (use parasternal views).

Surgical correction of congenital heart disease

Complete repairs

With effective correction there may be little echocardiographic evidence of repair. A full systematic study should be used and reports made of any residual functional effects on valve function, as well as disorders of left or right ventricle appearance or function. Residual shunts or abnormal vascular connections should be commented upon.

Shunts (Fig. 4.79)

These were designed to increase blood flow into the pulmonary artery to improve oxygenation but nowadays full repairs of defects are preferred.

Blalock–Taussig shunt

This shunt connects the subclavian or innominate artery to a branch of the pulmonary artery. The shunt can be made on the left or right. It can be seen in suprasternal views and both colour flow mapping and Doppler assessment can be attempted to identify stenosis or changes in flow.

Glenn shunt

The Glenn shunt (may be bilateral) anastomized the superior vena cava to the pulmonary artery either completely or to allow two-way flow.

Fontan procedure

This was used to bypass an abnormal right ventricle by directing flow from the systemic atrium to the pulmonary circulation. In fact there are a range of Fontan procedures and it can be difficult to evaluate with echocardiography without knowing the surgical details although assessing ventricular function and the circuit is essential.

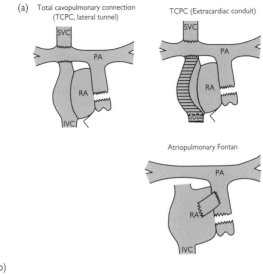

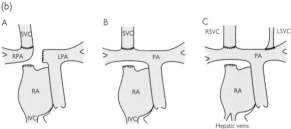

Fig. 4.79 (a) Types of Fontan operation. (b) Diagrams illustrating various types of Glenn shunt. A) Classical Glenn. B) Bidirectional Glenn. C) Bilateral bidirectional Glenn.

Reproduced from Myerson S, Choudhury Rand Mitchell A (2009) *Emergencies in Cardiology*, 2nd edn, Oxford University Press, Figures 16.10 and 16.11.

Transoesophageal examination

Introduction

- Transoesophageal echocardiography (TOE) has emerged over only the last 30 years. The first M-mode transoesophageal images were published in the 1970s by Dr Frazin, a cardiologist in Chicago, who attached a traditional probe onto the end of an endoscope. It did not catch on as a technique because the patient found it difficult to swallow the probe.

- By the early 1980s 2D imaging with superior, smaller probe technology had become realistic, significantly advanced by the introduction of the electronic, phased-array probe. The early probes were single plane and it was not until the 1990s that biplane probes became a reality. These were finally superseded by multiplane imaging, a move that provided the leap in functionality that we take for granted today.

- TOE uses all the same technology as transthoracic imaging. 2D echocardiography, colour and spectral Doppler can all be performed as well as tissue Doppler imaging and 3D reconstructions. However, transoesophageal imaging possesses a major advantage in that there is little tissue between the probe and the heart to degrade the image. This also means the probe virtually touches the heart so the ultrasound beam does not need to penetrate as far. Higher ultrasound frequencies can therefore be used (typically 5–7.5MHz) which enhances spatial resolution.

- A lot of the clinical applications have been driven by interest in intraoperative monitoring and this remains a key application of the technique. However, real-time imaging with unparalleled spatial and temporal resolution makes the image quality superior to all other modalities within the imaging window provided by the oesophagus. As the procedure is well tolerated, TOE has guaranteed usefulness for cardiology studies, particularly where detailed anatomical and functional imaging is needed.

- During the last few years real-time 3D transoesophageal echocardiography has become an important tool in particular to guide interventions.

Performing the study

- There are many different patients in whom TOE is requested, from patients who require elective monitoring of stable clinical problems such as aortic dissection to those with emergency haemodynamic problems. The background and approach to each study will therefore vary considerably. This chapter is written to provide a framework to perform an elective, or planned, transoesophageal echocardiogram in an awake patient.
- For intraoperative studies or those on Intensive Care Units the patient is already sedated or anaesthetized and, unless planned before an operation, may not have given consent. However, even in these situations the majority of the framework for performing a study is still relevant. All aspects of assessing indications and contraindications should be carried out, as well as preparation of machine, probe, and monitoring. The only real differences are usually the patient position (lying on their back), the presence of other things in the mouth (tracheal tubes), and depth of sedation (general anaesthetic or deep sedation).

Indications

There are generally accepted, evidence-based uses of TOE which have evolved in clinical situations where there is a need for high spatial and temporal resolution to assess pathology.

- Haemodynamic monitoring in anaesthetized patient:
  - Perioperative monitoring.
  - Intensive care monitoring.
- Evaluation of valve pathology:
  - Pre-surgical evaluation for repair of mitral or aortic valves.
  - Evaluation of cause of dysfunction.
- Intracardiac shunts.
- Cardiac embolic source:
  - Intracardiac shunts.
  - Left-sided thrombus—ventricle, left atrial appendage.
  - Left-sided valve abnormalities/masses/vegetations.
  - Aortic atheroma.
- Endocarditis:
  - Diagnosis.
  - Monitoring.
- Evaluation of prosthetic valve dysfunction.
- Congenital heart disease.
- Aortic dissection and aortic pathology.
- Cardiac masses (where transthoracic imaging inadequate).
- Imaging during procedures:
  - Percutaneous procedures—ASD/PFO closure, mitral balloon valvuloplasty.
  - Electrophysiology and pacing—transseptal puncture, lead placement.
  - Cardiothoracic surgery.[1]
- Transcatheter aortic valve implantation (TAVI).
- Poor transthoracic windows or inadequate image quality.

Reference

1 American Society of Anesthesiologists. Practice guidelines for perioperative transesophageal echocardiography. *Anesthesiology* 1996; **84**:986–1006.

Contraindications and complications

Consider contraindications before starting. Absolute contraindications tend to be oesophageal problems that make the procedure technically impossible and increase the risk of traumatic injury. The decision to go ahead despite relative contraindications depends on the importance of the clinical information to be gathered, whether there are alternative ways to gather the data and operator experience. During and after the procedure be vigilant for possible complications and ensure the patient is fully informed of these risks when taking consent.

Absolute contraindications
- Oesophageal tumours causing obstruction of the lumen.
- Oesophageal strictures.
- Oesophageal diverticula.
- Patient not cooperative.

Relative contraindications
- Oesophageal reflux refractory to medical therapy.
- Hiatal hernia.
- Odynophagia or dysphagia.
- Previous oesophageal or gastric surgery.
- Previous oesophageal or gastric bleed.
- Oesophageal varices: using a sheath is said to reduce the risk as the gel reduces the pressure of the probe tip. However, transgastric views are not advised and there must not have been a bleed in the preceding 4 weeks.
- Severe cervical arthritis.
- Profound oesophageal distortion.
- Recent radiation to head and neck.
- Significant dental pathology.

Complications
A study of complications in around 10,000 patients showed a very low incidence.[1] Failed intubation occurred in around 2%. All other complications had an incidence of <1%.
- Intubation problems—termination because of choking.
- Pulmonary problems—bronchospasm, hypoxia.
- Cardiac problems—ventricular extrasystole, tachycardia, atrial fibrillation, AV block, angina.
- Bleeding—from pharynx, related to vomiting, from oesophagus.
- Perforation—risk of perforation increases in small patients and in all conditions that make the oesophagus friable, e.g. prior radiation to head, neck or oesophagus, steroid treatment, gastro-oesophageal reflux disease, prolonged duration of probe in patient.
- Probe failure.

Antibiotic prophylaxis for TOE?

- Antibiotic prophylaxis is not recommended for any indication under current guidelines.
- It remains reasonable to consider antibiotics in occasional cases, for example a patient with a prosthetic heart valve and evidence of poor oral hygiene, in whom the study is being performed for an indication other than suspected endocarditis. In these individual cases, practice is governed by clinical common sense rather than evidence.

Reference

1 Daniel WG et al. Safety of transesophageal echocardiography. A multicenter survey of 10,419 examinations. *Circulation* 1991; **83**:817–21.

Information for the patient

For elective or planned studies patients should be provided with information or have a detailed verbal explanation. Informed consent is essential as it is a semi-invasive procedure and sedation is used.

Example information sheet

You have been asked to attend for transoesophageal echocardiography (TOE). A TOE is a test that allows the doctor to look closely at the heart without other organs obscuring the view. In order to carry out the procedure, the scope, which is a long flexible tube, is passed through the mouth and down the gullet.

Before the procedure

You should not have anything to eat or drink for at least 6 hours before the procedure. When you arrive you will be seen by a doctor who will take a medical history and after explaining the procedure, ask you to sign a consent form. If you have any concerns, please do not hesitate to ask, as we would like you to be as relaxed as possible. We will be pleased to answer any queries.

What happens during the procedure?

A blood pressure cuff will be attached to your arm and a small monitor placed on your finger to monitor the oxygen levels in the blood. The doctor will spray your throat with some local anaesthetic. A mouth guard is placed between your teeth to protect the tube and your teeth. You will be asked to turn onto your left side and the room's main lights will be turned off. Your sedation is then given through a small tube (cannula) which will be inserted into your arm. When you are sleepy the procedure will start. There will be several people looking after you including the doctor, a nurse and a technician. The procedure takes 10–20min to examine all areas carefully.

Benefits The benefits from TOE are that it can: define the nature of cardiac symptoms; decide which further therapeutic and diagnostic procedures you may have to undergo.

Risks

Risks from TOE are tiny. Usually the investigation is tolerated well; some patients may have some mild symptoms during the test (mostly coughing). Serious risks are very rare and include palpitations 0.75% (7 patients in every 1000), angina 0.1% (1 patient in every 1000), bronchospasm/hypoxia 0.8% (8 patients in every 1000), bleeding 0.2% (2 patients in every 1000), oesophagus perforation, extremely rare less than 0.01% (1 in every 10 000 patients). Your doctor would not recommend that you have a transoesophageal echocardiogram unless they felt that the benefits of the procedure outweighed these small risks.

After the procedure The sedation may last up to an hour. Your blood pressure and respiration will be checked and you may have an oxygen mask on while you are awake. The sedation has an amnesic effect so you should remember little of the procedure when you wake up.

Preparing for the study

Setting up the environment

- With the patient on their bed, ensure there is a blood pressure cuff on the arm and set to automatic monitoring every 5–10min. Check a baseline blood pressure.
- Set up stable ECG monitor on the machine.
- Monitor oxygen saturations and check a baseline saturation level.
- Provide supplemental oxygen, usually via nasal specs at 2L/min.
- Ensure suction is available and working.
- Check bed height and position so operator and nursing staff are not bending over the patient but stand upright during the procedure.
- Check relative position of machine, patient, and operator to ensure operator has a clear view of images.

Nursing

- The nurse should talk to the patient and check identity and consent.
- The nurse stands behind the patient or at the head of the bed to reassure the patient and support the head and mouth guard.
- During the procedure they should monitor haemodynamics and saturations and inform the operator if they change.
- They should monitor for secretions and give suction as required.
- After the procedure they should stay with the patient to ensure adequate recovery from the sedation.

Operator

- Check notes for indications and purpose of study. Check past medical history, allergies, and any contraindications.
- Make sure patient has been starved for at least 6 hours and has taken out any false teeth/loose bridges/loose teeth.
- Ensure the apparatus is ready: probe prepared (📖 p.354), attached, and selected; probe steering works; transoesophageal machine presets selected, ECG tracing and patient details on machine.
- Sedation drawn up (📖 p.358), local anaesthetic spray available, and IV cannula in arm ready for sedation.
- Ensure gel ready to be applied to probe.
- Then give local anaesthetic spray (📖 p.358).
- For the awake patient, ask them to roll onto their left side and ensure a stable position—often achieved if the patient brings their right leg over their left in a 'recovery position' arrangement. If in an ITU setting, ask if the patient is able to be rolled onto their left.
- Ensure the head of the bed is flat, the patient has their head on a pillow, and there is a mat under the head to absorb any secretions.
- For the awake patient, ask them to drop their chin onto their chest.
- Place the mouth guard between their teeth.
- Give sedation (📖 p.358) and start the intubation (📖 p.362).

Preparing for TOE—a 10-point plan

1. Put sheath on the probe.
2. Review referral form/notes for indication, contraindications.
3. Ask patient when was last meal (should be >6 hours before), previous problems with swallowing, known oesophageal disease, allergies.
4. Insert patient name and hospital number on scanner and ask patient to confirm.
5. Insert IV cannula.
6. Attach probe to the scanner, test steering and whether probe is accepted by the scanner.
7. Start blood pressure monitoring and pulse oximetry, nasal specs for oxygen supply (2L/min).
8. Apply local anaesthesia to patient's throat, then rotate patient into a left lateral decubitus position.
9. Put in mouth guard.
10. Give sedation.

Preparing and cleaning the probe

The probe can easily be damaged either externally (by chemicals or misuse) or by the patient (beware teeth!). There are also important health and safety issues about protecting the patient from the probe.

Checking the probe

Check over the probe at the start of the procedure. Look for evidence of damage to the coating and layers. There may be breaks or 'bubbling' in the coating. In extreme situations the underlying wire shielding may be exposed with a risk of current leak or heating to the patient. If you are concerned about the integrity of the probe use a different probe and contact the manufacturer.

Preparing and cleaning

There are 2 options for probe preparation and cleaning.

The probe is used without a cover
Glutaraladehyde

- In this case it is essential it is sterilized between cases. After the investigation the probe should be washed down with water and then immersed in a tube containing glutaraldehyde solution (licensed for endoscope disinfection) for a fixed period of time according to manufacturer guidelines.
- Gluttaraldehyde can cause allergies or breathing problems. Therefore ensure regular fresh air in the room where the probe is cleaned. Furthermore, the probe needs to be rewashed with water to ensure the solution is removed before the probe is used on the next patient.
- The handgrips and controls of the probe should be wiped with an alcohol-based agent. Alcohol should not normally be used to clean the transducer face at the tip of the probe.

The probe is used with a purpose-designed sheath

- Sheaths protect the probe from infection and provide electrical isolation from the patient.
- There are both latex and latex-free versions.
- To prepare, fill the sheath tip with the supplied gel using a syringe.
- Then feed the probe all the way into the sheath and fix the upper end with the supplied plastic clip.
- Avoid air bubbles in the gel around the transducer as these degrade image quality. Press them further up the sheath or pull and release the sheath tip to expel them away from the transducer.
- When performing a series of studies there is no need to carry out a complete disinfection between patients. After each investigation remove the sheath and wipe off any gel left on the probe. Then clean the probe with water and an alcohol-based agent.
- If the sheath breaks during the procedure or a perforation is seen afterwards, immerse the probe in disinfectant solution.
- In patients with a high infection risk (HIV, hepatitis B, etc.) disinfect the probe with a commercial solution after sheath removal and sterilize the controls with alcohol-based solutions.

Tristel sporicidal wipe

- This is a rapid action sporicidal wipe (Fig. 5.1) which is used to clean probes that have been used with sheaths.
- After removing the sheath, the first step is to clean the probe with the pre-clean sporicidal wipe. It is impregnated with a low-foaming surfactant system combined with triple enzymes, producing ultra-low surface tension for rapid cleaning.
- Then apply the sporicidal wipe which is initially activated with a foam pump.
- Next, application of the rinse wipe is the final step in the decontamination process. It is impregnated with deionized water and a low level of antioxidant which will remove and neutralize chemical residues from the probe surface.

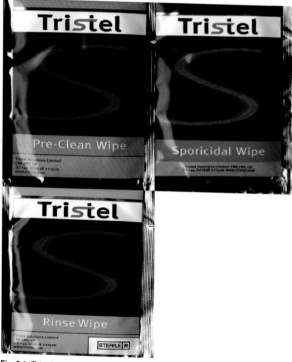

Fig. 5.1 Tristel sporicidal wipes. Following the procedure the probe is initially cleaned with the pre-clean wipe. The sporicidal wipe is then activated with a foam pump and used to clean the probe. Finally the rinse wipe is used to wipe the probe, neutralizing any remaining chemical residues.

Probe movements

A combination of probe movements is required to gather all the images (Fig. 5.2). For many of the views, changes in sector angle are the primary control, with physical movements used to optimize the image.

Withdrawal and advance

Moving the probe forward and backwards in the oesophagus is the simplest manoeuvre. The depth of the probe is best controlled with the hand nearest the patient's mouth. This hand can also judge the size of small movements forward and back relative to the mouth guard. The depth of probe insertion is marked on the probe in centimetres. This number should be used when images need to be annotated to record probe depth. It measures the distance from probe tip to front incisors.

Rotation (or turning)

The probe can be rotated clockwise or anti-clockwise within the oesophagus. This is achieved by twisting the handheld control section with one hand, and the probe near the mouth guard with your other hand. This movement is usually used to orientate the heart in the image plane and to look at the descending aorta.

Sector angle

On the controls there are usually 2 buttons side by side. These rotate the angle of the imaging plane forward and backward between 0° and 180°. The angle plane can also sometimes be changed directly from the ultrasound machine. The current angle plane is displayed on the screen.

Angulation (or retro-/ante-flexion)

The large wheel on the control panel moves a few centimetres of the transducer tip forwards and backwards. Angulation forwards is usually used to press the transducer against the oesophagus wall or stomach to improve contact and image quality. Angulation backwards can be effective at lengthening out the left ventricle.

Lateral motion

The small wheel on the control panel causes movement of the transducer tip from side-to-side. This is very rarely used and for the most part can be ignored. Occasionally with difficult images or abnormally positioned hearts small lateral motions may be helpful.

Position lock

Most probes have a lever behind the control wheels that locks the probe in position. For most studies this is not required and can be ignored. For long periods of monitoring—particularly in transgastric views intraoperatively—the lock can be used. However, there is an increased risk of traumatic injury with movement of the probe with the lock on. Care must be taken to remove the lock before the probe is repositioned.

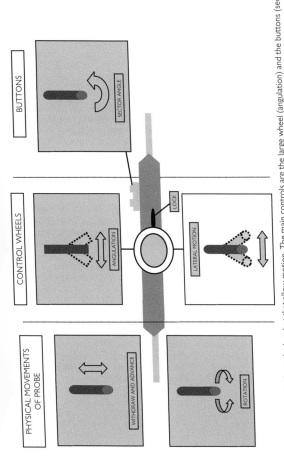

Fig. 5.2 Probe movements and the controls on the handset that allow motion. The main controls are the large wheel (angulation) and the buttons (sector angle). The small wheel and lock are rarely needed.

Anaesthetic, sedation, and analgesia

Local anaesthetic

- Start with a local anaesthetic Xylocaine® (lignocaine) spray.
- With the patient sitting up, spray several times onto the back of their throat. Ask them to hold the liquid for a few seconds and then swallow. Repeat the spray to ensure good anaesthesia.
- Warn the patient that the spray has an unusual taste, their mouth and throat will feel numb, and their swallow may feel strange or difficult.
- The spray will need 2–3min to have an effect.

Sedation and analgesia

There are no standard guidelines for TOE and it is possible to perform the study with no sedation. However, the following routines (see also Fig. 5.3) can be used (borrowed from other endoscopic procedures). A benzodiazepine provides sedation and amnesia, and an opioid analgesia. Remember that *'the difference between good and bad sedation is around three minutes'*, i.e. wait for the sedation to work.

- Ensure reversal agents are available and accessible (flumazenil for midazolam and naloxone for pethidine or fentanyl). Life support equipment should be accessible.
- Start with 25microgram IV fentanyl (or 25mg IV pethidine)—then give 2mg IV midazolam and this is usually sufficient for most patients. Aim for the patient to be *'drowsy but rousable'*. In certain patients and situations lower starting doses are advisable (see 📖 'Specific situations' p.358).
- Wait 3–5min then assess level of sedation (patient response, haemodynamics). If not adequate, give further bolus of 2mg IV midazolam.
- Repeat the *'wait and bolus'* regime until adequate sedation.
- Total sedation should not exceed 10mg midazolam and/or 75mg pethidine (or 100microgram fentanyl). Stop and consider a general anaesthetic at a later date.
- Once sedation is appropriate start intubation. If intubation is difficult because the patient is awake return to the sedation routine.
- During the procedure (after intubation) if the patient becomes distressed consider giving further boluses of sedation.

Specific situations

- In younger patients (and some older patients) increasing doses of midazolam can increase agitation and be counterproductive. Consider using more analgesia and less sedation from the outset.
- In older patients (particularly >80 years) oversedation is a problem so start with 1mg IV midazolam, withhold the opioid, and wait longer between boluses as the sedation may be slower to circulate.
- Use lower starting doses for those with significant left ventricular failure or respiratory disease, hypotension, or neurological impairment.

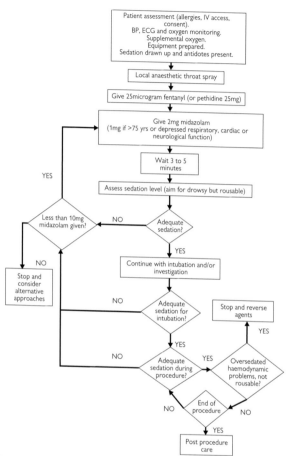

Patient assessment (allergies, IV access, consent).
BP, ECG and oxygen monitoring.
Supplemental oxygen.
Equipment prepared.
Sedation drawn up and antidotes present.

↓

Local anaesthetic throat spray

↓

Give 25microgram fentanyl (or pethidine 25mg)

↓

Give 2mg midazolam
(1mg if >75 yrs or depressed respiratory, cardiac or neurological function)

↓

Wait 3 to 5 minutes

↓

Assess sedation level (aim for drowsy but rousable)

↓

Adequate sedation?
— NO → Less than 10mg midazolam given?
— YES → (back to midazolam)
— NO → Stop and consider alternative approaches

Adequate sedation? — YES ↓

Continue with intubation and/or investigation

↓

Adequate sedation for intubation?
— NO → (back)
— YES ↓

Adequate sedation during procedure?
— NO → (back)
— YES → Oversedated haemodynamic problems, not rousable?
— YES → Stop and reverse agents
— NO ↓

End of procedure
— NO → (loop back)
— YES ↓

Post procedure care

Fig. 5.3 Flow chart for sedation protocol.

Sedation complications

Although by using low-dose conscious sedation with up-titration complications are relatively infrequent, it is always essential to be vigilant. Monitoring of the patient during the procedure is mandatory. Several expert bodies have produced guidelines for how to give sedation if you are not an anaesthetist. It is advisable to have a local policy for how to use sedation for TOE and an audit process so that problems or adverse events associated with the procedure are identified.

Peri-procedure

- Monitor for drops in blood pressure and saturations throughout the procedure. These are the commonest side effects of sedation.
- If hypotensive, patients may be mildly dehydrated as they are nil by mouth so consider IV fluids.
- Drops in saturations may be temporary at the start of sedation and can be corrected with increased supplemental oxygen.
- If there are ever any concerns about the level of sedation or degree of haemodynamic or respiratory changes, reverse the sedation and stop the procedure (if still ongoing).
- To reverse the midazolam give flumazenil. This is relatively short acting so after a period of time, if the sedative effects return, consider further boluses or even an infusion.
- To reverse the opioid give naloxone.
- In those with left ventricular failure, lying flat with sedation can precipitate acute failure so be alert for clinical signs and treat with diuretics etc. if necessary.
- Allergic reactions can occur with sedation so treat as appropriate.

Post-procedure

- After the procedure, the patient should be monitored until they are fully awake.
- If the procedure has been elective and the patient is going home afterwards they should be advised not to drive or operate heavy machinery for 24 hours.

Further reading

Mankia K et al. Safe combined intravenous opiate/benzodiazepine sedation for transoesophageal echocardiography. Br J Cardiol 2010; **17**:125–7.

Intubation

Intubation is a key skill to learn. Unless you intubate successfully the procedure can not start. The skills to perform successful intubation in elective studies with light sedation are broadly similar to those skills for intubation in intraoperative or Intensive Care settings. Everyone develops their own techniques but a standard procedure is as follows.

Intubation with light sedation

General

- Ideally have two people, one to hold the controls, and the other to hold the end of the probe and intubate. If on your own, lie the probe along the bed and concentrate on intubation. Some people can hold the controls in one hand and feed the probe with the other, but this requires an uncomplicated passage of the probe.
- Talk confidently and calmly to the patient. Guide them through the procedure and the swallows. After intubation reassure them and tell them to take gentle breaths through the nose. The attitude of the operator and how they relate to—and relax—the patient often determines the success of the procedure.

The routine

- The patient should be lying on their left side with their chin towards their chest. This encourages the probe to pass into the oesophagus (exactly what you try to avoid with chin-lift during resuscitation).
- Check the mouth guard is in position between the teeth.
- Wipe gel over the probe tip to about 40cm. Too much increases the risk of aspiration and too little makes probe movement difficult and uncomfortable for the patient.
- Check probe controls and put a curve on the end of the probe.
- Ensure the curve on the tip lines up with the expected curve into the back of the mouth then pass the probe through the mouth guard and onto the tongue.
- Ask the patient to swallow once to get the probe to the back of the mouth and then a second time to pass it into the oesophagus. The second step should be timed to coincide with the swallow.
- To direct the probe a finger can be placed in the mouth beside the mouth guard. This guides the probe into the back of the mouth. It is especially useful when learning, when the probe is not passing smoothly, or in the anaesthetized patient.
- When the probe is in the oesophagus stop and do not move anything for a few minutes while the patient settles.
- The operator should then remove one glove and get into position. One gloved hand controls the probe at the mouth guard and the other holds the controls. The operator usually stands facing the patient with their right hand at the patient's mouth and looks over their shoulder at the images. An alternative arrangement is to stand at right angles, with the left hand at the patient's mouth, facing the machine.

Intubation in the anaesthetized patient

- Use the same probe preparation and use a mouth guard.
- Ensure there is a curve on the probe, then use a finger to guide the tip into the back of the mouth.
- If the patient is on their back get someone to lift the chin towards the chest.
- The probe may pass smoothly into the oesophagus with light pressure. If there is resistance induce a reflex swallow with some forward pressure on the back of the tongue.
- If a tracheal tube is in place, passage of the probe into the oesophagus may be restricted by the tracheal tube. To overcome this, ask for the assistance of the anaesthetist, either to temporarily deflate the cuff or to manipulate the tracheal tube.

What to do if the probe does not pass or patient is agitated?

- You should not need to give more than a gentle steady force to the probe. If resistance is felt assume it has gone the wrong way.
- If you are not already using your finger to guide the probe, do so.
- Feel where the tip of the probe has gone. It may have doubled back on itself in the mouth or you may feel it heading up or down. Withdraw slightly, adjust the rotation and then try to advance again, with a swallow.
- If it is not clear where the probe has gone, withdraw entirely, check the curve on the probe and its direction, then restart.
- If the patient cannot swallow because they are too sedated use a finger to direct the probe.
- If the patient starts coughing think whether you may have passed the probe into the trachea. Withdraw the probe and start again.
- If the patient becomes very agitated, stop and consider whether to try again after more sedation and/or analgesia.
- In around 2% of cases intubation fails. Know when to stop. After two or three attempts have been unsuccessful consider getting help from a more experienced operator, if available. If the patient is becoming very agitated despite adequate sedation and analgesia, stop. If the investigation is essential, the study can always be rearranged with a general anaesthetic to ensure patient compliance and/or an anaesthetist to aid intubation.

Image acquisition

Standard acquisition

Acquisition of transoesophageal images should always be performed in a standardized way—with a set sequence of views. Virtually all the views have corresponding transthoracic views and therefore if you have prior training in transthoracic imaging think about these views to identify structures. As with performing a transthoracic study, all the views should be recorded for comprehensive data collection. Even when there is a specific question (e.g. exclusion of atrial clots before cardioversion) a full dataset should be acquired to ensure nothing is missed.

Optimize the views using small changes in transducer position

Adjust by angulation, moving the transducer up and down, and rotating the sector (tips will be given for each of the views). Don't move too fast and too much. Slight changes have a big impact on the image!

Most scan planes have several different structures

All structures cannot always be viewed in a single recorded loop. Slight adjustments of the probe position and/or sector may be needed and loops recorded for each structure.

If you get lost

If during a transoesophageal investigation you become disoriented find the 4-chamber view again. Reset the rotation to 0° and then try some rotation and repositioning of the probe until the 4 chambers come back into view.

The 'screenwiper' principle

The best initial sequence of views (scan planes) is summarized by the *screenwiper principle* (Fig. 5.4). This section describes how to collect transoesophageal data following the screenwiper principle.

- Starting from 0° the sector is moved across in steps to around 135° and then back again in a series of steps.
- At each step the view needs only minor modifications of probe position to optimize the image. This reduces major probe movements and minimizes patient discomfort.

Each view is examined in:
- 2D imaging.
- Then colour flow Doppler recordings.
- And, if needed, spectral Doppler recordings (PW and/or CW).

3D imaging allows the acquisition of real-time 3D information about cardiac structures and improves spatial orientation. 3D can be performed in selected views for example of the mitral valve. As with transthoracic echocardiography, a variety of acquisition modes can be used depending on the size of the volume of interest.

- Live 3D acquisition: allows the generation of live 3D images which are displayed in a pyramidal volume without the need for electrocardiographic gating.
- Live 3D zoom: allows the display of a magnified pyramidal volume (smaller than live 3D mode).
- Full volume acquisition: allows the segmental build up of a 3D image over several consecutive cardiac cycles and gives the largest volume images.
- 3D full volume colour acquisition.
- X-plane imaging: this provides 2 orthogonal views from the same heart beat. The initial image on the left is the baseline reference whilst the image on the right can be electronically rotated to any angle between 0–180°.

After the screenwiper is complete, additional views can then be used, as required, to look at pulmonary veins, transgastric views, the aorta, or any abnormal findings.

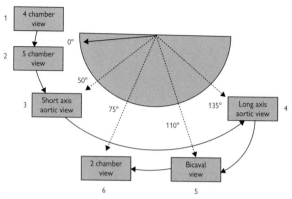

Fig. 5.4 'Screenwiper' principle showing sequence of sector angles for first 6 views. Once in position, the image can be optimized with slight variation in sector angle (usually <5°) followed by slight adjustments in depth and tilting as necessary.

Basic screenwiper study

1. 4-chamber view.
2. 5-chamber view.
3. Short axis aortic view (± right ventricle inflow/outflow).
4. Long axis aortic view.
5. Interatrial septal view.
6. Left atrial appendage view.

then further views

7. Left pulmonary venous view.
8. Right pulmonary venous view.
9. Pulmonary artery view.
10. Transgastric views.*
11. Descending aorta view.
12. Aortic arch view.

* Not necessary in all patients.

Four chamber view

This is the first view to acquire (Fig. 5.5) and is similar to the transthoracic 4-chamber view (but upside down). After intubation, advance the probe to around 35cm from the teeth.

Finding the view

- Rotation should be set at 0°.
- The atria will probably be the first feature you see.
- Turn the probe to swing all 4 chambers into view.
- Withdraw and advance the probe slightly to avoid the LVOT but keep a clear view of the mitral valve.
- If the LVOT is still seen, try adding up to 15°.
- If necessary, improve contact by probe angulation.

What do you see?

Use this view to assess
- Global and regional left ventricle function, and wall thickness.
- Right ventricle size and function.
- Mitral valve morphology (orifice, prolapse).
- Tricuspid valve morphology.

Use this view to measure
- Right and left ventricle size (although beware foreshortening).
- Mitral Doppler measurements.

Key features of view
- *Mitral valve:* key view for mitral valve to assess morphology and haemodynamics. A2 segment of anterior mitral leaflet (aML) and P3 segment of the posterior mitral leaflet (pML) seen. Colour flow mapping will show stenosis and/or regurgitation. Supplement with CW or PW Doppler as for transthoracic echocardiography.
- *Tricuspid valve:* lateral leaflet is better displayed than septal. Assessment is often limited by foreshortening. To get a better view of the tricuspid valve advance the probe slightly deeper into the oesophagus. Supplement with Doppler as required.
- *Left and right atrium:* the main cavity of both atria and the interatrial septum can be seen. However, fossa ovalis is not usually seen. Turn the probe slightly left and right to scan through the atria.
- *Left ventricle:* parts of the interventricular septum and the lateral wall are displayed. Often left ventricle is foreshortened and measurement of end-diastolic and end-systolic volumes may be inaccurate. Retroflex the probe to lengthen out the left ventricle but beware contact may be lost.
- *Right ventricle:* an impression of size and function of the right ventricle relative to the left is obtained, although there is a risk of foreshortening, as with the left ventricle.

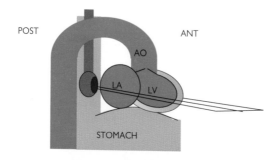

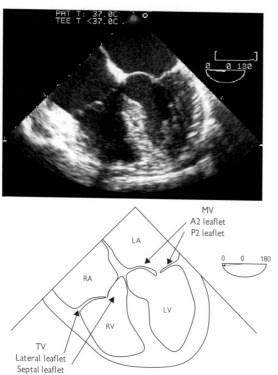

Fig. 5.5 Position of probe and classical image for a 4-chamber view. Without ante- or retro-angulation of the probe the left ventricle is usually foreshortened. See 📹 Video 5.1.

Five chamber view

This is the second view and is similar to the transthoracic apical 5-chamber view (Fig. 5.6). The main purpose is to get to the appropriate level for the aortic short axis view. However, an initial view of the LVOT is provided.

Finding the view
- Rotation should be set at 0°.
- From the 4-chamber view withdraw the probe very slightly until the LVOT comes into plane.

What do you see?

Use this view to assess
- LVOT obstruction.
- Aortic regurgitation.

Use this view to measure
- No specific measurements.

Key features of view
- Most of the features are as for the 4-chamber view.
- *LVOT*: look at the size of the outflow tract and use colour flow mapping within the tract to look for aortic regurgitation or flow turbulence due to obstruction.

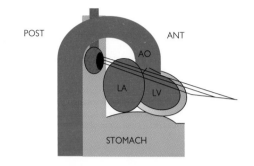

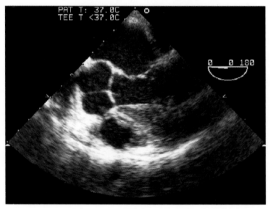

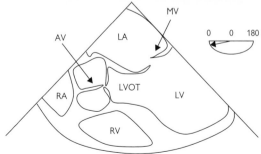

Fig. 5.6 Probe position for 5-chamber view with classic image. See ⛊ Video 5.2.

Short axis (aortic valve) view

An essential view. The perfect short axis view of the aortic valve, it can also provide information on the right heart and interatrial septum (Fig. 5.7). It is equivalent to the parasternal short axis.

Finding the view
- From the apical 5-chamber rotate the sector to around 50°.
- Optimize further with slight clockwise rotation of the probe.
- The probe may need to be withdrawn or advanced slightly to get the right scan plane. Focus on a clear view of the aortic valve.

What do you see?
Use this view to assess
- Aortic valve morphology and pathology.
- Perivalvular processes.
- Sometimes, tricuspid and pulmonary valves.
- Coronary artery origins can also be seen.
- Interatrial septum for patent foramen ovale.

Use this view to measure
- Left atrial diameter.
- Aortic valve orifice area and aortic root diameter.

Key features of view
- *Aortic valve:* the valve lies in the centre: left coronary cusp on the right, right coronary cusp at the bottom and non-coronary on the left. Colour flow identifies regurgitation and, by adjusting the image to go through the tips of valve, planimetry can be used to measure aortic valve orifice area.
- *Aortic root:* around the valve is the aortic root. Infection or aortic surgery can make this thickened or 'boggy'. Abscesses may also be seen.
- *Transverse sinus:* between the aortic root and the left atrium is the transverse sinus (part of the pericardial space). This may contain fluid.
- *Coronary arteries:* to display the coronary ostia withdraw the probe a few millimetres. Left main stem is at 2 o'clock and right coronary artery at 6 o'clock. The left coronary system can sometimes be tracked to, and beyond, the bifurcation. Colour flow and Doppler demonstrates flow.
- *Left atrium:* lying between the probe and the aortic valve, this is a standard view for linear measures of left atrial size.
- *Tricuspid valve:* this can sometimes be seen below and to the left of the aortic valve. Better views are obtained from the right ventricular inflow/outflow view.
- *Pulmonary valve:* this lies below and to the right of the aortic valve.
- *Interatrial septum:* the interatrial septum abuts the aortic root in the 10 o'clock position. The fossa ovalis is not usually seen but when looking for a patent foramen ovale this view is often very stable for shunt studies using colour flow or contrast.

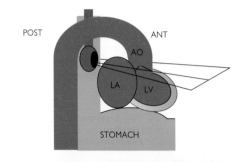

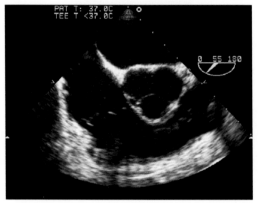

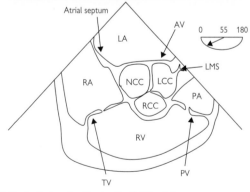

Fig. 5.7 Short axis view of aortic valve. See 📹 Video 5.3.

Short axis (right ventricle) view

This view may be included for better display of the pulmonary valve and is also called the *right ventricle inflow-outflow view* (Fig. 5.8).

It is very similar to the aortic view and can be skipped if the pulmonary valve has already been adequately displayed. It is equivalent to the parasternal short axis transthoracic view.

Finding the view

- From the short axis aortic view rotate the sector to around 70–80°.
- The probe may need to be withdrawn or advanced slightly to get the right scan plane. Focus on a clear view of the pulmonary valve.
- The optimal view will include the tricuspid and pulmonary valve with the right ventricle wrapped around the aortic valve—a right ventricular inflow–outflow view.

What do you see?

Use this view to assess
- Pulmonary valve morphology and pathology.
- Tricuspid valve morphology and pathology.
- Base of right ventricle.

Use this view to measure
- Right ventricle and outflow tract size.

Key features of view
- *Pulmonary valve:* this lies below and to the right of the aortic valve. Use colour flow to assess for regurgitation.
- *Tricuspid valve:* lies below and to the left of the aortic valve. Use colour flow to assess regurgitation and sometimes the valve is sufficiently aligned for CW Doppler measures.
- *Right ventricle:* the ventricle wraps around below the aortic valve and measurements of size at the base and in the outflow tract are sometimes possible.

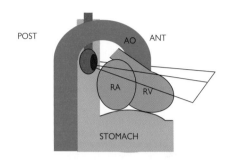

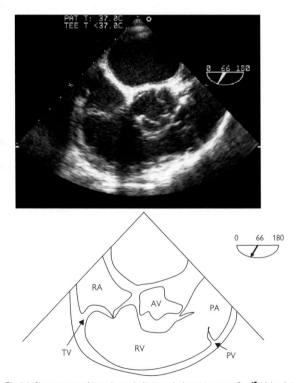

Fig. 5.8 Short axis view focused on right heart with change in sector. See 📷 Video 5.4.

Long axis (aortic valve) view

This view is equivalent to a transthoracic apical 3-chamber view or parasternal long axis view (Fig. 5.9). It is used to assess the aortic and mitral valves as well as left ventricle, outflow tract, and left atrium. In some people the mitral valve is not seen well as it lies more inferiorly. An adjusted long axis view will then be needed to assess the mitral valve (📖 p.418).

Finding the view
- From the short axis views rotate the sector to around 135°.
- Withdraw, advance, and turn the probe slightly to get the scan plane.
- Focus on a clear view of the aortic valve and ascending aorta.
- The optimal view will include 2 clear valve leaflets and a straight ascending aorta.

What do you see?
Use this view to assess
- Aortic valve morphology and pathology.
- Mitral valve morphology and pathology.
- Perivalvular processes.
- LVOT and membranous septum.
- Ascending aorta.

Use this view to measure
- Aortic root, sinuses, and ascending aorta.
- Left atrial size.

Key features of view
- *Aortic valve:* the right coronary cusp is seen at the bottom and non-coronary cusp at the top. Colour flow will demonstrate regurgitation and this can be a good view for identifying vegetations or masses.
- *Aortic root:* the entire aortic root, including sinuses of Valsalva, sinotubular junction, and ascending aorta should be visible for measurement.
- *Ascending aorta:* slight adjustment can often bring into view a lot of the proximal portion of the ascending aorta.
- *Mitral valve:* A2 and P2 segments of the valve are seen and can be used for colour flow and other Doppler measures. However, for proper visualization the probe may need to be advanced slightly.
- *Left atrium:* the atrium lies nearest the probe and linear size can be measured from probe to aortic root.
- *Left ventricle:* the septum (including the membranous septum below the aortic valve) and inferolateral wall can usually be seen to assess wall motion abnormalities.
- *Right ventricle:* the right ventricle outflow is just seen below the aortic valve and sometimes the pulmonary valve is partially visible.
- *Transverse sinus:* This lies between aortic root and left atrium and may contain fluid.

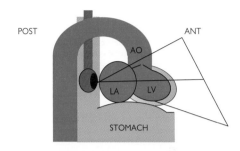

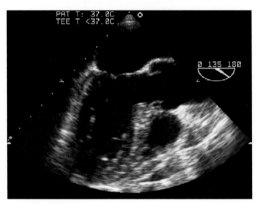

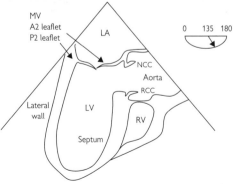

Fig. 5.9 Long axis view demonstrates aortic valve and left ventricle. See 📹 Video 5.5.

Long axis (mitral valve) view

This view is a slight adjustment of the long axis aortic view but focused on the mitral valve. If the views of the mitral valve were already optimal in the aortic long axis image this view can be skipped.

Finding the view

- From the long axis aortic view, at around 135°, advance the probe slightly.
- Focus on a clear view of the mitral valve and try and get an unforeshortened left ventricle.
- The optimal view will include 2 clear mitral valve leaflets.

What do you see?

Use this view to assess
- Mitral valve morphology and pathology.
- Left ventricular global and regional function.

Use view to measure
- Doppler measures of mitral regurgitation and stenosis.

Key features of view
- The features are similar to the long axis aortic view (except the aortic valve may be less clear).
- *Mitral valve:* A2 and P2 segments of the valve are seen. Colour flow can map regurgitation and assess flow convergence and vena contracta. The valve is also usually aligned for Doppler measures.

Atrial septum (bicaval) view

This is a unique transoesophageal view with no equivalent transthoracic image (Fig. 5.10). It is perfect for studying both atria and the septum.

Finding the view
- From the long axis views rotate the sector to around 110°.
- Turn the probe clockwise away from the left ventricle. You will see the septum come into view as a line across the screen.
- Withdraw, advance and turn the probe. Focus on a clear view of the septum, with the 'dip' of the fossa ovalis in the centre.
- The optimal view includes inferior and superior vena cavae on either side with the right atrial appendage visible on the right.

What do you see?

Use this view to assess
- Drainage of superior and inferior vena cava.
- Assessment for atrial septal defect and patent foramen ovale.
- Drainage of right upper pulmonary vein.
- Eustachian valve.

Use this view to measure
- The tricuspid regurgitation jet may be aligned for Doppler measures.
- A slightly adjusted view can be used to look at the right upper pulmonary vein flow.

Key features of view
- *Left and right atria:* the left atrium is nearest the probe.
- *Interatrial septum:* this is the most prominent feature and can be qualitatively assessed for thickness and atrial septal defects. Colour flow mapping and contrast provide more detailed information on interatrial shunts.
- *Inferior vena cava and Eustachian valve:* these lie on the left of the image and flow can be mapped with colour flow. The Eustachian valve is seen as a mobile strand originating from the orifice of the inferior vena cava.
- *Superior vena cava and christa terminalis:* these lie on the right of the image with the christa terminalis usually seen as a bright bar below the superior vena cava separating it from the right atrial appendage.
- *Right atrial appendage:* this is a wide-mouthed, shallow, trabeculated appendage lying on the right of the image below the superior vena cava. Atrial pacing wires may be seen hooking into the appendage.
- *Tricuspid valve:* the tricuspid valve may be seen in the far field. To optimize the valve image advance the probe. Colour flow can assess regurgitation and the valve is often aligned for Doppler measures.
- *Right upper pulmonary vein:* to see the vein the probe needs to be turned anticlockwise slightly to focus on the superior vena cava. The right upper pulmonary vein lies parallel to the superior vena cava. The vein is often aligned for Doppler measures. This view is used to look for abnormal pulmonary venous drainage.

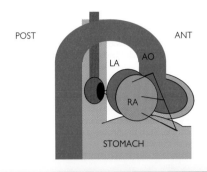

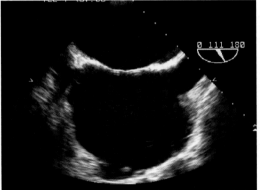

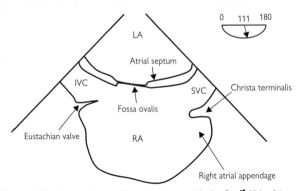

Fig. 5.10 Bicaval view with unusually prominent tricuspid valve. See ▣ Video 5.6.

Two chamber (atrial appendage) view

This view is important for several features of the left heart: mitral valve, left ventricular function and left atrial appendage (Fig. 5.11). The view is equivalent to the transthoracic apical 2-chamber view.

Finding the view

- Rotate back from the bicaval view to see mitral valve and left ventricle.
- Change the sector to around 75°.
- Withdraw and advance the probe to focus on a clear view of the mitral valve and left ventricle. Turn the probe to obtain the longest (unforeshortened) view of the left ventricle.
- To see the left atrial appendage clearly you may need to adjust the sector angle between 90° and 50°.
- The optimal view includes mitral valve, left atrial appendage, and an unforeshortened left ventricle. An unforeshortened left ventricle and left atrial appendage may not be visible in the same view and in this case separate images should be stored for each feature.

What do you see?

Use this view to assess

- Global and regional left ventricle function, wall thickness.
- Mitral valve morphology (orifice, prolapse).
- Left atrial appendage.
- Left upper pulmonary vein.

Use this view to measure

- Left ventricle diastolic and systolic dimensions.
- Ejection fraction.
- Mitral valve.

Key features of view

- *Left ventricle:* the inferior wall is on the left and anterior wall on the right. This is the preferred view for measurement of left ventricle size because the ventricle is less likely to be foreshortened with the sector at 70–90° (the plane can be made to cut through the apex by turning the probe). Regional abnormalities and papillary muscles can be assessed.
- *Mitral valve:* often a *commissural* view i.e. valve is cut along its commissure so that P1, A2, and P3 segments are seen. Colour flow and Doppler measures are possible. Long axis of valve ring can be assessed.
- *Left atrial appendage:* a curved finger heading down from the left atrium to the left of the mitral valve. Beware of variation in anatomy, multiple lobes or retroverted appendages. These will need assessment with atypical scan planes. Get an optimal image will slight variation in sector angle and probe position. The appendage is aligned for Doppler measures.
- *Left upper pulmonary vein and 'warfarin' ridge:* this lies above the left atrial appendage and is divided from it by the warfarin (or coumadin) ridge (seen as a bright bar on the right of the screen). Probe may need to be withdrawn slightly to view vein. Vein is aligned for Doppler measures.

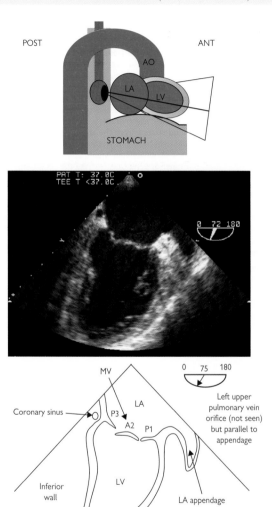

Fig. 5.11 2-chamber view cutting across mitral valve commissure. See ♨ Video 5.7.

Pulmonary vein views

Each pulmonary vein requires a separate view (Fig. 5.12).

Finding the views

Right upper pulmonary vein

- The right upper pulmonary vein is best seen in the adjusted atrial septal (bicaval) view (📖 p.380) lying parallel to the superior vena cava. This view also allows Doppler alignment.
- The vein can be identified starting from the apical 4-chamber 0° view. Rotate the probe to the right hand side of the image and withdraw slightly. The right upper pulmonary vein is seen adjacent to, and wrapping around, the superior vena cava. Varying the sector angle may between 0–20° can be useful to lengthen out the vein.

Right lower pulmonary vein

- The right lower pulmonary vein is best identified starting from the apical 4-chamber 0° view. Rotate the probe to focus on the right hand side of the image (as when finding the right upper pulmonary vein) and then advance the probe slightly. The vein should be seen just below the right upper pulmonary vein.

Left upper pulmonary vein

- The left upper pulmonary vein is best seen in the adjusted 2-chamber view (📖 p.382) lying parallel to, and above, the left atrial appendage. This view also allows Doppler alignment.
- The vein is also seen with sector set to 0°. Rotate the probe to focus on the left hand side of the image and withdraw slightly. Look for the vein orifice.

Left lower pulmonary vein

- To identify the left lower pulmonary vein start from the apical 4-chamber 0° view. Rotate the probe to focus on the left hand side of the image. The vein should be seen below the left upper pulmonary vein orifice.

What do you see?

Use these views to assess
- All 4 pulmonary veins.

Use these views to measure
- Pulmonary vein flow in upper pulmonary veins.

Identifying pulmonary veins

- At 0° the lower veins lie roughly perpendicular to the ultrasound beam (across the screen) while the upper veins lie parallel with the beam (pointing towards the probe).
- As the names suggest, the lower veins lie below the upper veins. If an upper vein is identified then advance the probe slightly to see the lower vein and vice versa.
- Colour flow mapping is very useful to identify the veins. The colour flow will demonstrate blood flow out of the veins into the atrium.

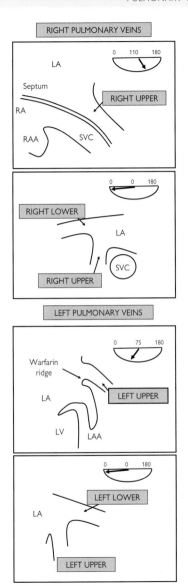

Fig. 5.12 Different viewing positions to identify pulmonary veins.

Coronary sinus view

Seeing the coronary sinus can be useful in some procedures such as electrophysiology studies or pacing device placement. It also allows assessment of congenital abnormalities such as a persistent left superior vena cava (Fig. 5.13).

Finding the view

- Start from a 4-chamber view at 0°.
- The coronary sinus wraps around and below the mitral valve, opening into the right atrium. Therefore advance the probe so that the image plane cuts below the mitral valve. This may be helped by some retroflexion of the probe.
- The optimal view has the coronary sinus perpendicular across the screen opening into the right atrium.

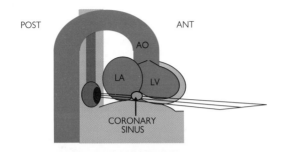

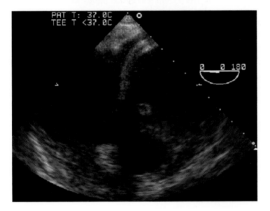

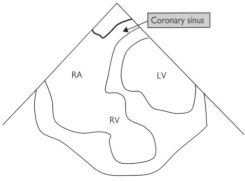

Fig. 5.13 Coronary sinus view. See 📹 Video 5.8.

Transgastric short axis views

Transgastric scanning can be quite uncomfortable to the conscious and mildly sedated patient. Transgastric views should be performed in well-sedated, compliant patients when further information is required. They can also be routinely performed intraoperatively. Short axis views are equivalent to transthoracic parasternal short axis views and can often be adjusted to create mid-papillary and mitral valve level views (Fig. 5.14). They can be particularly useful intraoperatively to monitor left ventricle function.

Finding the view

- From the 4-chamber view, with sector angle at 0°, advance the probe several centimetres. The patient may rouse slightly as you enter the stomach.
- Angulate the probe forwards hard to try and get it at right angles.
- Withdraw the probe so the transducer tip presses on the upper stomach wall, against the diaphragm, underneath the heart.
- Make slight adjustments by turning the probe, as well as withdrawing and advancing until the left ventricle is seen in short axis.
- Keep the probe angulated forward.
- By withdrawing and advancing the probe along the bottom of the heart it is theoretically possible to see the left ventricle at several levels, e.g. mid-papillary, mitral valve.
- The optimal view is an on-axis cross-section through the left ventricle.

What do you see?

Use this view to assess

- Global and regional left ventricle function, wall thickness.
- Mitral valve morphology.
- Can provide information on right ventricle size and function.
- Pericardial effusions may be seen.

Use this view to measure

- Left ventricle size and wall thickness.

Key features of view

- *Left ventricle (mid-papillary level):* with a clear short axis cut through the ventricle the septum, anterior, lateral, and inferior walls of the ventricle can be reviewed. This is an ideal view for measures of left ventricle size and thickness.
- *Mitral valve (mitral valve level):* a slight withdrawal of the probe from the mid-papillary level should bring the image plane up to the mitral valve. You should be able to scan through the chordae up to the leaflet tips. Use colour flow to highlight regurgitation jets.
- *Right ventricle:* the right ventricle can be seen as a crescent around one side of the left ventricle. This view can give an impression of right ventricle size and function.

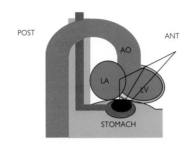

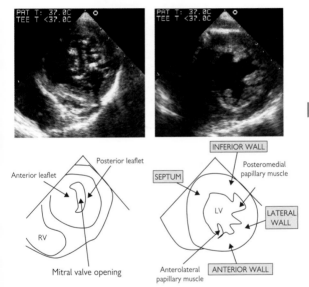

Fig. 5.14 Transgastric short axis views at mitral valve (left) and mid ventricle (right) levels. See 📹 Video 5.9 and 📹 Video 5.10.

Transgastric long axis view

The long axis view provides an unparalleled view of the mitral subvalvular apparatus (Fig. 5.15).

Finding the view

- From the short view rotate the sector angle to 90°.
- Keep hard probe angulation.
- Make slight adjustments by turning the probe until the left ventricle is seen in long axis.
- The optimal view should include the mitral valve, subvalvular apparatus, and left ventricle.

What do you see?

Use this view to assess
- Global and regional left ventricle function, wall thickness.
- Mitral valve morphology.
- Subvalvular mitral apparatus.

Use this view to measure
- Left ventricle size and wall thickness.

Key features of view
- *Left ventricle:* similar to the 2-chamber view the inferior wall is nearest the probe and anterior walls in the far field. Foreshortening occurs easily. This can provide information on wall thickness as well as global and regional function.
- *Mitral valve and subvalvular apparatus:* a commissural view, the leaflet anatomy is not always clear but the subvalvular apparatus can be incredibly detailed. The different order chordae tendinae as well as both papillary muscles can be reviewed. Colour flow can map regurgitation.
- *Left atrium and left atrial appendage:* the left atrium is present but not usually in great detail. You may notice the left atrial appendage in the far field.

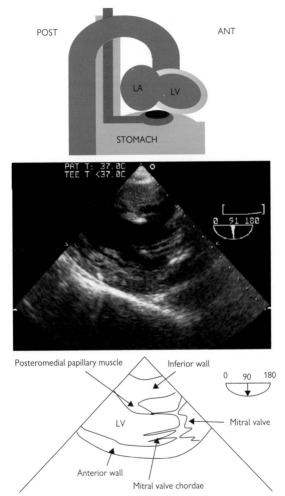

Fig. 5.15 Transgastric long axis view of left ventricle. See 📹 Video 5.11.

Transgastric long axis (aortic) view

The long axis view can be modified slightly to bring the LVOT into the image for Doppler measures across the aortic valve (Fig. 5.16).

Finding the view

- From the long axis view rotate the sector angle to 110°.
- Keep hard probe angulation.
- Make slight adjustments by turning the probe until the LVOT is seen in the far field. Colour flow may help to identify flow through the aortic valve.
- The optimal view should include the LVOT aligned in the far field aligned for Doppler measures.

What do you see?

Use this view to assess

- Doppler measures of aortic valve velocities.

Use this view to measure

- Aortic and LVOT velocities.

Key features of view

- *Aortic valve and LVOT:* the aortic valve may be seen close to the mitral valve in the far field. Colour flow mapping may make this more apparent. The valve and outflow tract is aligned in this view for Doppler measures.

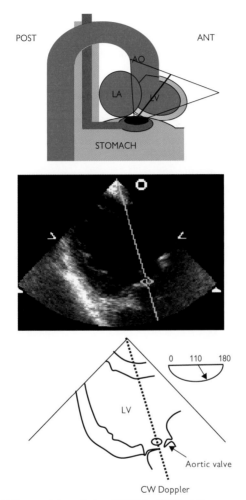

POST

ANT

AO

LA

LV

STOMACH

0   110   180

LV

Aortic valve

CW Doppler

Fig. 5.16 Transgastric long axis view of LVOT. See 🎥 Video 5.12.

Transgastric right ventricular view

This is similar to the left ventricular long axis view but can be difficult to find. However, if available it can give a useful assessment of the right ventricle and inflow (Fig. 5.17).

Finding the view
- From the transgastric long axis left ventricle view turn the probe clockwise.
- The right ventricle should appear in long axis similar to the left ventricle.
- The optimal view should include the tricuspid valve, subvalvular apparatus, and right ventricle.

What do you see?
Use this view to assess
- Tricuspid valve morphology.
- Subvalvular tricuspid apparatus.

Use this view to measure:
- No specific measurements.

Key features of view
- *Right ventricle:* this is an unusual 2-chamber view of the right ventricle and atrium but can give an impression of right-sided chamber size.
- *Tricuspid valve and subvalvular apparatus:* as with the mitral views the subvalvular apparatus is usually detailed. Colour flow can map regurgitation and there can be a qualitative assessment of tricuspid valve function. As the right ventricle is relatively difficult to see with transoesophageal imaging this may provide a good window to look for tricuspid valve pathology, e.g. vegetations and masses.
- *Right atrium:* the right atrium can be viewed.

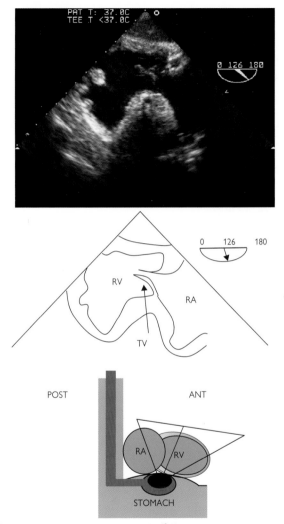

Fig. 5.17 Transgastric right ventricle view. See 🎥 Video 5.13.

Deep transgastric view

Deep transgastric views are only really required when Doppler information is needed about the aortic valve and transthoracic imaging is not possible. The view tries to recreate a transthoracic apical 5-chamber view (Fig. 5.18).

Finding the view
- From the transgastric long axis view advance the probe further into the stomach.
- Set the sector to 0°.
- Ensure full angulation of the probe and good contact with the stomach wall.

What do you see?
Use this view to assess
- Global and regional left ventricle function.
- LVOT and aortic valve.

Use this view to measure
- Left ventricle function.
- Aortic and LVOT velocities (if seen – may need some sector angle adjustment).

Key features of view
- *Aortic valve and LVOT:* the aortic valve lies in the far field and may be highlighted by colour flow mapping. The primary purpose of this view is to align the valve and outflow tract for Doppler measures.
- *Left ventricle:* similar to the 4-chamber view. The septum and lateral wall are seen.

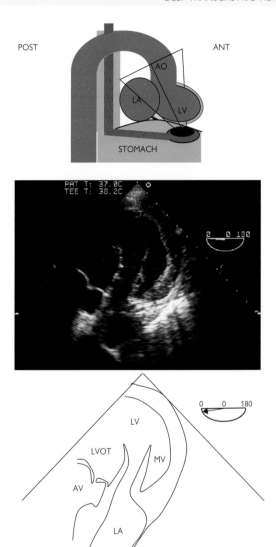

Fig. 5.18 Deep transgastric view. See 📹 Video 5.14.

Pulmonary artery view

A view to study the pulmonary arteries. Can be useful to assess size of artery or look for large pulmonary emboli (Fig. 5.19).

Finding the view
- Start from the short axis aortic view. The sector may need to be reduced slightly to 40°.
- Withdraw the probe slowly until you have a short axis view of the ascending aorta.
- The probe may need to be angulated forward gently to demonstrate the pulmonary artery.

What do you see?
Use this view to assess
- Ascending aorta for dissection or dilatation.
- Pulmonary artery.

Use this view to measure:
- Aortic and pulmonary artery size.

Key features of view
- *Pulmonary arteries:* the right pulmonary artery is seen wrapping around the aorta and lies between the aorta and probe. The main pulmonary artery is seen to the side of the aorta. The left pulmonary artery is not visible.
- *Ascending aorta:* a short segment of the ascending aorta can usually be seen to assess dilatation, dissection, and atheroma.
- *Superior vena cava:* the superior vena cava is seen in cross-section close to the aorta and right pulmonary artery.

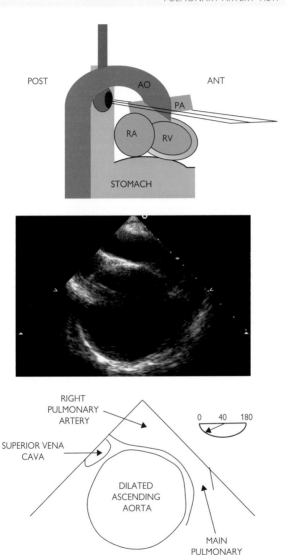

Fig. 5.19 View of the pulmonary artery.

Aortic views

The final views are usually the aortic views (Fig. 5.20). They can be important for monitoring dissection or studying atheroma. They can also be used to assess aortic flow in aortic regurgitation. The only limitation is that TOE can not see the distal ascending aorta and proximal part of the aortic arch as the air-filled left bronchus obscures the view.

Finding the view

- The ascending aorta is seen in the pulmonary artery view. Obtain the short axis aortic view at 50° and then withdraw the probe slowly to scan up the aorta as far as images are maintained.
- For descending aorta and aortic arch, start from the 4-chamber view with a sector angle of 0° and turn the probe slowly so that it starts to face posteriorly.
- It is usually best to turn the probe anti-clockwise until the circular aorta is seen.
- Decrease the depth so that the aorta fills the screen and you usually also need to reduce the gain slightly.
- The probe may then be withdrawn slowly to scan up the aorta. As the aorta curls around the oesophagus some slight turning will be required as the probe is withdrawn.
- The optimal view is a cross-section through the aorta. A long axis view can also be useful and is achieved by changing the sector angle to 90°.

What do you see?

Use this view to assess

- Aortic dissection or dilatation.
- Atheroma and thrombus.
- Aortic flow, e.g. in aortic regurgitation.

Use this view to measure:

- Aortic size.
- Aortic flow.

Key features of view

- *Descending aorta:* there is good depiction of the aortic walls and their layers as well as thickening and gross atherosclerosis. If measurements are made, annotate images with the depth of the probe so that serial measures are possible.
- *Aortic arch:* at the top of the descending aorta the aortic cross-section will disappear and the vessel opens out into the arch. The origin of the left subclavian artery may be seen. By changing the sector angle to 90° at this point a cross-section can be maintained.
- *Ascending aorta:* a short segment of the ascending aorta can usually be seen to assess dilatation, dissection, and atheroma.

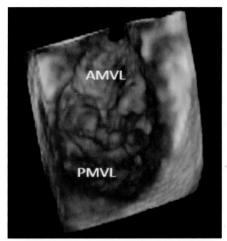

Fig. 5.22 Live 3D acquisition of mitral valve. Subsequent rotation and cropping to allow visualization of the valve from the LV apex. AMVL = anterior mitral valve leaflet; PMVL = posterior mitral valve leaflet. See ⏣ Video 5.18.

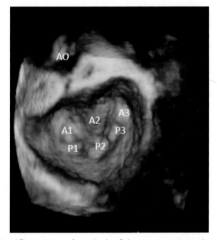

Fig. 5.23 Live 3D acquisition of mitral valve. Subsequent rotation and cropping to allow visualization of the valve from the left atrium and identification of the anterior (A) mitral valve leaflet scallops and posterior (P) mitral valve leaflet scallops; Ao = aorta. See ⏣ Video 5.19.

3D aortic valve

3D imaging of the aortic valve is useful for highlighting the mechanism of pathology and also to guide aortic valve interventional procedures (Fig. 5.24).

Finding the view
- From the mid oesophageal the short axis 50–70° view is used.

Image acquisition modes
- 3D imaging of the aortic valve can be difficult because of its anterior position and thin pliable cusps.
- All 3D acquisition modes can be used although multiple images may need to be recorded when using zoom mode to ensure entire coverage of the valve.
- In full volume mode, colour Doppler can be used to acquire a 3D colour image across the valve.

What do you see?
Use aortic valve views to assess
- Aortic valve morphology and pathology.

3D applications for imaging the aortic valve
- It is becoming increasingly used to guide TAVI (📖 p.464).
- Imaging of prosthetic aortic valves using 3D acquisition modes can be very useful, allowing a detailed assessment of the valve and any coexisting pathology (e.g. areas of dehiscence).

Use view to measure
- 3D colour full volume data sets can be rotated and cut in different planes and used to quantify the origin of the regurgitant jet(s) as well as estimate the vena contracta and regurgitant orifice area.
- As 3D datasets can be viewed from multiple angles and cropped in different planes, it allows estimation of the smallest true AV orifice by planimetry (Fig. 5.25), aortic ring, LVOT, and proximal aorta.

Key features of view
- Anatomy of aortic valve

3D aorta

Image acquisition modes
- All 3D imaging modes can be used depending on the size of the region of interest which is being examined.

What do you see?
Use aortic valve views to assess
- Aorta and root pathology e.g. dissection/atheroma.

3D applications for imaging the aorta
- 3D imaging of the aortic root can provide detailed assessment of complex anatomical pathologies, e.g. aneurysm, aortic dissection.

Use view to measure
- The extent of dissection/thrombus/atheroma if present.

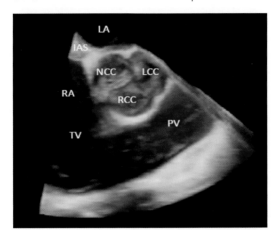

Fig. 5.24 Live 3D TOE short axis view of the aortic valve when closed. View shows non-coronary cusp (NCC), right coronary cusp (RCC), left coronary cusp (LCC), LA (left atrium), inter atrial septum (IAS), right atrium (RA), tricuspid valve (TV), and pulmonary valve (PV). See 📹 Video 5.20 and 📹 Video 5.21.

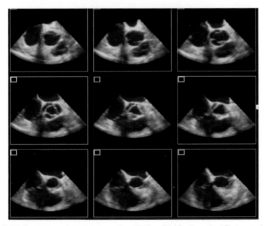

Fig. 5.25 Post-processing systems such as Phillips QLAB allow the 3D view to be sliced down over several planes. Multiple slices seen here from aortic valve short axis view. See 📹 Video 5.22.

3D tricuspid valve

3D imaging of the tricuspid valve can be difficult because of the valve's thin leaflets and also its anterior position (Fig. 5.26).

Finding the view
• From the 4-chamber 0° view or transgastric RV view, rotate the probe so that the tricuspid valve is focused on.

Image acquisition modes
• From the 4-chamber view, 3D datasets of the tricuspid valve can be acquired.
• All 3D acquisition modes can be used although multiple images may need to be recorded when using zoom mode to ensure entire coverage of the valve.
• In full volume mode, colour Doppler can be used to acquire a 3D colour image across the valve.

What do you see?
Use view to assess
• Tricuspid valve and annulus morphology and pathology.

3D applications for imaging the tricuspid valve
• Acquisition of 3D datasets allows post-processing and the tricuspid valve to be rotated to be viewed from the surgical view of the right atrium.
• 3D imaging allows the TV to be viewed from the atria and gives an appreciation of its relationship to the MV and AV.

Use view to measure
• 3D colour full volume data sets can be rotated and cut in different planes and used to quantify the origin of the regurgitant jet(s) as well as estimate the vena contracta and regurgitant orifice area.
• As 3D datasets can be viewed from multiple angles and cropped in different planes, it allows estimation of the smallest true TV orifice by planimetry.

Key features of view
• Rotation and viewing through different planes allow all the valve leaflets and to be viewed.

3D pulmonary valve

• As the pulmonary valve is the most anterior of all valves and also the thinnest, 3D TOE is limited and it is difficult to obtain adequate 3D views.

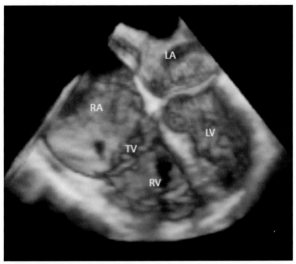

Fig. 5.26 Full volume 3D 4-chamber acquisition showing closed tricuspid valve (TV), right atrium (RA), right ventricle (RV), left atrium (LA), and left ventricle (LV). See 📹 Video 5.23.

3D left ventricle

3D imaging of the left ventricle can be used to help quantify LV function or to confirm the presence of pathology (e.g. apical thrombus) (Fig. 5.27).

Finding the view
- From the 4 chamber 0° view or 2 chamber 90° view, optimize the depth settings and ensure that the ventricle is not foreshortened.

Image acquisition modes
- Full volume acquisition mode is used to enable the best chance of capturing the entire ventricle.
- Close inspection of the full volume datasets is necessary following acquisition to review the image quality and to also exclude the presence of stitch artefacts.

What do you see?
Use view to assess
- Left ventricle

3D applications for imaging the left ventricle
- Post-processing packages allow the ventricular volumes and ejection fraction to be estimated from the 3D datasets (Fig. 5.28).
- The 3D datasets can be rotated and cropped to review images of the left ventricle from the short axis plane.
- Assessment of regional LV function and synchrony.

Use view to measure
- Left ventricular volumes.
- Ejection fraction.

Key features of view
- Left ventricle.

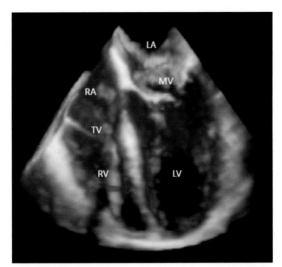

Fig. 5.27 Full volume 3D LV 4-chamber acquisition showing closed tricuspid valve (TV), right atrium (RA), right ventricle (RV), left atrium (LA), mitral valve (MV), and left ventricle (LV).

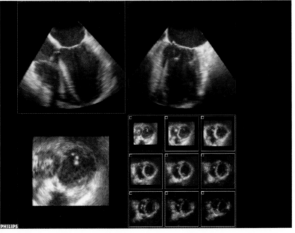

Fig. 5.28 Full volume 3D LV 4-chamber acquisition with post-processing on Phillips QLAB islice. iSlice allows the LV to be viewed in 2 orthogonal views with multiple short axis slices taken over regular intervals (bottom right panel).

3D interatrial septum

3D imaging of the interatrial septum has become invaluable not only for confirming dimensions of atrial septal defects but also to demonstrate the spatial relationship of defects to surrounding structures (Fig. 5.29). These views are also used to guide percutaneous atrial septal interventional procedures.

Finding the view
- The optimal view is obtained from the bicaval 110° view.

Image acquisition modes
- Using full volume or zoom modes allows detailed assessment of the interatrial septum from the bicaval view.

What do you see?
Use views to assess
- Interatrial septum.
- Right atrium.
- Left atrium.
- SVC.
- IVC.

3D applications for imaging the interatrial septum
- Acquisition of 3D datasets allows post-processing and the interatrial septum to be rotated to be viewed from either the left or the right atrium.
- 3D TOE allows a visually superior understanding of the atrial septal anatomy and of pathology compared to 2D TOE.
- It is becoming increasingly used to guide percutaneous closure of atrial septal defects.

Use view to measure
- As 3D datasets can be viewed from multiple angles and cropped in different planes, it allows the size of defects and their relationship to surround structures to be better appreciated.
- 3D colour full volume data sets can be used to view the flow of blood across defects.

Key features of view
- Interatrial septum and defects.
- The relationship of the interatrial septal defects to the MV, AV, SVC, IVC.

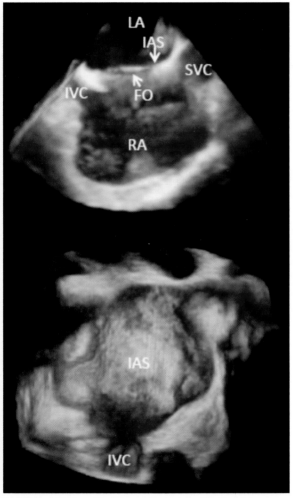

Fig. 5.29 Top: full volume 3D acquisition of atrial septum from bicaval view showing interatrial septum (IAS), fossa ovalis (FO), left atrium (LA), inferior vena cava (IVC), superior vena cava (SVC), and right atrium (RA). Bottom: En face view of the interatrial septum which has been rotated and cropped to show its orientation with regards to the IVC. See 📹 Video 5.24.

X-plane

The use of X-plane imaging during TOE provides the operator with further anatomical information and can also be useful as guidance during interventional procedures. X-plane allows 2 high resolution images of the heart to be displayed simultaneously in real time (Fig. 5.30).

Finding the view
- Obtain the appropriate 2D view.
- Optimize the 2D image settings.
- Select X-plane mode. Live imaging provides 2 orthogonal views from the same heart beat. The initial image on the left is the baseline reference whilst the image on the right can be electronically rotated to any angle between 0–180°.
- When happy acquire the image.
- X-plane images can be acquired with and without the use of colour Doppler.

Use this view to
- Examine the left atrial appendage anatomy and for pathology (e.g. thrombus).
- When high spatial and temporal resolution is needed e.g. valve vegetations.

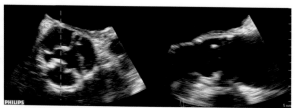

Fig. 5.30 X-plane image acquisition of the aortic valve. After selecting X-plane, the left hand image will display the current live image. Adjusting the angle cursor (red dashed line) will alter the angle of acquisition of the second image on the left hand side. See 📹 Video 5.25.

Transoesophageal anatomy and pathology: valves

Mitral valve

TOE is one of the most important tools for the assessment of mitral valve disease and allows superb visualization of the mitral valve. The modality is particularly good for systematic reviews of the different valve segments. Mitral valve anatomy is described on 📖 p.106. Briefly, there are 2 leaflets each with 3 segments (or scallops)—a large anterior and a crescent-shaped posterior leaflet. Assessment of stenosis and regurgitation follows the same criteria as for transthoracic imaging (📖 pp.110 and 116) but TOE allows a more detailed study of the pathology underlying regurgitation or stenosis.

Normal findings

Views

- The mitral valve is sliced through in virtually all the mid-oesophageal views and the 'screenwiper' principle allows rotation through the valve in multiple planes (Fig. 6.1). The mid-oesophageal views also allow alignment of Doppler and colour flow across the valve. The minimum views are the mid-oesophageal views at around 0°, 135°, 90°, and 80°.
- The transgastric views provide additional information in both the short axis 0° (pulled back slightly) and the long axis 90° view for the subvalvular apparatus.

Normal findings

- 4-chamber 0° view: this classically includes A2, A1, and P1 segments of the valve (however, there is a tendency to cut more through A2 and P2 if the LVOT is seen and the papillary muscles are not evident).
- Long axis 135° view: equivalent to the apical 3-chamber view this gives a good stable view of A2 and P2.
- 2-chamber 75° view: stable 'commissural' view to see P1 and P3 either side of A2. Rotation of the probe allows you to swing more towards the anterior or posterior leaflet. Slight adjustment of sector angle will bring in the left atrial appendage and localize A1/P1 next to the appendage.
- Transgastric short axis view or 'fish mouth' view has the A3/P3 segments nearest the probe. The 90° view can be used to look at the papillary muscles and chordae.

Identifying mitral valve leaflets and segments

There are rigorous descriptions of which leaflets are seen in which view. Initially standard views allow good orientation but as you become more familiar you can play with these by slight adjustments of the probe to cut through the 3D structure at any point. There are 2 tips to identify the segments and leaflets:

- The anterior leaflet is nearest the septum/LVOT and usually appears larger than the posterior leaflet.
- The segments are numbered so that A1 and P1 are nearest the left atrial appendage.

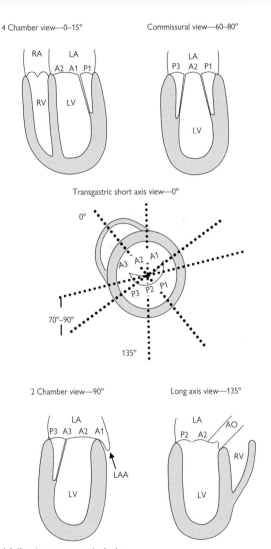

4 Chamber view—0–15°

Commissural view—60–80°

Transgastric short axis view—0°

2 Chamber view—90°

Long axis view—135°

Fig. 6.1 Key views to assess mitral valve.

Mitral regurgitation

TOE should be used to assess mitral regurgitation when:
- TTE is inconclusive or technically difficult.
- To define the underlying mechanism for planning mitral valve surgery.

TOE is particularly useful to visualize where the regurgitant jet passes through the valve. Higher transducer frequencies and multiple views result in more reliable measurements of both vena contracta and flow convergence. However, the different transducer frequency, pulse repetition frequency, and gain also mean they appear larger on transoesophageal images than transthoracic images.

Assessment

Appearance
- Start in the 4-chamber 0° view and map the regurgitation with colour flow. Scan through the valve at different angles to establish the shape, direction, and pattern of the jet. Comment on:
  - Where the regurgitation passes through the valve, e.g. perforation, failure of coaptation, prolapse of a leaflet scallop.
  - Direction of eccentric jets (anterior or posterior). Remember anteriorly-directed suggests posterior valve pathology and vice versa.
  - How far back the jet extends (involving pulmonary veins?).
  - If there are several jets comment on each.
- Use transgastric long axis 90° view to look at subvalvular apparatus (Fig. 6.2). Comment on: papillary muscle and chordae with reference to shortening and rupture.
- Report associated features, e.g. atrial size, ventricle size, and function.

3D TOE MR
- As the probe is much closer in TOE and with higher resolution, live imaging can often be used rather than full-volume acquisition.
- Studies have demonstrated greater accuracy than 2D TOE in identifying the position of the prolapse (see 📖 p.428).
- Excellent resolution is possible.
- As well as being used for assessment of regurgitation, 3D TOE can guide placement of clips for transcutaneous treatment of mitral regurgitation.

3D colour flow Doppler
- This allows assessment of MR especially eccentric jets (Fig. 6.5).
- Acquisition does require multiple cycles and there may be problems with artefacts on reconstruction, especially with AF.
- 2D PISA assessment is based on the assumption of a hemispherical 3D shape. However, this is not always the case and all planes can be assessed with 3D TOE (Fig. 6.3).
- The origin of paravalvular leaks can be difficult to identify. However, this can be made easier using 3D TOE.

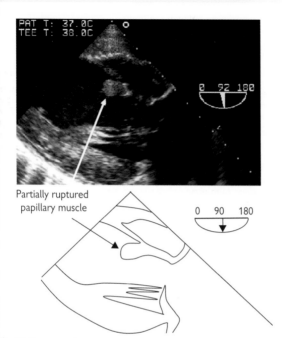

Partially ruptured
papillary muscle

Fig. 6.2 Transgastric long axis view demonstrates subvalvular apparatus. In this
example there is a partial papillary muscle rupture.

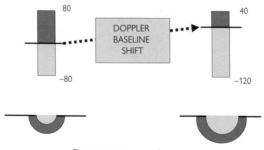

Flow convergence zone becomes
larger and more clearly defined

Fig. 6.3 Flow convergence radius is more clearly defined with Doppler baseline shift.

Grading severity

Assess severity on vena contracta, flow convergence, pulmonary venous flow, and valve structure. Colour jet area can also be used (Table 6.1).

Colour Doppler jet area

This can be difficult to assess with TOE because sector width often does not include the whole of the atrium. Proportional jet area is therefore difficult to judge. 4-chamber 0° and long axis 135° views may give the best impression.

Vena contracta

TOE provides excellent views and resolution for measurement of colour flow through the valve.

- In mid-oesophageal views choose the plane which cuts through the jet
- Zoom in on the colour flow through the mitral valve and record a loop. Identify the image with maximal flow through the valve.
- The vena contracta is the narrowest region of the regurgitant jet (usually as it passes through the valve). Report the diameter.

Pulmonary venous flow

TOE provides a unique opportunity to visualize directly all 4 pulmonary veins and measure pulmonary vein flow (Fig. 6.4). The contralateral pulmonary vein to an eccentric jet (i.e. left pulmonary veins for an anteriorly directed jet and vice versa) should be used to avoid changes in flow due to washing of the jet into the vein.

- In 4-chamber 0° view rotate to the left to identify the left-sided veins (📖 p.384). Advance or withdraw the probe to bring them into view. The left upper pulmonary vein usually points towards the probe and left lower pulmonary vein is perpendicular. To help with identification place colour flow by the edge of the atrium and look for the jets of the veins draining into the atrium. Slight changes in the plane angle can optimize the view. Right-sided veins are identified in the same way but with rotation to the right. Again the right upper pulmonary vein points towards the probe and lower vein is perpendicular.
- Alternative views are: (1) 110° bicaval view rotated to the left - right upper pulmonary vein lies parallel to the septum (2) 2-chamber 75° (left atrial appendage) view, in which the left upper pulmonary vein lies parallel to the left atrial appendage.
- Place the pulsed wave Doppler sample volume around 1 cm into the chosen vein (Fig. 6.4).
- Look at the systolic and diastolic components of the spectral trace and comment if the systolic wave is blunted or reversed relative to the diastolic wave (normally the same direction, with systolic dominant).

Supportive measures

These can be measured as for transthoracic imaging (📖 p.122).

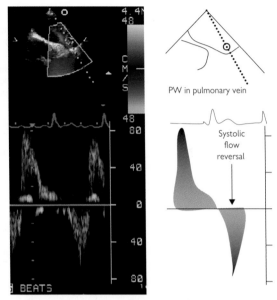

Fig. 6.4 Pulmonary venous flow with an example of abnormal systolic flow reversal.

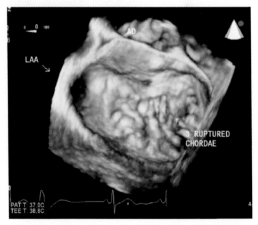

Fig. 6.5 Live 3D acquisition of mitral valve with P1 prolapse. The image has been cropped and rotated to be seen from the left atrium. AV aortic valve, the anterior (A) mitral valve scallops and posterior (P) mitral valve leaflet scallops are seen. See ▣ Video 6.1.

Carpentier (functional) classification

The Carpentier classification (Type 1 to 3) is sometimes used to report the functional basis for mitral regurgitation. This categorizes cause according to leaflet motion. It is relevant to different surgical approaches.

- Normal leaflet motion (Type 1):
  - Annular dilatation causes regurgitation due to failed coaptation.
  - Leaflet perforation (e.g. from endocarditis).
- Excessive leaflet motion (Type 2):
  - Prolapse of leaflet edge beyond the plane of the annulus.
  - Mitral valve prolapse, rupture/dysfunction of the papillary muscle.
- Restricted leaflet motion (Type 3):
  - Leaflet edge remains below the plane of the annulus during systole. Usually secondary to rheumatic disease, left ventricle dilatation, posterior wall infarction.

Table 6.1 Parameters to assess mitral regurgitation

Specific signs of severity

	Mild	Severe
Vena contracta	<0.3cm	>0.7cm
Jet (Nyquist 50–60cm/s)	<4cm or <20% left atrium Small & central	>40% left atrium large & central or wall impinging and swirling
PISA r (Nyquist 40cm/s) None/minimal	(<0.4cm)	Large (>1cm)
Pulmonary vein flow	–	Systolic reversal
Valve structure	–	Flail or rupture

Supportive signs of severity

	Mild	Severe
Pulmonary vein flow	Systolic dominant	
Mitral inflow	A-wave dominant	E-wave dominant (>1.2 m/s)
CW trace	Soft & parabolic	Dense & triangular
LV and LA	Normal size LV if chronic MR	Enlarged LV & LA if no other cause

Report as *moderate* if signs of regurgitation are greater than *mild* but there are no features of *severe* regurgitation.

Mitral valve prolapse

The clear images of valve leaflets allow identification of the morphology of mitral valve prolapse. Description of mitral valve prolapse is a common indication for TOE because of its clinical importance to determine whether a valve can be repaired or will need to be replaced. The commonest prolapse is of the P2 segment of the posterior leaflet. This is amenable to a standard repair procedure.

Assessment of prolapse

- Start by studying the regurgitation. Comment on appearance and severity. Take particular note of the direction of the jet as a guide to the predominant leaflet prolapse (Fig. 6.6). Anteriorly-directed suggests posterior leaflet prolapse and vice versa. Also comment on changes in left atrial and ventricular size and function.
- Then use the 'screenwiper' principle to scan through the mitral valve at 0°, 135°, 110°, 80° (Fig. 6.7). Ensure each segment has been studied (Fig. 6.6). Comment on which segments prolapse. If the tips of the segment reflect back into the left atrium then report this as 'flail' (important when planning the operation).
- Remember that both leaflets, or more than one segment, may be prolapsing. Report all the abnormalities.
- A transgastric 0° short axis view can be used to confirm the segment prolapse and the long axis 90° view should be used to look at the subvalvular apparatus to identify chordae or papillary muscle rupture.

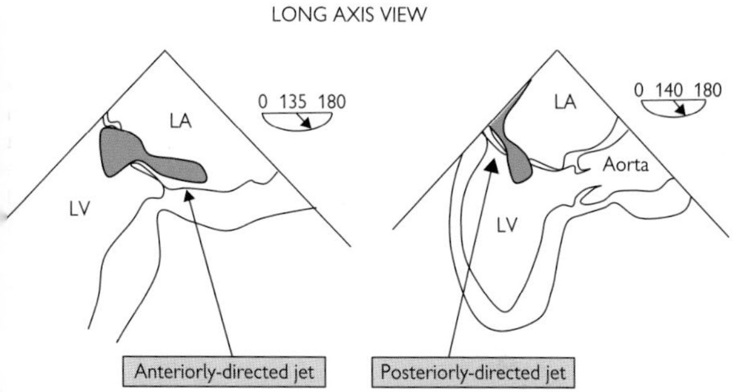

LONG AXIS VIEW

Fig. 6.6 Examples of mitral valve prolapse in 135° long axis views. Left figure shows an anteriorly-directed jet due to posterior leaflet prolapse and the right figure a posteriorly-directed jet.

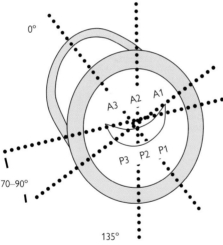

Fig. 6.7 The short axis figure demonstrates which scallops are seen in the three key views. The 4-chamber 0° and long axis 135° views are particularly good for studying the central scallops (A2 and P2). The 2-chamber view with sector variation between 70–90° can be very useful for looking at the side scallops (A1/P1, A3/P3).

3D assessment of prolapse

The use of 3D echocardiography has lead to improvements in the understanding of normal MV anatomy and the cause for mitral valvular pathology.

- Set up a 3D volume from the oesophageal position. Ensure from the biplane view that it includes all the mitral valve and in particular the area you suspect is prolapsing.
- Once the volume position and image quality is optimized, acquire a 3D dataset. Live 3D or 3D zoom image mode acquisition is ideally suited to imaging of the mitral valve as the image volume usually is sufficient for good coverage of the valve and there is adequate spatial and temporal resolution without the limitation of stitching artefacts seen with full volume acquisition. However, you may want to acquire a full volume as well for later post-processing.
- Rotate, crop, and set gain settings to focus on the mitral valve.
- View the valve from the left atrium and assess valvular morphology in detail. Identify individual scallops (remember A1 and P1 lie near the left atrial appendage, which should be visible as a round opening in the left atrial wall) (Figs. 6.8, 6.11).
- Confirm your impression from the 2D images of the extent of prolapse (number of scallops, width of prolapsing scallop) and confirm the cause of the prolapse e.g. ruptured chordae.
- In particular, use the global 3D view to resolve any uncertainties about the number of affected scallops and position of pathology, as well as ensuring there are no other areas of pathology on the mitral valve that were missed on the 2D sequential views.
- 3D colour flow mapping may be useful to confirm the position of small areas of prolapse (Fig. 6.9).
- The images can then be post-processed to create a model of the mitral valve to aid surgery.

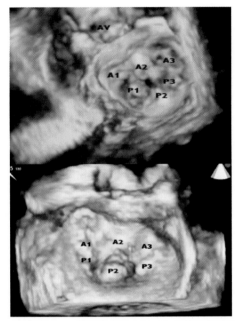

Fig. 6.8 Live 3D acquisition of mitral valve with P1 prolapse (above) and P2 prolapse (below). The image has been cropped and rotated to be seen from the left atrium. AV aortic valve, the anterior (A) mitral valve scallops and posterior (P) mitral valve leaflet scallops are seen. See 🎬 Video 6.2, 🎬 Video 6.3, 🎬 Video 6.4.

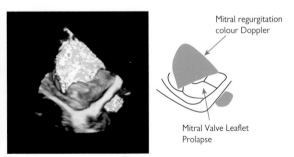

Fig. 6.9 3D colour Doppler acquisition of mitral regurgitation due to mitral valve leaflet prolapse. See 🎬 Video 6.5.

Post-processing of 3D datasets to create mitral valve model

- 2D echocardiography only allows the mitral valve annulus to be measured in 2 perpendicular planes. There may be difficulties in choosing the appropriate sites for annulus measurement due to poor spatial resolution.
- The advent of complex post-processing software such as TomTec and Phillips mitral valve quantification have allowed extraction of modelling data from 3D volumes (Fig. 6.10).
- A series of 2D sections are obtained from the 3D data and the operator defines the annulus and commissures and traces the leaflets. The post processing software then generates a valve model.
- Different parameters of the mitral valve can then be quantified according to a number of presets.

These advances have improved the understanding of the complex geometry of the mitral annulus and has added to the surgical decision-making process.

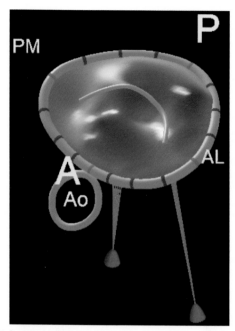

Fig. 6.10 Reconstructed 3D image of mitral valve prolapse. The areas of maximal prolapse are shown in red. A = anterior; P = posterior; PM = posteromedial; AL = anterolateral; Ao = aorta.

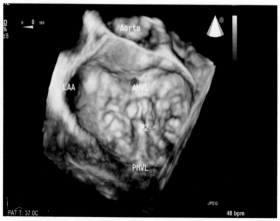

Fig. 6.11 Live 3D view showing left atrial appendage (LAA) and surgical view of mitral valve from left atrium.

Mitral stenosis

TOE is not routinely used to assess mitral stenosis but stenosis should be commented upon and graded if seen during a study. Assessment may be needed if there are poor transthoracic windows or if the valve is being assessed for percutaneous intervention with balloon valvotomy (📖 p.444). TOE is also used intraoperatively during percutaneous interventions on the mitral valve.

Appearance

Remember to comment on mobility, calcification, and chordae. Comment on associated valvular lesions, left atrium, and right heart.

Grading severity

Grade severity on planimetered area (📖 p.434) supported by pressure half time and pressure gradient, see Table 6.2.

Pressure half-time and pressure gradient:

- In any oesophageal view with good alignment through the valve align the CW Doppler through the mitral valve orifice.
- For pressure half-time, measure the slope of the E-wave diastolic flow on the spectral trace (Fig. 6.12). Trace the Doppler waveform to obtain mean pressure gradient. Remember:

Table 6.2 Parameters to assess mitral stenosis

	Mild	Moderate	Severe
MV area (cm^2)	>1.5	1.0–1.5	<1.0
MV pressure half-time (ms)	<150	150–220	>220
Mean pressure gradient (mmHg)	<5	Variable	>10
TR velocity (m/s)	<2.7	Variable	>3

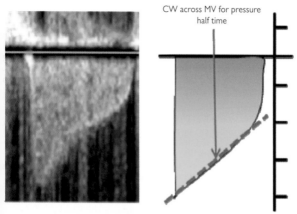

CW across MV for pressure
half time

Fig. 6.12 Pressure half-time measured in a long axis view.

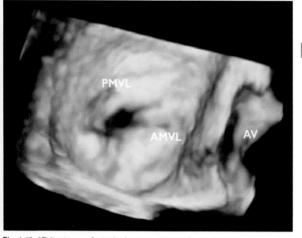

Fig. 6.13 3D live image of mitral valve in a patient with mitral stenosis. Image captured at end-diastole highlighting the small central mitral valve orifice. PMVL = posterior mitral valve leaflet; AMVL = anterior mitral valve leaflet; AV = aortic valve. See 📹 Video 6.6.

$$Mitral\ valve\ area = 220/pressure\ half\text{-}time$$

Planimetry
- A transgastric 0° view provides a short axis 'fish mouth' view of the mitral valve. The probe may need to be withdrawn and advanced slightly to optimize the image and ensure the *leaflet tips* are being imaged. Identify the maximum opening in diastole and trace along the inner edge of the leaflets. Report the surface area of the orifice.

3D planimetry
- 3D TOE can aid in mitral stenosis assessment as planimetry of the mitral valve orifice can be performed on a 3D acquisition whereby the true leaflet tip orifice can be selected within a multiplanar reconstruction (Fig. 6.13).
- Set up a 3D volume from the oesophageal position ensuring that all of the mitral valve is seen in the biplane view. Minor adjustments may be needed to find the optimal view especially in the presence of drop out shadowing which can be seen in calcific mitral stenosis (Fig. 6.14).
- When happy with the probe position, acquire the 3D image.
- Rotate, crop, and set gain settings to focus on the mitral valve and view the valve from the left atrium.
- The dataset can be exported for post-processing. The mitral valve will be displayed in 2 orthogonal views. The cropping plane can then be adjusted to cut through the narrowest end-diastolic MV orifice (Fig. 6.15).

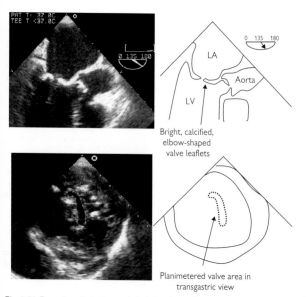

LA

Aorta

LV

Bright, calcified,
elbow-shaped
valve leaflets

Planimetered valve area in
transgastric view

Fig. 6.14 Examples of mitral stenosis in 4-chamber and transgastric views.
Note planimetered surface area in short axis view.

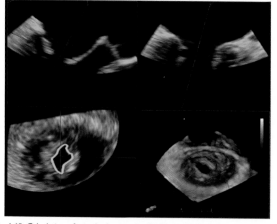

Fig. 6.15 Calculation of mitral valve area by QLAB 7.1 (Phillips). Two orthogonal
views of the mitral valve (top left quadrant and top right quadrant) following 3D
zoom mode live acquisition (bottom right quadrant). Following alignment of the
mitral valve orifice, the valve area can be traced (bottom left quadrant).

Mitral valve preoperative assessment

Transoesophageal echocardiographic assessment of the mitral valve is essential before surgery. The key surgical decision in the patient with mitral regurgitation is whether the valve is to be repaired or replaced. With mitral stenosis the request for imaging is usually to assess suitability for valvotomy or to determine severity of stenosis and effects on the left ventricle and other valves.

What the surgeon wants to know

Mitral regurgitation

The main objectives prior to mitral valve surgery are to define:

- Underlying anatomic details of the mitral regurgitation. Include a full assessment (📖 p.420) and ensure comments on:
  - Severity.
  - Central or eccentric.
  - If prolapse, which scallops are affected and whether flail elements.
- Size of annuloplasty ring likely to be needed if repaired or size of valve if replaced. Report:
  - Mitral annulus size in 2 orthogonal planes.
  - Leaflet length.
- Presence and location of annulus calcification. There is a risk of annulus leak if in an area of repair.
- If regurgitation secondary to endocarditis, comment on complications of the endocarditis: fistulae from left ventricle to aorta, right ventricle or left atrium; mitral valve annulus abscess; other valve involvement in endocarditis (typically aortic or tricuspid valve).

3D mitral valve preoperative assessment

3D TOE is eminently suited to mitral valve assessment (Fig. 6.16). Both a 3D zoom and full volume acquisition can be used to precisely quantify leaflet anatomy, annulus geometry, and region of prolapse, which can aid surgical planning.

3D image acquisition of the mitral valve has the applications:

- Allows the visualization of the mitral valve from both the atrial and ventricular aspect providing views familiar to the surgeon.
- In the assessment of certain types of mitral valve prolapse 3D TOE accurately identifies involved segments.
- In mitral stenosis 3D TOE can provide detailed assessment of the leaflets and their commissures as well as subvalvular apparatus.

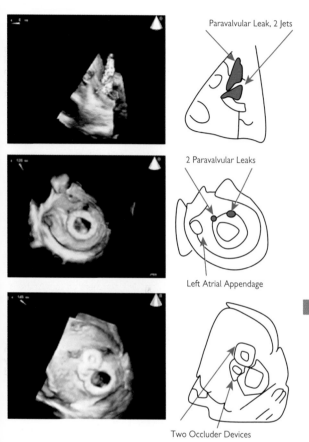

Fig. 6.16 3D TOE prosthetic valve assessment. See 🎥 Video 6.7, 🎥 Video 6.8, 🎥 Video 6.9. Surgical view showing bioprosthesis in mitral position with paravalvular leak (top and middle). Same value with 2 Amplatz occluder devices (bottom) to close leaks.

Mitral stenosis
- Underlying anatomical details of the mitral stenosis. Include a full assessment (📖 p.432) and ensure comments on:
  - Severity.
  - Pathological basis: rheumatic or degenerative.
- Assess suitability for valvuloplasty (📖 p.444).
- Size of replacement valve likely to be needed. Report:
  - Mitral annulus size (in both valve axes if possible).

For all mitral surgery
- Left atrial size. A dilated left atrium (>50 mm) provides good surgical exposure of mitral valve directly through a left atrial incision. If the left atrium is normal size or only mildly increased the surgeon may need an alternative surgical approach (e.g. transatrial septum).
- Assessment of cardiac function. Significant left ventricle dysfunction caused by mitral regurgitation encourages mitral valve repair rather than replacement.
- Reports of other valve disease, particularly the aortic valve.

Preoperative versus intraoperative assessment

The severity of mitral regurgitation may be underestimated during intra-operative TOE. Preload, afterload, and inotropic state of the heart are reduced during general anaesthesia. Therefore, all patients undergoing valve surgery should have transoesophageal imaging prior to surgery. Assessment of the valve intraoperatively should take into account the preoperative information and changes in conditions due to the anaesthesia. Volume loading and inotropic agents can sometimes be used to mimic haemodynamics comparable to those without anaesthesia.

Factors that make mitral valve repair unfavourable

- Annular calcification. It is most common in the posterior annulus and can extend into the myocardium and leaflets.
- Marked mitral ring dilatation (>5cm in the 2-chamber view).
- Extensive leaflet disease (3 or greater prolapsed or flail segments seen).

Risk of systolic anterior motion of mitral valve post-repair

If repair is planned then it is important to assess, before surgery, the risk of postoperative systolic anterior motion of the anterior leaflet and consequent obstruction of the LVOT. This causes obstruction in ~15% of patients after mitral valve repair. The following findings in the preoperative examination are associated with an increased risk of postoperative systolic anterior motion of the anterior leaflet and should be reported if present:

- Excess mitral leaflet tissue. Particularly elongated anterior leaflet causing an increase in slack leaflet available to obstruct the outflow tract.
- Anteriorly-displaced papillary muscles.
- Non-dilated left ventricle.
- Narrow mitral-aortic angle.
- More anterior position of the leaflet coaptation point due to relatively large posterior mitral leaflet: Anterior to posterior leaflet ratio <1.
- Distance from the coaptation point to the septum <2.5cm.

In high-risk cases the surgical approach may be modified. In patients with an excessive posterior leaflet a sliding leaflet plasty can be carried out after resection of the P2 segment. Another option is the use of a rigid ring to increase the anterior–posterior diameter—in particular if the coaptation line is displaced anteriorly after resection of excessive tissue.

MitraClip®

The MitraClip® is a device which allows percutaneous edge-to-edge repair for mitral regurgitation (Fig. 6.17). There are several anatomical features which are assessed echocardiographically when determining the suitability for the MitraClip®.

Contraindications

- Mitral valve orifice <4cm² with secondary mitral regurgitation.
- Endocarditis.
- Cardiac mass/thrombus.
- Active rheumatic valve disease.
- Mitral stenosis.
- Previous mitral valve replacement.
- Unsuitable leaflet anatomy (calcification and/or cleft affecting leaflets in the potential deployment zone).
- The presence of a flail leaflet when: the width of the flail segment ≥15mm or the flail gap is ≥10mm; bileaflet flail.

Anatomic suitability

- A TOE is carried out pre device deployment to carefully analyse the anatomy of the interatrial septum and the mitral valve leaflets, annulus, chordae, and subvalvular apparatus (Fig. 6.18).
- The presence of an atrial septal defect/patent foramen ovale and the thickness of the atrial septum should be noted. These will determine the ease with which the transseptal puncture is performed.
- All standard mitral valve views should be obtained with and without colour Doppler in order to identify the area of maximal MR as well as the anatomy of each leaflet at that position.
- The grasping zone of the MitraClip® is ideally at the junction of A2:P2. Adverse factors which may hinder device deployment should be noted: leaflet thickness; leaflet calcification; chordal fusion/calcification or calcification of the subvalvular apparatus below the maximal area of MR.

Degenerative MR (see Fig. 6.18)

- *Flail gap*: should be taken in the 135° long axis, 0° 4-chamber or 90° 2-chamber view where the flail gap is largest. (Needs to be <10mm.)
- *Flail width*: should be taken in transgastric short axis where the flail width is largest. (Needs to be <15mm.)

Functional MR

- *Coaption depth*: should be taken in 0° 4-chamber view where coaption depth is greatest. (Needs to be <11mm.)
- *Coaption length*: should be taken in 0° 4-chamber view where length is shortest. (Needs to be >2mm.)

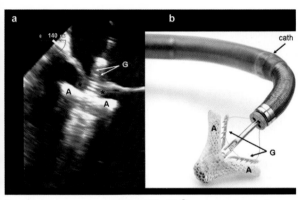

Fig. 6.17 Appearance of a non-deployed MitraClip® a. transoesophageal echocardiogram with the clip across the mitral valve leaflets (LVOT view) and the leaflets inserted into the V between the arms of the clip (ventricular aspect of the valve, A) and the grippers (atrial aspect of the valve, G). Both leaflet tips should be clearly seen in this position (*) prior to closure of the clip and grasping the leaflet.

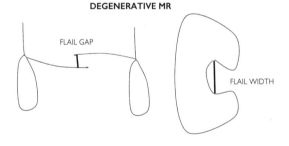

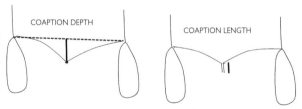

Fig. 6.18 How to measure key criteria for Mitral Clip® suitability.

Procedure

Transseptal puncture

- The bicaval view, short axis view and 4-chamber view of the atrial septum should all be obtained to demonstrate the anatomy. The trans-septal catheter tip can be watched moving into the fossa ovalis causing tenting (Fig. 6.19).
- Generally the puncture should be 3–4cm from the mitral valve although this should be modified according to the site and mechanism of the pathology.
- Following successful puncture, views are obtained to help the safe navigation of the catheter and then guidewire into the left upper pulmonary vein (avoiding the left atrial appendage).

Introduction of guide catheter and MitraClip®

- Using a modified short axis view the guide catheter/dilator are introduced. The guide catheter has echogenic markers on it helping to identify when it has crossed the interatrial septum.
- The dilator and guidewire are withdrawn and the MitraClip® inserted until visible in the mid LA.
- The MitraClip® is navigated to a position where it straddles the MV. An LVOT view will demonstrate the MitraClip® above the MV.

Crossing the mitral valve

- Using a combination of the LVOT and bicommissural views the clip is positioned directly over the target area of the MV. Biplane echocardiography can be useful to confirm this position in 2 orthogonal views.
- Correct position is confirmed using colour Doppler and the clip should ideally bisect the regurgitant jet equally.
- The clip is advanced into the LV and the superior aspect of the gripper arms should be clearly identified below the MV leaflets.
- Live 3D TOE images can also help confirm the positioning and that the clip is perpendicular to the closure line of the valves (Fig. 6.20).

MitraClip® insertion and grasping

- Once the positioning of the clip has been confirmed it is retracted towards the MV leaflets. Echocardiography is pivotal to ensure that there is no distortion to the valvar/subvalvar apparatus and that perpendicularity is maintained.
- The moment of grasp should be recorded to ensure that a suitable amount of leaflet is held within each arm of the clip.

Confirmation of leaflet grasping and device deployment

- Adequate grasp is confirmed by visualizing the anterior and posterior mitral valve leaflets from the LVOT and 4-chamber views.
- It is important to note the leaflet insertion point and leaflet movement is adequate.
- When happy with adequate leaflet grasping the clip arms are closed to approximately 60° and final images are performed to demonstrate the accurate placement of the clip, the reduction in the degree of MR and the absence of mitral stenosis.

- The MitraClip® is then fully deployed and the valve reassessed to determine the haemodynamic success of the procedure, any potential requirement for a second clip, and the size of the residual defect from the transeptal puncture.

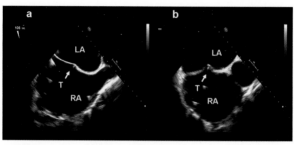

Fig. 6.19 Positioning of catheter for transseptal puncture. Tenting (T) of the inter-atrial septum at the fossa ovalis caused by the transseptal catheter is clearly seen, with the two views allowing superoinferior adjustment (a, bicaval) and antero-posterior adjustment (b, modified short axis aortic). LA = left atrium, RA = right atrium, T = tenting.

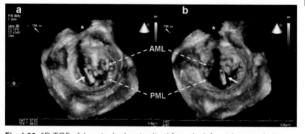

Fig. 6.20 3D TOE of the mitral valve visualized from the left atrial aspect during positioning of the MitraClip® above the valve leaflets to ensure perpendicularity with the closure line of the valve.

Mitral valve balloon valvotomy

TOE is performed routinely to assess suitability for percutaneous valvotomy for treatment of mitral stenosis. Contraindications to intervention that should be reported include:
- Left atrial appendage thrombus.
- Moderate mitral regurgitation or greater.
- Severe aortic or tricuspid valvular disease.

Echocardiographic scoring of mitral valve morphology can be preformed to predict successful outcome. The commonest is the Wilkin's scoring based on 4 features each scored 1–4, giving a minimum score of 4 and maximum of 16. The lower the score the more suitable the valve for balloon valvotomy. A score of >8 suggests poor long-term outcome with percutaneous intervention.

Leaflet mobility

1 Highly mobile with restriction of leaflet tips only.
2 Mid portion and base of leaflets have reduced mobility.
3 Valve leaflets move forward in diastole mainly at the base.
4 No or minimal forward movement of the leaflets in diastole.

Valvar thickening

1 Leaflets near normal (4–5mm).
2 Mid leaflet thickening, pronounced thickening of the margins.
3 Thickening extends through entire leaflet (5–8mm).
4 Pronounced thickening of all leaflet tissue (8–10mm).

Subvalvar thickening

1 Minimal thickening of chordal structure just below the valve.
2 Tickening of chordae extending up to 1/3 of chordal length.
3 Thickening extending to the distal 1/3 of chordae.
4 Extensive thickening and shortening of all chorda extending down to the papillary muscles.

Valve calcification

1 A single area of increased echo brightness.
2 Scattered areas of brightness confined to the leaflet margins.
3 Brightness extending into the mid portion of the leaflets.
4 Extensive brightness through most of the leaflet tissue.

3D TOE during balloon valvotomy?

Balloon mitral valvuloplasty is usually performed with echocardiography guidance—3D TOE is ideal for monitoring transseptal puncture, balloon placement, inflation, and effects on the valve.

Doppler indices are inaccurate post-valvuloplasty and 3D planimetry allows a more accurate assessment of procedural success (with the best correlation with invasive monitoring) or immediate complications.

Mitral valve repair

Postoperative assessment

Assessment of mitral valve repair should be based on:

Residual regurgitation

Despite competent valve at surgical inspection and leak test by the surgeon there may still be significant valvular regurgitation in the beating, volume-loaded heart. This may be due to ischaemic wall dysfunction or systolic anterior motion of the mitral leaflet. Use standard 2D and colour images to assess severity, location, and likely underlying mechanism. 3D image can provide much more precise location and mechanisms of residual regurgitation.

- Moderate to severe residual regurgitation usually requires surgical revision or conversion to valve replacement.
- Para-annulus leak can occur after repair if there was a large posterior leaflet resection. Even mild degrees of para-annulus leak usually require further surgical revision to avoid postoperative haemolysis.

New stenosis

After repair of the mitral valve the repaired leaflet usually appears thickened, shortened, and almost immobile. Use CW Doppler to assess trans-mitral pressure gradient and pressure half-time. However, pressure half-time method may be inaccurate immediately postoperative (the method assumes that the left atrial and ventricular compliance do not affect the pressure decline, but up to 72 hours after surgery compliance is altered). Interpret orifice area taking into account heart rate and stroke volume. Stenosis is often due to under-sized annuloplasty.

Systolic anterior leaflet motion/left ventricle outflow obstruction

Systolic anterior leaflet motion/left ventricle outflow obstruction can be due to mitral valve repair with or without concomitant basal septal hypertrophy, but also can be caused by haemodynamic factors. Inotropic agents, vasodilators, and low volume states provoke systolic anterior leaflet motion/ left ventricle outflow obstruction in susceptible patients and have to be discontinued before considering re-intervention. In some patients beta-blockers may be useful. To demonstrate systolic anterior motion of the mitral leaflet use the aortic long axis 135° view. 2D and M-mode images can demonstrate abnormal leaflet movement. However, Doppler measurements have to be performed in gastric views, which may be difficult in theatre and the peak gradient of outflow tract should be differentiated from the mitral regurgitation jet.

Consider whether effects can be reduced by changes in cardiac physiology (improved left ventricle cavity size and diastolic filling): increase left ventricle filling, stop/reduce positive inotropic drugs, commence beta-blockade, pace the ventricle. Monitor effectiveness of medical treatments with repeat echocardiography. If medical management fails surgical revision of repair or valve replacement may be indicated.

Left ventricular function

Hypo- or akinesis of the lateral and inferoposterior wall can be due to circumflex artery injury if sutures are too deep into the mitral ring. New impaired posterior wall contraction is most likely due to air embolism into the right coronary which is usually reversible with or without additional cardiopulmonary bypass support.

Aortic valve

Aortic valve competence can be impaired by deep suture placement in the mitral anterior annulus or significant reduction of mitral annulus in patients who has minimal aortic cusp coaptation reserve before the mitral valve repair.

De-airing

During cardiopulmonary bypass air can be trapped in pulmonary veins, the left ventricle apex, or left atrial appendage. This air is mobilized by the surgeon before coming off bypass and enters the left ventricle and aorta. As it is expelled it resembles the typical pattern of agitated saline (as might happen if there was a massive right-to-left shunt during contrast echocardiography). Remaining air can be scanned for after de-airing.

Mitral valve replacement

Post-operative assessment

Mechanical valve dysfunction is more likely with: over-sized prosthesis; small left ventricle cavity; excessive subvalvular apparatus, double valve replacement; anatomical mechanical prosthesis orientation. Bioprostheses dysfunction may be due to: distorted annulus due to over sizing or suture looping of cusps. The key features to assess immediately after replacement are:

Valve prosthesis regurgitation

Use colour flow to look for normal prosthesis wash jets (closing jets) and differentiate from paravalvular regurgitation. If present consider:

- Severity: for biological valves mild central jet is normal. Small degrees of paraprosthetic regurgitation (mechanical and biological valves) immediately after surgery often improve with protamine administration. If moderate to severe central regurgitation and restricted prosthetic cusp opening/closing, surgical intervention is normally indicated. 3D image is highly recommended for identifying the location and mechanism of regurgitation.

Valve prosthesis opening

Use 2D and 3D imaging to look for symmetrical, synchronized opening and closing of prosthesis leaflets (Figs. 6.21 and 6.22). Look for functional stenosis (measure prosthesis mean gradient and effective orifice area). If abnormal opening consider:

- Relation between prosthetic valve and subvalvular apparatus: with mechanical bileaflet prostheses, opening and closing may be reduced or restricted because the leaflets impinge on the subvalvular apparatus (posterior leaflet may be preserved in valve replacement).
- Left ventricle filling and contraction: If not adequately filled or poorly contracting, re-evaulate when filling status and contraction are brought to normal level. If prosthesis still dysfunctional surgical intervention is advisable.

LVOT obstruction

Assess valve movement with 2D and 3D imaging and colour flow mapping in the outflow tract. PW Doppler in the outflow tract can be used in transgastric views. Obstruction may be due to septal hypertrophy combined with a high profile prosthesis intruding into the outflow tract.

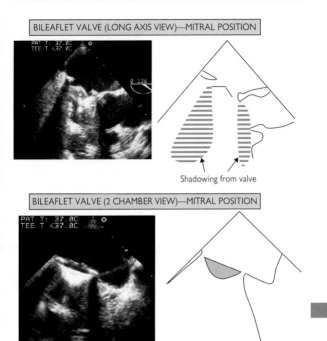

BILEAFLET VALVE (LONG AXIS VIEW)—MITRAL POSITION

Shadowing from valve

BILEAFLET VALVE (2 CHAMBER VIEW)—MITRAL POSITION

Fig. 6.21 Examples of mechanical mitral valve prostheses in long axis and 2-chamber views. See 🎞 Video 6.10.

Cardiac function

After mitral surgery use 2D imaging to re-assess global and regional left and right ventricular function. With acute correction of regurgitation, left ventricular ejection fraction can be expected to drop (e.g. from 60–70% to 40%) due to sudden reduction in left ventricular stroke volume, without proportional reduction in left ventricular cavity size, combined with a variable degree of underlying impaired contractile function. Mitral valve replacement for mitral regurgitation has more adverse physiological effects on left ventricular function than repair.

- If left ventricular filling is adequate but cavity is dilated and global ejection fraction is <30% consider inotropic support and monitor response with echocardiography until stable haemodynamics.
- If there is a new lateral or inferoposterior wall motion abnormality, consider whether the circumflex artery could have been damaged. Large posterior wall hypokinesis can be caused by air embolism, additional support may be required.
- Always consider other general causes for acute severe deterioration in global cardiac dysfunction after cardiopulmonary bypass.

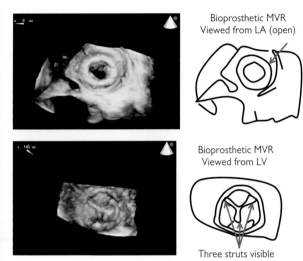

Bioprosthetic MVR
Viewed from LA (open)

Bioprosthetic MVR
Viewed from LV

Three struts visible

Fig. 6.22 3D prosthetic valve views. See 📷 Video 6.11 and 📷 Video 6.12.

Aortic valve

Very good views of the aortic valve can be obtained with TOE because there is only the left atrium, which is a clear fluid-filled window, between the valve and the probe. Aortic valve anatomy is described on 📖 p.132 but essentially comprises of 3 cusps and associated sinuses of Valsalva, named after the coronary arteries that derive from them (right, left, non-coronary).

TOE is indicated to study the aortic valve when transthoracic images are of insufficient quality or better spatial resolution is needed to provide complete assessment of valve pathology, for example vegetations, aortic root abscesses, aortic valve area and prosthetic valve function.

Normal findings

Views

- The best views to see the aortic valve are the 50° short axis view and 135° long axis view (Fig. 6.23). These can be supported by the 5-chamber 0° left ventricular outflow view.
- Additional information is obtained from transgastric views which provide better alignment for Doppler. The aortic valve can be studied with a transgastric long axis 110° view and the deep transgastric 0° view.

Aortic valve

- *5-chamber 0° left ventricular outflow view*: this provides a limited first view of the left ventricular outflow and with colour flow can be used to judge whether there is any aortic regurgitation.
- *Short axis 50° view*: this is the first clear view and is similar to the transthoracic parasternal short axis but upside down. A classic Y-shaped cross-sectional view of the cusps is seen (left on the right, right on the left and non nearest the probe). To optimize the image try slight rotation or movement of the probe up and down. Get all 3 cusps in view, of equal size. Withdraw the probe further to bring the coronary arteries, sinotubular junction, and then ascending aorta into view. Advance the probe to see the LVOT. Colour flow mapping allows positioning of aortic regurgitant jets. This view also allows the stenotic valve area to be measured.
- *Long axis 135° view*: this view is similar to the transthoracic parasternal long axis. Right and non-coronary cusps are seen (non-coronary nearest the probe and right nearest the right ventricle). Use the view to measure aortic root, sinotubular junction, and valve annulus.
- *Transgastric 110° long axis view*: this view allows the outflow tract to be aligned with Doppler. The aortic cusps are sometimes seen in the far field but it can be difficult to get a clear image. Colour flow can help to pick out the outflow tract.
- *Deep transgastric view*: this is an alternative to align the Doppler with the outflow tract and valve. It provides an equivalent view to the transthoracic apical 5-chamber but is difficult to obtain. If there are good transthoracic windows it will not add more information.

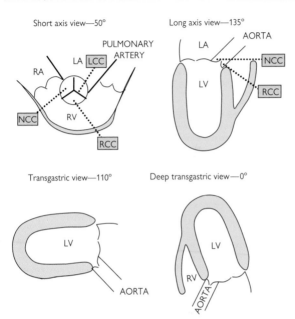

Fig. 6.23 Key views to assess the aortic valve (NCC = non-coronary cusp; RCC = right coronary cusp; LCC = left coronary cusp).

Aortic stenosis

Evaluation of aortic stenosis with TOE follows the same routine as for transthoracic but with more emphasis on 2D imaging to assess valve pathology. The criteria to determine severity (Table 6.3) are the same as transthoracic echocardiography (Table 3.3).

Assessment

Bear in mind the potential causes of aortic stenosis:

- In all the views look for evidence of calcification.
- In the 50° short axis view look at number of cusps.
- Look at associated structures—aortic root dilatation etc.

Grading severity

2D-imaging

In 50° short axis view and 135° long axis view look at valve motion. If the valve appears to open normally aortic stenosis is unlikely to be present. In the 135° long axis view, if the cusps separate by >12mm aortic stenosis is mild or better.

Planimetered valve orifice

- In 135° long axis view obtain a clear image of all cusp edges.
- Move the probe back and forth until the cusp tips in systole are seen in plane.
- Zoom onto the valve and store a loop. Scroll through the loop and try and identify the largest opening during systole.
- Trace along the inner edge of the cusps.
- Report the surface area of the orifice.

Problems with planimetered measures:

Shadowing from heavy calcification can make it difficult to get an accurate area or it may be difficult to the get the open tips in systole in plane with the probe.

Doppler assessment

Both the velocity across the valve and continuity equation require aortic valve vti (or peak flow), LVOT vti (or peak flow), and LVOT dimension. It is often easier and more accurate to do this with TTE but can also be done during a transoesophageal examination.

- Use a transgastric 110° long axis or deep transgastric view to line up the CW Doppler with the aortic valve and aorta (Fig. 6.24).
- Acquire a spectral recording and trace the aortic vti.
- In the same view acquire a PW Doppler in the LVOT and trace the vti.
- Measure the LVOT diameter in the 135° long axis view.
- Report the peak velocity or use the standard continuity equation:

$$\text{valve area} = \text{LVOT area} \times \text{LVOT vti/aortic vti}$$

Table 6.3 Parameters to assess aortic stenosis

	Mild	Moderate	Severe
Peak velocity (m/s)	2.0–2.9	3.0–4.0	>4.0
Peak gradient (mmHg)	<35	35–65	>65
Mean gradient (mmHg)	<20	20–40	>40
Valve area (cm^2)	>1.5	1.0–1.5	<1.0

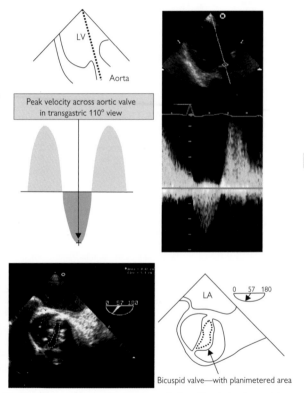

Fig. 6.24 Measurement of aortic stenosis severity from Doppler in a transgastric 110° view (top) and planimetered area in a short axis 50° view (bottom).

Aortic regurgitation

In evaluation of aortic regurgitation with TOE there is more emphasis on 2D imaging to assess cause. Doppler criteria to determine severity (Table 6.4) are as for transthoracic (Table 3.4).

Assessment

Bear in mind potential causes of regurgitation and study both valve and aortic root (📖 p.310).
- In all the views look for evidence of abnormal valve motion.
- In the 50° short axis view look at the valve and position of regurgitation. Study the sinuses and aortic root.
- In the 135° long axis view look at the aortic root dimension and check for dissection.
- Comment on the location and direction of jet. 3D imaging can be of use for identification of the origin of regurgitation jets around the aortic valve. For this 3D colour flow mapping is required.

Grading severity

Colour flow Doppler
- Aortic regurgitation can first be identified in the 5-chamber 0° view although this may not give you an idea of severity.
- The 50° short axis view with colour flow provides an impression of where the regurgitation is and the area of the jet relative to the LVOT.
- The 135° long axis view with colour flow provides the most information to assess severity. This view can be used to assess vena contracta and jet width relative to LVOT (Fig. 6.25).

3D colour flow mapping
- To collect a 3D colour flow dataset (Fig. 6.26) use the oesophageal window with the 3D volume optimized to include the aortic valve.
- It is often easiest to start with your optimized 2D long axis 135° view or 50° short axis view of the aortic valve before switching to the biplane view to set up the 3D volume.
- Remember that the colour flow mapping full volume acquisitions tend to be over more heartbeats and therefore are more prone to stitching artefacts.
- Large jets are often more complex and therefore more difficult to characterize on 3D. The easiest jets to localize are thin, long jets or multiple small jets. 3D can be very useful to identify the presence of multiple jets in a single global view that may have been missed, or thought to be the same jet, on sequential 2D views.

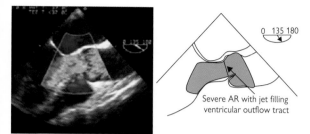

Severe AR with jet filling
ventricular outflow tract

Fig. 6.25 Broad vena contracta filling outflow tract (bottom) consistent with severe regurgitation. See 🎥 Video 6.13.

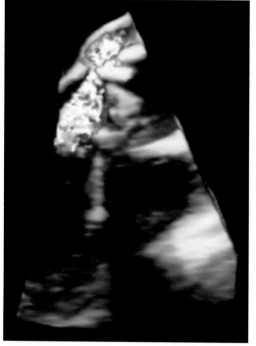

Fig. 6.26 3D colour Doppler of paraprosthetic aortic regurgitation. See 🎥 Video 6.14.

Aortic flow reversal
- In the 90° long axis aortic view PW Doppler with some correction for angle will allow assessment of aortic flow in diastole. Some diastolic flow reversal is normal. Holodiastolic flow reversal is associated with severe aortic regurgitation (Fig. 6.27).

Continuous wave Doppler
- For CW assessment of aortic regurgitation a transgastric 110° long axis view or deep transgastric view is required to align the Doppler signal.
- Look at density of signal, deceleration slope and peak velocity. However, these are less accurate with TOE because of technical limitations in alignment.

Table 6.4 Parameters to assess severity of aortic regurgitation

Specific signs of severity		
	Mild	**Severe**
Vena contracta	<0.3cm	>0.6cm
Jet (Nyquist 50–60cm/s)	central, <25% of LVOT	central, >65% of LVOT
Descending aorta	No or brief early diastolic flow reversal	Holodiastolic flow reversal

Supportive signs of severity		
	Mild	**Severe**
Pressure half-time	>500ms	<200ms
Left ventricle	Normal LV	Moderate or greater (only for chronic lesions) LV enlargement (no other cause)

Report as *moderate* if signs of regurgitation are greater than *mild* but there are no features of *severe* regurgitation.

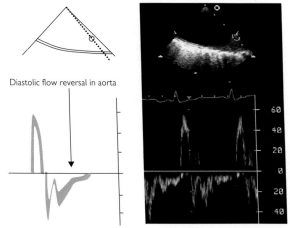

Diastolic flow reversal in aorta

Fig. 6.27 Abnormal aortic flow reversal consistent with severe regurgitation.

Aortic valve preoperative assessment

Thorough preoperative assessment allows careful planning of surgery on the aortic valve. Aortic valve replacement is the most frequently performed valve surgery with an increasingly elderly population. Preoperative information should include data on the valve, the left ventricle, and the aorta.

What the surgeon wants to know

General

Before all types of aortic surgery the basic information needed is:

- Aortic valve cusp morphology and function.
- Aortic root size (look for abscesses if endocarditis present).
- Aortic annulus size (to judge prostheses size if replacement planned).
- Evidence of sinotubular junction dilatation (if >25% bigger than aortic annulus then aortic homograft or stentless bioprosthesis may be contraindicated).
- Ascending aortic dimension and geometry (ascending aorta dilatation >45mm may require replacement).
- Descending aorta size and flow velocity.
- Anatomy and dynamics of LVOT (in surgery for stenosis check for a subaortic stenosis to account for gradient).
- Coronary ostia size, location, and flow velocity (check for ostial stenoses and coronary sinus calcification that might complicate coronary reimplantation in aortic root replacement).
- Left ventricle cavity size, function, and degree of hypertrophy.

Bicuspid valves

In young patient with bicuspid aortic valve pay particular attention to:

- Concomitant abnormalities in LVOT.
- Coronary anatomy.
- Aortic root, arch, and descending aortic structure.

Aortic remodelling

In aortic root remodelling check native valve can be preserved. Look at:

- Aortic cusp morphology and mobility.
- Aortic sinus geometry.

3D aortic valve preoperative assessment

- Assessment for suitability and guiding transcatheter aortic valve implantation, see p.464.

Aortic valve replacement

Postoperative assessment

Assessment of an aortic valve replacement should be based on:

Valve prosthesis opening

With 2D, 3D imaging (and if appropriate M-mode) look at valve opening and closing (Fig. 6.28). Assess velocity across the aortic valve with CW Doppler from a transgastric view. Expect a mean gradient of <15mmHg.

Valve prosthesis regurgitation

Check for regurgitation with colour flow. There may be small closing jets or some mild paraprosthetic regurgitation particularly before protamine is given. If regurgitation is seen, determine severity and location (trans- or paraprosthetic). If bioprosthetic valve implanted, consider whether due to annulus distortion. Paravalvular regurgitation is more likely with a severely calcified aortic annulus, infected aortic valve or redo aortic valve surgery.

Endocarditis

If surgery was for endocarditis ensure any abscesses or fistulae that were present have been excluded or closed.

Cardiac function

For all surgery, determine global and regional cardiac function using standard techniques (📖 p.480). Expect an ejection fraction of 40–60% if normal before surgery. If significant impairment consider causes as for mitral valve surgery (📖 p.447) and in particular consider whether there has been damage to coronary artery ostia.

Coronary arteries

Check for proximal coronary obstruction or occlusion. In short axis views assess proximal coronary lumen size and flow velocity. Acute coronary obstruction can be due to acute thrombus, emboli, prosthesis mal-position and/or oversizing, or abnormal coronary anatomy in congenital aortic valve disease. Depending on the degree and location of coronary ostia obstruction, it can cause failure to wean off cardiopulmonary bypass at the outset or delayed onset of cardiac arrest by the time of chest closure.

De-airing

During cardiopulmonary bypass air can be trapped in pulmonary veins, the left ventricle apex, or left atrial appendage. This air is mobilized by the surgeon before coming off bypass and enters the left ventricle and aorta. As it is expelled it resembles the typical pattern of agitated saline (as might happen if there was a massive right-to-left shunt during contrast echocardiography). Remaining air can be scanned for after de-airing.

Other

Monitor for LVOT obstruction and systolic anterior motion of mitral valve (see 📖 p.446). If there has been septal myectomy check for a ventricular septal defect.

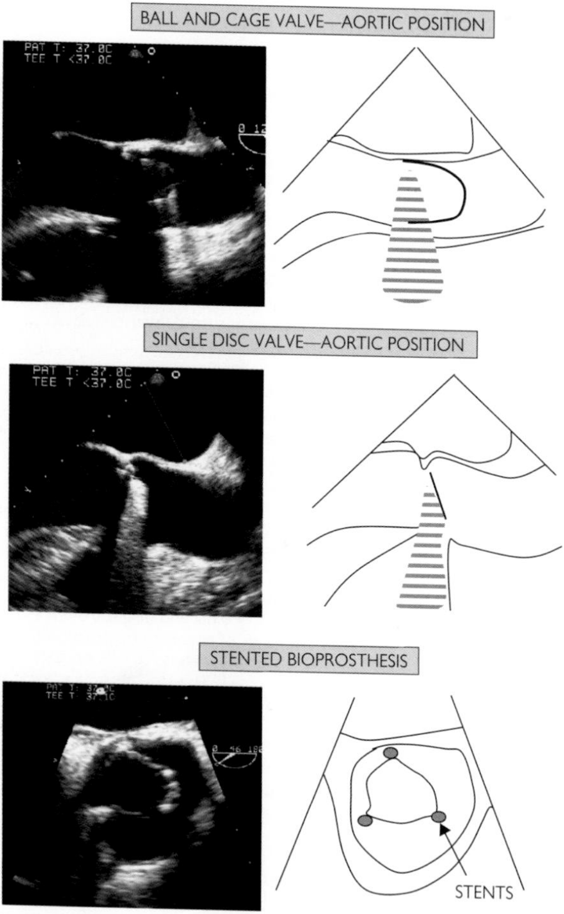

BALL AND CAGE VALVE—AORTIC POSITION

SINGLE DISC VALVE—AORTIC POSITION

STENTED BIOPROSTHESIS

STENTS

Fig. 6.28 Examples of prosthetic valves in the aortic position. Top figure is a long axis view of a ball-and-cage valve and the middle figure of a single disc valve. The bottom figure is a short axis view of a stented bioprosthesis. See ▣ Video 6.15 and ▣ Video 6.16.

TAVI

Assessment of patient suitability for transcatheter aortic valve implantation (TAVI) requires detailed imaging including echocardiography. A full study is performed either with TTE or TOE but often both.

Assessment before TAVI

The study needs to include information on:

Aortic valve

The information needed by the operator relates to the severity of aortic stenosis to confirm that TAVI is required, the anatomy to determine whether the valve is suitable for percutaneous closure, and the presence of other pathology that may influence patient outcome. The report should include:

- Whether the valve is tricuspid valve or bicuspid (bicuspid valve currently a contraindication).
- The true severity of aortic stenosis: aortic valve area <1cm^2 or <0.6cm^2/m^2. Accurate planimetry of the valve based on careful 2D or 3D alignment with leaflet tips should be included.
- Extent and location of valve calcification: possibility of coronary obstruction by displaced calcification.
- Size and shape of aortic sinuses and sinotubular junction.
- Aortic annulus size: measure annulus size in a parasternal long axis view or from a 3D dataset from hinge point to hinge point of valve leaflets—crucial for correct device sizing (Fig. 6.29).
- Report on the presence of left ventricular septal hypertrophy: prominent septal bulge may complicate device positioning.
- Try and determine location of coronary ostia and height from annulus (coronary height). Table 6.5: assess risk of coronary obstruction by device.

General

Assess ventricle and other valves:

- Assess left ventricular hypertrophy and function and cavity size: particularly important for transapical approach.
- Assess right ventricular function and estimate pulmonary pressure: risk of RV deterioration during procedure.
- Mitral valve anatomy and function: significant mitral regurgitation is a relative contraindication.
- Aortic calcification: extensive descending aorta atheroma may increase embolic risk.
- Presence of pleural and pericardial effusions: to allow early identification of any complications.

In patients with significant left ventricular dysfunction and aortic stenosis a dobutamine stress echo may be helpful in clarifying both the severity of the aortic stenosis and the degree of left ventricular hibernation.

Importance of annulus size

Current TAVI devices (Edwards Sapien® and Medtronic CoreValve®) are suitable for annulus sizes ranging from 18–27mm (Table 6.5). If there is concern over measurement accuracy then comparison with data from angiography, computed tomography, and magnetic resonance aortography may be required to decide on eventual device size.

The degree of valvular calcification and LVOT size are also important factors in correct device sizing. Undersizing the prosthesis may lead to paravalvular regurgitation, oversizing may lead to poor stent expansion, coronary obstruction or root rupture.

Table 6.5 TAVI devices

Device	Annulus range	Sinus of Valsalva	Sinotubular junction	Coronary height
CoreValve® 26mm	20–23mm	≥27mm	≤40mm	≥14mm
CoreValve® 29mm	24–27mm	≥28mm	≤43mm	≥14mm
Edwards Sapien® 23mm	18–21.5mm	N/A	N/A	≥10mm
Edwards Sapien®	21.5–24.5mm	N/A	N/A	≥11mm

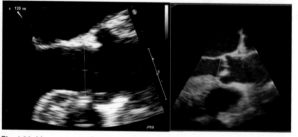

Fig. 6.29 Measurement of aortic annulus size by 2D (left) and 3D (right) TOE.

Assessment during TAVI

Peri-procedural echocardiography, usually with TOE (although both ICE and TTE have been used), is key to ensuring accurate valve deployment and excluding any complications (Fig. 6.30).

TAVI procedure steps

Crossing the aortic valve

- Assess position of wire across valve—usually in commissure between non- and right-coronary cusps.
- Exclude pericardial effusion due to wire perforation of left ventricle.
- Assess degree of aortic regurgitation once wire and catheter across valve.

Balloon aortic valvuloplasty

- Confirm balloon position across aortic valve.
- Assess degree of expansion of balloon.
- Quantify aortic regurgitation post valvuloplasty.
- Assess change in aortic valve motion—sufficient to allow passage of prosthesis?

Prosthesis positioning and deployment

- The exact position of the prosthesis depends on the type used but both require precise placement to within 1mm to ensure correct function.
- Full expansion of the balloon during deployment should be noted.
- Degree and extent of any paravalvular regurgitation post deployment—rarely a second balloon inflation may be needed.

Assessment of any complications

The echocardiographer must be alert to potential complications and continuously monitor for:

- Decline in left or right ventricular function following rapid pacing or prosthesis deployment.
- Pericardial effusion and tamponade due to ventricular or annulus perforation.
- Prosthetic dysfunction due to stuck leaflets.
- Paravalvular regurgitation.
- Aortic injury or dissection.
- Coronary obstruction.
- Thrombus formation on wires and sheaths.

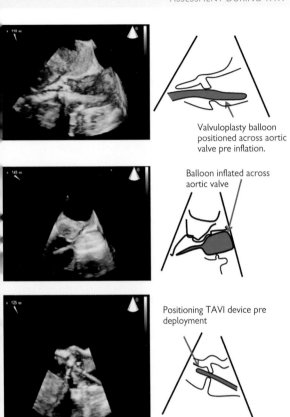

Valvuloplasty balloon positioned across aortic valve pre inflation.

Balloon inflated across aortic valve

Positioning TAVI device pre deployment

Fig. 6.30 The use of TOE during TAVI. See Video 6.17, Video 6.18, Video 6.19, and Video 6.20.

Tricuspid valve

The tricuspid valve is often included in a transoesophageal study but unless the indication is a study of endocarditis, is not the primary focus. Generally the right heart is more difficult to study with TOE because it lies furthest from the probe.

Normal findings

Views

- The best views are: 4-chamber 0°; bicaval 110°; short axis 80° (right ventricular inflow/outflow); and right ventricle transgastric 90°.

Findings

- *4-chamber 0° view*: the tricuspid valve lies on the left and the probe may need to be advanced slightly to optimize the image.
- *Bicaval 110° view*: usually used to study the atrial septum, if the probe is advanced slightly, the tricuspid valve often comes into view in the far field. This view usually gives good alignment for Doppler studies.
- *Right ventricle 80° short axis view*: the aortic valve appears in cross-section in the centre of the view with the right ventricle wrapped around in the far field. This view gives a good image of both tricuspid and pulmonary valves with tricuspid valve on the left.
- *Transgastric 90° long axis view*: from a standard long axis view of the left ventricle, clockwise rotation of the probe to the right can sometimes bring the right ventricle with the tricuspid valve and subvalvular apparatus clearly into view.

Tricuspid regurgitation and stenosis

Assessment of regurgitation

Assess regurgitation on appearance and severity according to the standard transthoracic guidelines (📖 p.158). Vena contracta (Fig. 6.31), PISA, CW tracing, valve structure, and right heart size are usually possible with TOE, whereas jet area and hepatic vein flow are not. See Table 6.6.

Assessment of stenosis

Assess stenosis on appearance (leaflet thickening or restriction) and severity according to the transvalvular gradient. Remember: severe tricuspid stenosis is associated with a gradient of 3–10mmHg.

Table 6.6 Parameters to assess tricuspid regurgitation

	Mild	Severe
Jet (Nyquist 50–60cm/s)	<5cm^2	>10 cm^2
Vena contracta	–	>0.7cm
PISA r (Nyquist 40cm/s)	<0.5cm	>1cm
Hepatic vein flow	Normal	Systolic reversal
Valve structure	Normal	Abnormal
CW trace	Soft & parabolic	Dense & triangular
RV/RA/IVC	Normal size	Usually dilated

Report as *moderate* if signs of regurgitation are greater than *mild* but there are few features of *severe* regurgitation.

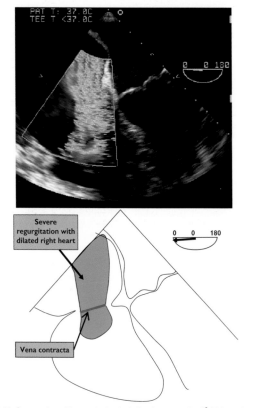

Fig. 6.31 Severe tricuspid regurgitation in 4-chamber view. See 📹 Video 6.21.

Pulmonary valve

Both transthoracic and transoesophageal imaging tend to have limited views of the pulmonary valve. There are no consistent views in TOE that allow Doppler alignment through the valve apart from modified transgastric views in some patients.

Normal findings

Views and findings

- The most useful views are based on the short axis 50–80° (right ventricular inflow/outflow) view. This is a short axis view through the aortic valve in which the pulmonary valve is seen lying behind and slightly to the right of the aortic valve. The image may be optimized by changing the angle slightly from between 50° and 90° until the leaflets of the pulmonary valve are seen opening and closing. Short axis views of the pulmonary valve are now possible using X-plane in this view and aligning the second plane through the valve.

Pulmonary regurgitation and stenosis

Assessment of regurgitation

Colour flow mapping of the pulmonary valve identifies small regurgitant jets in most people—usually to one edge near the aortic valve. If there appears to be more regurgitation than normal, comment on size, site, and severity. Grade severity as *mild*, *moderate*, or *severe* based on colour flow mapping criteria (📖 p.172). It may also be possible to use PW Doppler in the pulmonary artery to look for holodiastolic flow reversal consistent with severe pulmonary regurgitation. Remember to comment on the right heart. See Table 6.7.

Assessment of stenosis

Pulmonary stenosis is usually valvular and congenital (e.g. related to rubella, Noonan's, or tetralogy of Fallot). Comment on valve appearance and appearance of related structures (i.e. pulmonary artery, right heart). It is difficult to align Doppler measures across the pulmonary valve with TOE but the degree of opening using 2D/3D may be used as an estimate of severity. See Table 6.8.

Table 6.7 Parameters to assess pulmonary regurgitation

	Mild	Severe
Jet size on colour flow	<10mm long	Large with wide origin
CW density and shape	Soft & slow	Dense & steep
Pulmonary valve	Normal	Abnormal
Pulmonary artery flow	Increased	Greatly increased compared to systemic
Right ventricle size	Normal	Dilated

If features suggest more than *mild* regurgitation but no features of *severe* grade as *moderate*.

Table 6.8 Parameters to assess pulmonary stenosis

	Mild	Moderate	Severe
Peak gradient (mmHg)	10–25	25–40	>40
Valve area (cm^2)	>1.0	0.5–1.0	<0.5

Endocarditis

TOE has better sensitivity and specificity than TTE for identifying vegetations. The higher spatial and temporal resolution can identify smaller vegetations with rapid movement. Image quality is also better to identify complications of endocarditis: aortic root, fistulae, and valve dysfunction such as leaflet perforation. Remember a normal echocardiogram, including TOE, never excludes endocarditis.

Assessment

Use a full systematic examination with focus on both left and right-sided valves. Report on:

Vegetations

- Vegetations tend to appear as masses on valves (rarely, septum and chamber walls (Fig. 6.32). Focus on each valve (aortic, mitral, tricuspid, and pulmonary valve) and vary position slightly while watching for 'flicking' bright objects attached to valve. Record loops and scroll through frame-by-frame to pick out any abnormal mobile elements.
- If one is seen, move probe position and see if you can see it in multiple planes. Consider possible differential diagnoses, e.g. fibrin strand (Lambl's excrescence), chordae (perhaps ruptured).
- If vegetation, also look for 'seeded' vegetations where the vegetation (or its associated regurgitant jet) touches other valves or walls (e.g. outflow tract, septum and aorta).
- Report: location, number, size, functional effect.

Abscess

Look particularly at valve rings (but also study leaflets) focus on aortic root and mitral valve. The aortic root can be seen particularly well so look for thickening, 'boggy' appearances or frank abscesses. If after valve surgery, remember there may be some normal inflammation associated with the operation. Report position, size, functional effects (compression) and whether the abscess has now opened into a cavity (if so, say which).

Fistulae

These can usually be best seen with TOE. Suspect a fistula if there is a known abscess, a new murmur has been heard or there has been a sudden haemodynamic change in the patient. Use colour flow mapping to look for abnormal flow and cavity jets. Fistulae can be between any adjacent cavities where there has been infection e.g. around valves, aorta to right heart.

Valve dysfunction

If there is a vegetation give details of functional effect on valve. Even if you have not seen a vegetation look for suspicious valve dysfunction in a systematic manner and report.

Pericardial effusion see 📖 p.298.

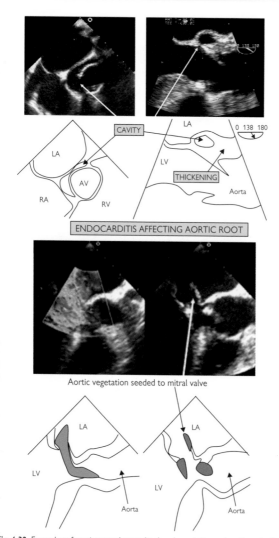

CAVITY

LA

0 138 180

LA

THICKENING

AV

LV

RA

RV

Aorta

ENDOCARDITIS AFFECTING AORTIC ROOT

Aortic vegetation seeded to mitral valve

LA

LA

LV

LV

Aorta

Aorta

Fig. 6.32 Examples of aortic root abscess (top) and vegetations of aortic and mitral valves (bottom). See 📹 Video 6.22 and 📹 Video 6.23.

Transoesophageal anatomy and pathology: chambers and vessels

Left ventricle

TTE usually provides sufficient information to assess the left ventricle and should be the echocardiographic modality of choice. With TOE the left ventricle is in the far field and it can be difficult to obtain unforeshortened views. Transgastric imaging allows accurate measures from stable short axis views. Nevertheless, during a transoesophageal study assessment should be made of the left ventricle, even if limited, to gain an impression of left ventricular size and function and help interpretation of other findings.

Anatomy is described on ☐ p.192. Briefly, the left ventricle is a muscular cavity with a septum dividing it from the right ventricle. The ventricle has anterior, inferior, lateral and inferolateral (or posterior) walls.

Indications for transoesophageal imaging

TOE is indicated when transthoracic windows are poor, in particular situations such as in Intensive Care Unit or Cardiac Recovery, or when intraoperative evaluation of cardiac function is needed during cardiac surgery.

Normal findings

Views

The key views to assess the left ventricle are the 4-chamber 0°, long axis 135°, 2-chamber 80°, and transgastric 0° short axis view (Fig. 7.1).

Findings

- *4-chamber 0° view*: equivalent to the apical 4-chamber but usually with marked foreshortening of the left ventricle. The septum is on the left and lateral wall on the right. To realign the plane through the apex try probe retroflexion until the apex comes into view. The probe may lose contact with oesophagus on retroflexion.
- *Long axis 135° view*: equivalent to the parasternal long axis it is often easier to align through the apex with gentle rotation. The septum (anterior portion) is seen by the left ventricular outflow and the posterior (inferolateral) wall is on the left.
- *2-chamber 70–90° view*: equivalent to an apical 2-chamber view. The inferior wall is on the left and anterior wall on the right. This is a preferred view for measuring left ventricle size.
- *Transgastric short axis 0° view*: the best view to confidently assess left ventricle function and obtain systolic and diastolic measures of cavity size and wall thickness. Equivalent to a parasternal short axis view. Advancing and withdrawing the probe may make it possible to scan through the left ventricle in cross section from apex to mitral valve. The walls of the ventricle are the opposite order to the parasternal short axis, i.e. inferior wall lies nearest the probe and anterior in the far field with septum on the left and lateral wall on the right.

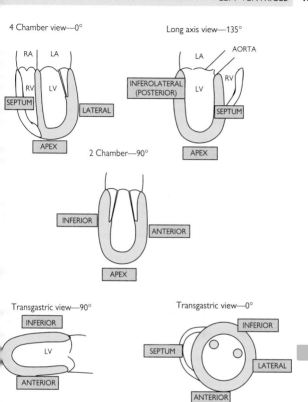

Fig. 7.1 Key views to assess the left ventricle.

Left ventricular size and mass

Report quantitative measures of size (Tables 7.1 and 7.2) if measurements are possible and include a general summary: *normal, mild, moderate, or severe* dilatation; *normal, mild, moderate, or severe* hypertrophy. Both linear and volumetric measures are possible with TOE. Use 2D measures as it is not usually possible to align an M-mode cursor unless transgastric views are obtained. Start with an overview of the ventricle in all views to gather an impression of appearance, size, and function.

Linear measures

2D-imaging

- Optimize a transgastric 0° view at the mid-papillary level and record a loop (Fig. 7.3).
- Identify the end-diastolic frame (widest ventricle). Measure from the inferior wall endocardial border to the anterior wall endocardial border in a line at right angles to each wall. Report the *left ventricular end-diastolic diameter*. Scroll through to identify the end-systolic frame (smallest ventricle) and use the same technique to measure the *left ventricular end-systolic diameter*.
- M-mode, although not usually done, is technically possible in this view.
- The 2-chamber 80° view gives another window to measure left ventricular diameters from anterior to inferior walls (Fig. 7.2).
- Left ventricular hypertrophy can be assessed with measures of wall thickness from the transgastric 2D images at end-diastole in the septum and posterior wall.

Volumetric measures

Simpson's method

Simpson's method of discs can be used if the oesophageal views allow planes to be set up through the apex. It relies on a good 4-chamber 0° view that is not foreshortened.

- In the 4-chamber 0° view optimize an image of the left ventricle, with clear endocardial border and enough depth to include the apex.
- Record a loop. Trace around the border in diastolic and systolic frames to obtain *left ventricular end-diastolic* and *end-systolic volumes*.
- Measure left ventricular length from apex to middle of mitral valve in the same view to obtain *left ventricular long axis*.
- For biplane measures repeat the process using an optimized 2-chamber 80° view.

Area–length equation

This method (📖 p.200) can be used based on a transgastric 0° short axis mid-papillary level view.

Mass

All the equations and models from TTE (📖 p.210) can be applied. Ideally use the transgastric 0° view (equivalent to parasternal short axis). For measurements based on apical 4- and 2-chamber views use the respective 4-chamber 0° and 2-chamber 80° views. Transoesophageal evaluation is reasonably accurate, but tends to report slightly higher left ventricular mass.

SYSTOLE   DIASTOLE

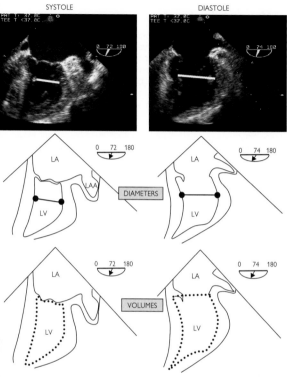

Fig. 7.2 Measures of left ventricle size in 2-chamber view.

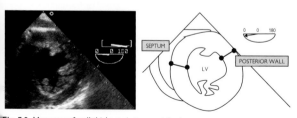

Fig. 7.3 Measures of wall thickness in transgastric view.

Left ventricular function

Assessment of left ventricular function with TOE is often needed in the context of Intensive Care or intraoperatively. Assessment has clinical importance and should be as comprehensive as possible. Minimal requirements are: left ventricular size and shape; systolic function including regional differences. Diastolic function assessment from transmitral and pulmonary vein flow is possible.

Global systolic function

As with transthoracic imaging an eyeball assessment of function is often used and quoted as *normal, mild, moderate,* or *severe impairment.* However, a visual gauge should, when possible, be backed up by quantification. Use the same equations as for transthoracic imaging (📖 p.226) based on the equivalent measures. The transoesophageal views for measurement of left ventricular diameters are the 4-chamber 0°, 2-chamber 80°, and transgastric views. Left ventricular diameters in transgastric views are measured from anterior wall to inferior wall in a line perpendicular to the long axis of the ventricle, at the junction of the basal and middle thirds of the long axis. Left ventricular volumes are traced as for transthoracic imaging—with care to avoid using foreshortened images. Doppler-based measures e.g. dP/dT (📖 p.232) can be used from the oesophageal views of mitral regurgitation.

Regional systolic function

The usual requirement for regional assessment is to determine wall movement in coronary artery territories (Fig. 7.4). The standard 16-segment model can be applied to transoesophageal images and technically wall motion scores are possible although not normally quoted.

Wall motion

- Use 4-chamber 0°, long axis 135°, 2-chamber 80°, and transgastric 0° views. Avoid foreshortening. Endocardial border definition is usually very good.
- Look at the segments and decide whether normal, hypokinetic (excursion <5mm), akinetic (excursion <2mm), or dyskinetic (endocardium moves out in systole). If you are unsure look for thickening >50% between diastole and systole. If present report as normal or hypokinetic.
- Remember, most commonly:
  - Left anterior descending artery supplies: mid and apical septum and lateral wall in 4-chamber 0° view; anterior wall and apex in 2-chamber 80° view, and septum and apex in long axis 135° view.
  - Left circumflex artery supplies: basal and mid segments of posterior (inferolateral) wall in long axis 135° view and basal lateral wall in four chamber 0° view.
  - Right coronary artery supplies: inferior wall in 2-chamber 80° view and basal septum in 4-chamber 0° view.
  - Transgastric short axis view has right coronary territory nearest the probe, left anterior descending territory in the far field, left circumflex territory supplying the posterior wall (on the right).

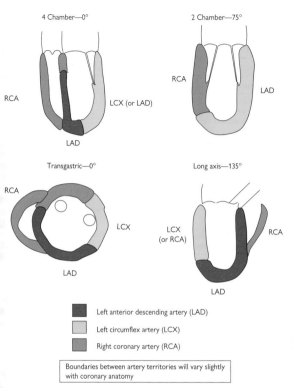

4 Chamber—0°

2 Chamber—75°

RCA

LCX (or LAD)

LAD

RCA

LAD

Transgastric—0°

Long axis—135°

RCA

LCX

LCX
(or RCA)

RCA

LAD

LAD

◼ Left anterior descending artery (LAD)

◻ Left circumflex artery (LCX)

◼ Right coronary artery (RCA)

Boundaries between artery territories will vary slightly
with coronary anatomy

Fig. 7.4 Coronary supply to left and right ventricle.

Left ventricular ranges (Table 7.1)

Table 7.1 Left ventricular ranges in women[1]

	Normal	Mild	Moderate	Severe
LV dimension				
LV d diameter, cm	3.9–5.3	5.4–5.7	5.8–6.1	>6.1
LV d diameter/BSA, cm/m²	2.4–3.2	3.3–3.4	3.5–3.7	>3.7
LV d diam/height, cm/m	2.5–3.2	3.3–3.4	3.5–3.6	>3.7
LV volume				
LV d vol, mL	56–104	105–117	118–130	>130
LV d vol/BSA, mL/m²	**35–75**	**76–86**	**87–96**	**>96**
LV s vol, mL	19–49	50–59	60–69	>69
LV s vol/BSA, mL/m²	**12–30**	**31–36**	**37–42**	**>42**
Linear method: fractional shortening				
Endocardial, %	27–45	22–26	17–21	<17
Mid-wall, %	15–23	13–14	11–12	<11
2D method: Ejection fraction, %	>54	45–54	30–44	<30
Linear method				
LV mass, g	67–162	163–186	187–210	>210
LV mass/BSA, g/m²	**43–95**	**96–108**	**109–121**	**>121**
LV mass/height, g/m	41–99	100–115	116–128	>128
LV mass/height², g/m²	18–44	45–51	52–58	>58
Relative wall thickness, cm	0.22–0.42	0.43–0.47	0.48–0.52	>0.52
Septal thickness, cm	**0.6–0.9**	**1.0–1.2**	**1.3–1.5**	**>1.5**
Posterior wall thickness, cm	**0.6–0.9**	**1.0–1.2**	**1.3–1.5**	**>1.5**
2D method				
LV mass, g	66–150	151–171	172–182	>182
LV mass/BSA, g/m²	**44–88**	**89–100**	**101–112**	**>112**

BSA, Body surface area; d, diastolic; s, systolic.
Bold rows identify best validated measures.

Table 7.2 Left ventricular ranges in men[1]

	Normal	Mild	Moderate	Severe
LV dimension				
LV d diameter, cm	4.2–5.9	6.0–6.3	6.4–6.8	>6.8
LV d diameter/BSA, cm/m²	2.2–3.1	3.2–3.4	3.5–3.6	>3.6
LV d diam/height, cm/m	2.4–3.3	3.4–3.5	3.6–3.7	>3.7
LV volume				
LV d vol, mL	67–155	156–178	179–201	>201
LV d vol/BSA, mL/m²	**35–75**	**76–86**	**87–96**	**>96**
LV s vol, mL	22–58	59–70	71–82	>82
LV s vol/BSA, mL/m²	**12–30**	**31–36**	**37–42**	**>42**
Linear method: fractional shortening				
Endocardial, %	25–43	20–24	15–19	<15
Mid-wall, %	14–22	12–13	10–11	<10
2D method: Ejection fraction, %	>54	45–54	30–44	<30
Linear method				
LV mass, g	88–224	225–258	259–292	>292
LV mass/BSA, g/m²	**49–115**	**116–131**	**132–148**	**>148**
LV mass/height, g/m	52–126	127–144	145–162	>163
LV mass/height², g/m²	20–48	49–55	56–63	>63
Relative wall thickness, cm	0.24–0.42	0.43–0.46	0.47–0.51	>0.51
Septal thickness, cm	**0.6–1.0**	**1.1–1.3**	**1.4–1.6**	**>1.6**
Posterior wall thickness, cm	**0.6–1.0**	**1.1–1.3**	**1.4–1.6**	**>1.6**
2D method				
LV mass, g	96–200	201–227	228–254	>254
LV mass/BSA, g/m²	**50–102**	**103–116**	**117–130**	**>130**

BSA—Body surface area; d, diastolic; s, systolic.
Bold rows identify best validated measures.

Reference

1 Recommendations for chamber quantification: A report of the American Society of Echocardiography Guidelines and Standards Committee and the Chamber Quantification Writing Group, developed in conjunction with the European Association of Echocardiography. *J Am Soc Echocardiogr* 2000; **18**:1440–63.

Right ventricle

The right ventricle is more difficult to see with TOE than transthoracic imaging because it lies distant to the probe. However with an appropriate combination of views it is possible to make a reasonable assessment of right ventricular size and function. Briefly the anatomy consists of a free wall and the interventricular septum. The cavity is crescent-shaped and wrapped around the left ventricle. Inflow is through the tricuspid valve and outflow through the pulmonary valve.

Normal findings

Views

- The key views are: 4-chamber 0° view and short axis 50–80° view (right ventricular inflow/outflow view) (Fig. 7.5). These can be supplemented by transgastric 90° long axis view with the probe rotated clockwise away from the left ventricle.

Findings

- *4-chamber 0° view:* rotation to the right focuses on the right atrium with the right ventricle furthest from the probe. The right ventricular free wall and septum can be seen. This view permits some assessment of size although the right ventricle is often foreshortened.
- *Short axis 50–80° view:* this is also known as the right ventricular inflow/outflow view and allows assessment of the more basal areas of the right ventricle free wall, as well as, the tricuspid and pulmonary valves.
- *Transgastric 0° view:* this permits a short axis view through the left ventricle. The right ventricle will be seen wrapping around the left ventricle (equivalent to a parasternal short axis). This view can be used to look for septal motion to assess right ventricle overload.
- *Transgastric 90° view (right ventricle):* rotating the probe away from the standard left ventricle view may demonstrate the right ventricle. The tricuspid subvalvular apparatus is visible.

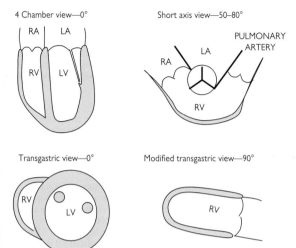

4 Chamber view—0°

RA | LA

RV | LV

Short axis view—50–80°

PULMONARY ARTERY

LA

RA

RV

Transgastric view—0°

RV

LV

Modified transgastric view—90°

RV

Fig. 7.5 Key views to assess the right ventricle.

Right ventricular size

The complex shape of the right ventricle makes assessment complex and it may be difficult to support a qualitative impression with quantitative measures. Assessment is similar to transthoracic imaging (📖 p.264). Use several views and comment on wall thickness, cavity size, and outflow tract size (Fig. 7.6).

Wall thickness

- Use 4-chamber 0° view and comment on thickness of the free wall at the level of the tricuspid valve chordae tendinae. Do not include epicardial fat or coarse trabeculations in the measurement.

Cavity size

Qualitative

- Use 4-chamber 0° view and look at mid-cavity diameter. Right ventricular size is *normal* if <2/3 left ventricular size, *mildly dilated* if slightly smaller than left ventricle, *moderately dilated* when the same size, and *severely dilated* if larger than the left ventricle.
- Alternatively, look at the apex and report as *mildly dilated* if >2/3 of the way to the left ventricular apex, *moderately dilated* if it reaches the left ventricular apex, and *severely dilated* if it extends past the left ventricle.

Quantitative

- Use the 4-chamber 0° view optimized to avoid foreshortening. Measure *right ventricular length*, *tricuspid annulus diameter*, and *mid cavity diameter* (Table 7.3).
- Use right ventricular inflow/outflow 80° view to measure *right ventricular outflow diameter*, *pulmonary valve diameter*, and *pulmonary artery diameter*.

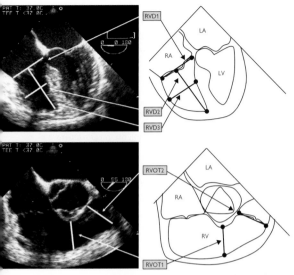

Fig. 7.6 Measures of right ventricular size. These are equivalent to the transthoracic measures (📖 p.264). RVD1 = tricuspid annulus diameter, RVD2 = mid cavity diameter, RVD3 = right ventricle length, RVOT1 = diameter of basal part of right ventricle, RVOT2 = diameter of outflow tract at pulmonary valve. A further measure can be made of pulmonary artery diameter.

Right ventricular function

The right ventricle contracts in both the long and short axis. The long axis assessment of the free wall is the easiest way to gauge right ventricular function.

Assessment

- Use a 4-chamber 0° view.
- Make a qualitative judgement of global function as *mild*, *moderate*, or *severe* impairment based on whether there is less than the accepted 25mm movement of the tricuspid annulus towards the apex but not a major reduction in movement (*mild*), no movement (*severe*), or something in between (*moderate*).
- If you want to quantify the global assessment, measure right ventricular length in diastole and systole and calculate fractional shortening:

$$\frac{\text{RV diastolic length} - \text{RV systolic length}}{\text{RV length in diastole}}$$

(normal is >35% fractional shortening)
- For regional assessment look at the basal, mid, and apical segments of the free wall in the same 4-chamber view and report them as hypokinetic, akinetic, or dyskinetic. As with the left ventricle you should be able to see right free wall thickening to corroborate a statement of normal or hypokinetic motion.

Right ventricular ranges (Table 7.3)

Table 7.3 Right ventricular ranges

	Normal	Mild	Moderate	Severe
RV dimension				
Basal RV diameter, cm	2.0–2.8	2.9–3.3	3.4–3.8	>3.8
Mid RV diameter, cm	2.7–3.3	3.4–3.7	3.8–4.1	>4.1
Base–apex length, cm	7.1–7.9	8.0–8.5	8.6–9.1	>9.1
RVOT diameter				
Above aortic valve, cm	2.5–2.9	3.0–3.2	3.3–3.5	>3.5
Above pulmonary valve, cm	1.7–2.3	2.4–2.7	2.8–3.1	>3.1
PA diameter				
Below pulmonary valve, cm	1.5–2.1	2.2–2.5	2.6–2.9	>2.9
RV area and fractional area change				
RV diastolic area, cm^2	11–28	29–32	33–37	>37
RV systolic area, cm^2	7.5–16	17–19	20–22	>22
Fractional area change, %	32–60	25–31	18–24	<18

In relation to Fig. 7.6 apical 4-chamber view: basal RV = RVD1, mid RV = RVD2, base–apex = RVD3.

In relation to Fig. 7.6 parasternal short axis view: aortic valve to free wall = RVOT1, level of pulmonary valve = RVOT2, pulmonary artery = PA1.

Left atrium

The transoesophageal probe lies directly behind the left atrium and provides excellent views of inflow from all pulmonary veins, outflow across the mitral valve, left atrial appendage, and atrial septum. Any left atrial masses are therefore seen much better with transoesophageal than transthoracic imaging.

Normal findings

Views

- The key views are: 4-chamber 0° view, 2-chamber 75° view, long axis 135° view, and bicaval 110° view.
- Further views are needed to look at the pulmonary veins (🕮 p.494).

Findings

- *4-chamber 0° view:* the left atrium lies directly in front of the probe and may allow measurements of left atrial size.
- *Long axis 135° view:* again the left atrium lies in front of the probe and can be measured.
- *2-chamber 75° view:* with slight adjustments this is perfect for assessment of the left atrial appendage.
- *Bicaval 110° view:* the standard view for assessment of the septum.

Left atrial size

Left atrial size is difficult to assess with TOE because the imaging sector does not normally include the whole of the atrium. Volumes are therefore unreliable particularly if the atrium is dilated. Linear measures are possible but may miss longitudinal changes (Fig. 7.7).

Assessment

- Give a qualitative judgement of size based on size relative to the left ventricle. If the left atrium entirely fits into the 4-chamber 0° view it is likely to be small. If it appears similar in size to the left ventricle it is probably severely dilated. There may be supportive qualitative changes of dilatation, such as spontaneous contrast to suggest slow blood movement in a large cavity.
- Use quantitative measures of area in the 4-chamber 0° view if the boundaries of the left atrium can be seen. Trace around the border to estimate left atrial size and use equations as for transthoracic imaging (🕮 p.280).
- Simple linear measures are usually sufficient in the long axis 135° view or short axis 50° view. Measure the distance between the probe and the left atrial wall by the aortic valve. Remember that quantitative measures are likely to be unreliable and should be interpreted taking into account other echocardiographic findings and qualitative assessment of atrial size.

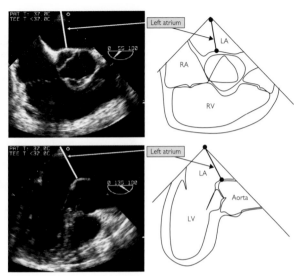

Fig. 7.7 Positions to make linear measures of atrial size.

Left atrial appendage

The left atrial appendage is the most common site for left atrial thrombi in at risk patients, e.g. those with atrial fibrillation, and is therefore of great clinical relevance, for instance when planning cardioversion or looking for source of emboli.

Normal findings

Views

- The key view is the 2-chamber view (Fig. 7.8).
- However, the left atrial appendage can have a variable shape so this key view will need to be adjusted in patients being assessed for cardiac source of emboli, if the left atrium is enlarged or atrial fibrillation is found. Once the left atrial appendage is spotted in the 2-chamber view, adjust the scan angle and move the probe up and down to scan through the whole appendage.
- It can be useful to study the appendage at ~90° to this view to see the pectinate muscles in more detail. The scan plane can be rotated to ~140° while maintaining the appendage in the centre of the image.

Findings

- *2-chamber view:* the left atrial appendage lies on the right, curving around the edge of the mitral valve. Parallel to the appendage and nearer the probe is the left upper pulmonary vein. The appendage and vein are separated by a bright ridge of tissue known as the warfarin or coumadin ridge. This can accumulate fat and may appear bulbous.

Assessment

To assess the appendage:

- Identify the appendage (in some people it can be absent or have been removed/tied/stapled during cardiac surgery).
- Scan through at different planes to identify shape, orientation and number of lobes (usually one lobe but bilobed appendages occur in around 10%). Retroverted appendages (pointing towards the probe) can occur. Inverted appendages are a rare complication of surgery and appear as a mobile mass in the left atrium below the pulmonary vein.
- Look for evidence of thrombus or rarely tumours. Differentiate abnormal masses (e.g. thrombus) from pectinate muscles normally present in the appendage. Thrombus is normally associated with low flow. If it is not clear whether there is a mass, colour flow mapping can demonstrate flow down to the apex, or left-sided ultrasound contrast can opacify the appendage (a mass will remain dark).
- X-plane imaging can be very useful to 'scan' through the appendage.
- Measure filling and emptying velocities (Fig. 7.8). Place PW Doppler cursor 1cm into the appendage and record a trace. Normal velocities are >40cm/s. Low velocities are associated with atrial fibrillation or atrial stunning and should make you suspicious that there may be a clot. Less than 20cm/s indicates a higher risk of clots. Atrial flutter is associated with regular velocities, occurring at a faster rate than the ventricular rate. Look for spontaneous contrast in the atrium or 'smoking' out of the appendage if velocities appear low.

Spontaneous contrast

Spontaneous contrast in the left atrium appears 'smoke-like'. It is classified as *mild* or *severe* (based on a qualitative assessment of quantity) and may be located in the left atrial appendage, or both appendage and atrium. Usually spontaneous contrast in the left atrium indicates increased risk of thrombosis. It is due to sludging of the red blood cells and is found when intracardiac velocities decrease. In particular, a dilated left atrium and atrial fibrillation cause spontaneous contrast. Anticoagulation does not affect spontaneous contrast. The higher the frequency of the transducer the better spontaneous echo contrast is displayed.

Differentiating pectinate muscle from thrombus

Pectinate muscle
- Strand-like
- Can span the appendage
- Adherent
- Not mobile

Thrombus
- Generally rounded
- May fill the appendage
- Adherent or pedunculated
- Can be mobile
- Often associated with spontaneous contrast

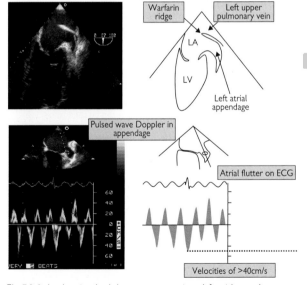

Fig. 7.8 2-chamber view (top) demonstrates prominent left atrial appendage, warfarin ridge and pulmonary vein. PW trace (bottom) demonstrates velocities in appendage consistent with atrial flutter. See Video 7.1, Video 7.2, Video 7.3.

Pulmonary veins

Normal anatomy
There are normally 4 pulmonary veins that drain blood from the pulmonary circulation to the left atrium—2 on the left (lower and upper) and 2 on the right (lower and upper). They all lie at the back of the atrium. Variations in anatomy include only 1 pulmonary vein on 1 side, usually because the upper and lower veins have joined proximally, or significant differences in the size of each vein.

Normal findings
Views
The transoesophageal probe lies behind the atria between the 4 pulmonary veins. To see all 4 pulmonary veins modifications of standard views are required. The key views are the 4-chamber 0° view, 2-chamber 75° view, and bicaval 110° view (Fig. 7.9).

Findings
- *4-chamber 0° view:* all 4 veins can usually be tracked down in this view. Start from the 4-chamber view and rotate to right or left then advance or withdraw the probe to bring each vein into view. The upper pulmonary veins on both sides point towards the probe and are best aligned for Doppler measures. The lower pulmonary veins lie perpendicular to the probe.
- *2-chamber 80° view:* in this view the the left upper pulmonary vein lies parallel to the appendage, nearer the probe.
- *Bicaval 110° view:* by rotating the bicaval view the right upper pulmonary vein can be brought into view as it drains into the left atrium parallel to the septum and superior vena cava.

How to optimize pulmonary vein views

- *4-chamber 0° view:* if the veins are not obvious, colour flow mapping placed in the near field on the left or right can be used to highlight the inflow.
- If the veins are seen but not clearly aligned, rotation of probe angle between 0° and 90° may help to improve the view.

Assessment
Pulmonary veins are often needed for flow assessment relevant to left atrial pressure, particularly in mitral regurgitation (📖 p.120). Their anatomy may also be relevant to procedures that use the pulmonary veins as landmarks, such as ablation for atrial fibrillation.
- Comment on whether:
  - All 4 are seen or whether there are more or less than 4.
  - They are in standard locations.
  - There is any discrepancy in size.
- Report pulmonary vein flow patterns.

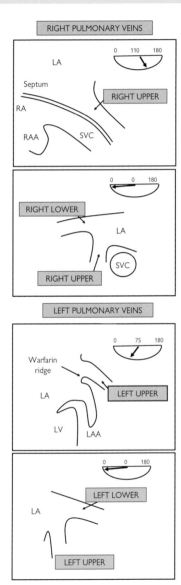

Fig. 7.9 Diagram highlighting the 3 sectors which can be used to identify all 4 pulmonary veins. LA = left atrium, RA = right atrium, RAA = right atrial appendage, SVC = superior vena cava, LV = left ventricle.

Right atrium

There are good views of the right atrium with TOE because of its relative proximity to the probe. Right atrial inflow from both superior and inferior vena cavae as well as coronary sinus are also straightforward to image. More detailed studies of the right atrial appendage, Eustachian valve and atrial septum are possible.

Normal findings

Views

- Key views are 4-chamber 0° view and bicaval 110° view.
- A transgastric view is possible with rotation of the probe from a standard transgastric 90° long axis view of the left ventricle. This will normally bring into view the right ventricle and with some withdrawal of the probe may allow views of the right atrium and tricuspid valve.

Findings

- *4-chamber 0° view:* equivalent to the apical 4-chamber, rotation of the probe to the right allows focused study of right atrium and a qualitative assessment of size.
- *Bicaval 110° view:* this is the best view to see the whole of the right atrium with inferior cava draining on the left and superior vena cava on the right. The right atrial appendage is invariably present just below the superior vena cava. The Eustachian valve (if present) will be seen at the ostium of the inferior superior cava usually directed towards the fossa ovalis. The atrial septum lies parallel to the probe and the fossa ovalis is usually seen as a 'dip' in the middle of the septum. Use this view to assess the atrial septum.

Right atrial size

- Assess right atrial size qualitatively based on the 4-chamber 0° view (Fig. 7.10). Judge size relative to the left atrium and right ventricle. Normally the 2 atria are roughly the same size.
- The simplest quantitative assessment is the linear measure of the *minor axis* in a 4-chamber 0° view (linear measure from middle of right atrial lateral wall to mid atrial septum). Volumes have not been validated but can be attempted as for transthoracic imaging.

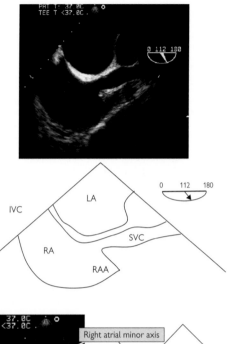

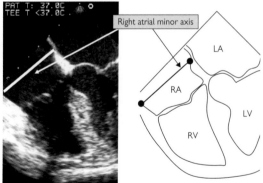

Fig. 7.10 A bicaval view (top) provides excellent depiction of the right atrium. Thrombus, pacing wires, and lines can be seen in the atrium. The 4-chamber view (bottom) can be used for limited measures of the right atrium.

Right atrial features

These usually do not represent pathological findings, but may be mistaken for abnormalities:

Eustachian valve

Best seen in the bicaval 110° view (Fig. 7.11). The Eustachian valve is a membranous structure originating from the junction of the inferior vena cava and right atrium. It represents a remnant from fetal circulation where placental oxygenated blood coming from the inferior vena cava has to be diverted through the foramen secundum into the left heart. Thus the blood flow coming from the inferior vena cava hits the fossa ovalis. This has implications for contrast application via injections into the arm veins: there is usually a wash-out of contrast close to the fossa, which may impair contrast passage. Size can be highly variable. Rarely thrombosis or endocarditis can be attached to the valve.

Chiari network

The Eustachian valve may reach the interatrial septum and have net-like perforations. This is a Chiari network (Fig. 7.11). The Eustachian valve forms from the regression of one of the valves of the sinus venosus and if this is incomplete a Chiari network is formed. Echocardiographically a network of small strands may be seen—sometimes with a broad base, which can be attached to different parts of the right atrium.

Thebesian valve

Like the Eustachian valve this does not represent a real valve. It is a muscle and/or fibrous band at the orifice of the coronary sinus in the right atrium. It can be seen in views displaying the orifice of the coronary sinus.

Christa terminalis

Separates the smooth part of the right atrium from the pectinated muscle of the right atrium. In the bicaval view the *christa terminalis* is displayed as a ridge at the junction of the right atrium and superior vena cava. When pulling back from a 4-chamber view the christa terminalis can be seen as a bright protrusion of the lateral atrial wall. Further pulling back shows how this structure continues into the superior vena cava.

Coronary sinus

To see the coronary sinus use a 4-chamber 0° view. Advance the probe slightly and retroflex slightly to look below the mitral valve. The coronary sinus should appear across the image draining to the right atrium.

The sinus can enlarge if there is anomalous drainage of a persistent left superior vena cava. Anomalous drainage can be demonstrated by injecting agitated saline into a *left-sided* arm vein. Because the left-sided vena cava drains into the coronary sinus the contrast comes through the coronary sinus into the right atrium.

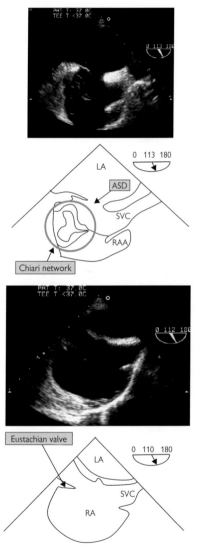

Fig. 7.11 Example of Chiari network (top) and Eustachian valve (bottom) in bicaval views. See 📷 Video 7.4, 📷 Video 7.5, 📷 Video 7.6.

Atrial septum

The atrial septum divides the left and right atrium and embryologically has 2 distinct elements—the primum and secundum septum, which fuse after birth. Abnormal development or closure of the septum is fundamental to the emergence of septal defects. TOE is uniquely suited to study the septum because it can be viewed through the left atrium in several planes suitable for colour flow and continuous wave Doppler, as well as, contrast studies.

Normal findings

Views

The key views are 4-chamber 0° view, short axis 50° view, bicaval 110° view (Fig. 7.12).

Findings

- *4-chamber 0° view:* in the 4-chamber view the septum is close to the probe and rotation to the left can be used for an initial assessment. Atrial septal defects are usually first evident in this view and colour flow mapping can identify left to right flow patterns. The atrial septum normally bows slightly towards the right atrium but in ventilated patients there is a mild systolic bowing towards the left both during inspiration and expiration. If right atrial pressure exceeds left atrial pressure it will bows towards the left.
- *Short axis 50° view:* here the septum extends from the aortic valve ring, in a line at 10 o'clock. The primum septum is evident closest to the valve and this view can be used for stable contrast studies.
- *Bicaval 110° view:* the standard view to study the septum as it lies parallel to the probe. The fossa ovalis is usually easily seen as a depression. This view should be used for colour flow and contrast studies.

Assessment

Assess the septum in all views using 2D. Look for:
- Lipomatous hypertrophy (bright thickening of the septum that spares the fossa ovalis).
- Septal defects or an appearance of layers in the septum suggestive of a patent foramen ovale.
- Atrial septal aneurysms. The septum should move by >10mm either towards right or left atrium.

Then use colour flow over the septum in the bicaval view:
- A septal defect will be seen as interatrial flow. Also, screen for patent foramen ovale—a small colour flow jet may be seen in the fossa ovalis into the atrium during a short part of the cardiac cycle.

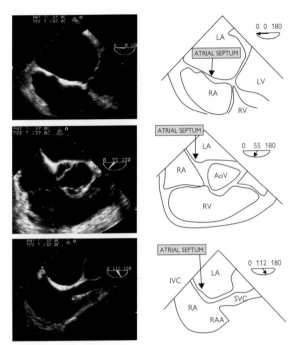

Fig. 7.12 Key views to assess the atrial septum. 4-chamber 0° view (top), short axis 50° view (middle), bicaval 110° view (bottom).

Atrial septal defects and patent foramen ovale

Requests for TOE in people with suspected atrial septal defects and patent foramen ovale are usually because:
- There is a high suspicion from transthoracic imaging of a defect.
- The patient is being evaluated for intervention.
- The study is to look for an embolic source.

Assessment

As for transthoracic imaging (📖 p.288) initial assessment should be with 2D imaging to look for obvious defects, followed by colour flow mapping. If a septal defect is seen, Doppler can be used to quantify the shunt size. Finally, agitated saline contrast injections should always be used if the septal defect or foramen ovale has not clearly been seen.

2D and colour flow mapping

Use all 3 views but in particular the bicaval view. Look for gaps and then overlay the colour flow to look for flow (most likely to be left to right). Comment on:
- Defect position including proximity to aortic valve and likely classification (primum or secundum) (Figs. 7.13 and 7.14).
- Defect size in several directions.
- Direction and timing of flow from colour flow mapping.
- Associated cardiac defects (particularly relevant for primum defects).

Doppler quantification of shunt

See transthoracic imaging (📖 p.288). Doppler quantification is not normally needed for patent foramen ovale. Shunt quantification using measurement of Qp and Qs is often limited with TOE because alignment of the Doppler beam to flow through the pulmonary valve is difficult. However measurement of the diameter of the pulmonary artery or right ventricle outflow tract and of the left ventricle outflow tract is more reliable than on transthoracic images. Pulmonary and aortic vti can be determined separately with transthoracic imaging.

Agitated saline contrast versus colour flow mapping

In patent foramen ovale or septal defects the left-to-right shunt can be detected by colour flow mapping. In most patients a right-to-left shunt is present when right atrial pressure increases, for instance during Valsalva manoeuvre. However, it may be difficult to display these right-to-left shunts with colour Doppler. In these cases contrast echocardiography is indicated (📖 p.506). Contrast echocardiography is also needed, when colour flow mapping does not reveal a shunt, since contrast echocardiography appears to be more sensitive.

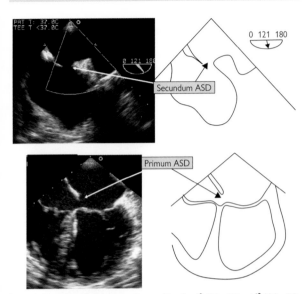

Fig. 7.13 Examples of atrial septum abnormalities. See 📹 Video 7.7 and 📹 Video 7.8.

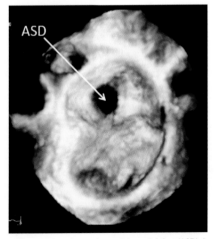

Fig. 7.14 Live 3D acquisition of secundum atrial septal defect (ASD), Image rotated and cropped so defect is visualized form the left atrium. See 📹 Video 7.9.

Secundum atrial septal defect—device closure

TOE is indicated to guide transcatheter closure of secundum defects. 3D TOE can provide more detailed assessment of the defect during the interventional procedure. The key features to record before the procedure to plan closure are:

- Size in different scan planes (many ASDs are not circular!).
- Presence of multiple defects.
- Presence of interatrial septal aneurysm.
- Size of rim of normal tissue between defect and adjacent structures for device to fit over. In particular look at rim close to aortic valve.
- Assess for thrombus in left atrial appendage.
- Other cardiac abnormalities (must assess pulmonary veins and ensure a structurally normal heart).

During the procedure monitor and advise on:

- Guidewire position while crossing the defect.
- Defect size for device sizing.
- Positioning of closure device during deployment.
- Residual shunt after closure.
- Development of thrombus.
- Any impingement on valves.

After the procedure and during follow-up look for:

- Device position.
- Residual shunts.
- Clots or other abnormalities on the device.

Primum atrial septal defect

Primum septal defects are usually well displayed with TTE. During a transoesophageal study the beginning of the defect will be seen in the hinge-points of the mitral and tricuspid valves, which arise from the same level. A 4-chamber 0° view is usually ideal. TOE (Fig. 7.15) is useful for a comprehensive assessment of the pathology, which often includes defects of the proximal interventricular septum, mitral and tricuspid valve insufficiency (including cleft anterior mitral leaflet).

Sinus venosus defect

Sinus venosus defects are very difficult to display using transthoracic 2D echocardiography. A superior sinus venosus defect is best displayed in a modified bicaval view with the probe slightly rotated to the right. There will often be communication between the pulmonary vein and the superior vena cava opposite to the sinus venosus defect. The abnormal drainage of the right upper pulmonary vein can also be displayed in a 0° view pulled back from the standard flour chamber image to show a short axis view of the superior vena cava and ascending aorta.

Inferior sinus venosus defects are less common and may be associated with abnormal drainage of the right lower pulmonary vein.

Coronary sinus defects are between the coronary sinus and the left atrium. Coronary sinus views are needed to display the shunt, which may be difficult to see.

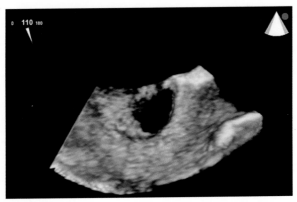

Fig. 7.15 3D transoesophageal view of atrial septal defect.

Contrast study for intracardiac shunts

The 3 elements to ensure a good contrast study looking for an atrial shunt are identical to those for transthoracic imaging (Fig. 7.16). The sedation with transoesophageal imaging complicates the Valsalva manoeuvre but does not make it impossible and the manoeuvre must be used.

1. A stable image

The bicaval 110° view aligns the septum across the image and therefore provides good views of contrast flow. An alternative view is the short axis 50° view at aortic valve level. The Valsalva manoeuvre causes movement of the heart up and down. The 50° view tends to be more stable with this movement as the septum is in line with the image plane.

2. Good quality contrast

The contrast should be 8mL of saline, 1mL of air, and (ideally) 1mL of blood from the patient mixed in 2 connected syringes until 'frothy'. Use syringes with locks to avoid them bursting off. Inject rapidly through a venflon inserted into the right antecubital vein (if the patient is lying on their left side this arm will not be compressed and be uppermost). This will ensure the fastest transit of contrast to the heart (ensure the blood pressure cuff does not inflate on this arm during the procedure). Good contrast should completely and rapidly opacify the right atrium. Sometimes rapid flow from the inferior vena cava causes mixing and partitioning of contrasted and uncontrasted blood in the right atrium. As the inferior vena cava directs blood at the foramen ovale the mixing tends to keep contrast away from the septum. If this persists despite fast boluses then an alternative is to inject contrast via a femoral vein.

3. A good Valsalva

If further studies are needed after rest injections always do the study with a Valsalva. The critical time is when the patient relaxes, when right-sided pressures transiently elevate relative to left. The patient takes a breath and bears down hard. Inject the contrast and when it fills the right atrium tell them to relax. If there is a shunt a few bubbles appear in the left atrium and left ventricle within 5 beats of the patient relaxing. If bubbles appear later this suggests a pulmonary arteriovenous malformation. This procedure is entirely feasible during transoesophageal imaging with a compliant patient. To improve compliance lighter sedation can be used and/or the shunt study can be near the end of the examination (as sedation becomes lighter). Assistance can be given by asking the patient to press against a hand placed on the stomach.

Image acquisition

Set the system to capture 10 cardiac cycles and start acquisition on contrast injection. Look back through the loop searching for bubbles. Repeat the study with more contrast until you are happy all 3 elements of the study are perfect.

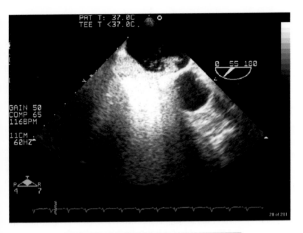

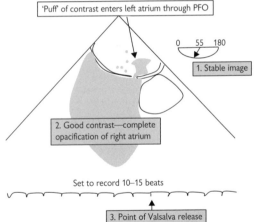

'Puff' of contrast enters left atrium through PFO

0   55   180

1. Stable image

2. Good contrast—complete opacification of right atrium

Set to record 10–15 beats

3. Point of Valsalva release

Fig. 7.16 The 3 key elements of an agitated saline contrast study. See 📹 Video 7.10.

Ventricular septum

The ventricular septum can be difficult to see entirely with transoesophageal imaging and therefore it is not indicated for assessment of the septum. However, it is normal to assess the septum routinely during a study and comment if abnormalities are identified incidentally. TOE provides reasonable views of the proximal septum and can be efficient for membranous septal defects. More apical defects, as often occur post-ischaemia, are difficult to see.

Normal findings

Views

The key views are the 4-chamber 0° view and the long axis 135° view (Fig. 7.17). These can be supplemented by the short axis 50° view to look at septum around the aortic valve. The transgastric short axis 0° view can also be useful.

Findings

- *4-chamber 0° view:* the septum lies between the left and right ventricle. With an unforeshortened view it may be possible to see to the apex but the views are not aligned for colour flow mapping. The view gives good depiction of the proximal septum. Withdrawal to the 5-chamber view allows imaging of the septum below the aortic valve.
- *Short axis 50° view:* with a slight advance of the probe the membranous and outlet septum just below the aortic valve can be seen.
- *Long axis 135° view:* this also demonstrates the septum close to the aortic valve.
- *Transgastric view:* this gives equivalent information to the parasternal short axis view and provides information on the muscular (trabecular) septum in the mid-ventricle.

Assessment

Assess the septum in all views with 2D and then overlay colour flow to look for defects. If there is evidence of hypertrophy, particularly in the outflow tract, then colour flow can also be used to look for subaortic valve flow acceleration.

- If comments on the septum are required then report septal thickness (this can be measured from transgastric views) and comment on any irregular thickening of the septum.
- To identify a ventricular septal defect first look in 2D for evidence of a 'gap' then use colour flow to identify definite flow across the septum. If there is a gap measure the size in two different directions/planes. Finally, if Doppler alignment is possible consider calculation of a shunt. However, if a septal defect is sufficient to cause major shunts these can often be seen most easily with transthoracic imaging.

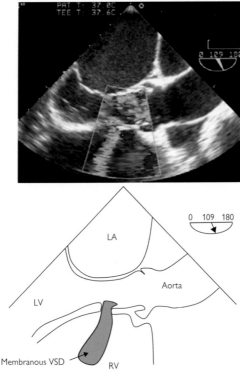

Fig. 7.17 Example of a large perimembranous ventricular septal defect seen in a long axis 135° view. A left to right shunt is demonstrated with colour flow mapping. See 📷 Video 7.11.

Pericardium

TTE usually gives all the information needed to assess the pericardium. However, the pericardium should be assessed routinely during transoesophageal studies. TOE can be useful in perioperative cardiac patients to assess localized collections or because of poor postoperative windows. Assessment of the pericardium should follow the same routine as with transthoracic imaging.

Normal findings

Views

Part of the pericardium can be seen (and should be assessed) in all views.

Findings

Pericardial surfaces

The surfaces are usually a thin white line around the heart (normal 1–2mm thick). Transoesophageal imaging is more accurate for assessing thickness than transthoracic but should not be relied upon.

Pericardial space

The space, if it contains fluid, is a black, lucent area associated with the pericardial surfaces (normally <0.5cm, although small effusions can have significant effects post surgery).

Transverse and oblique sinuses

TOE is good for studying the *transverse* and *oblique sinuses*. The *transverse sinus* lies between left atrium and aorta/pulmonary trunk (Fig. 7.18).
- Use atrio-ventricular short axis 50° view and then long axis 135° view.
- Fluid or haematoma in the sinus appears as space—shaped like a crescent or triangle—between ascending aorta and left atrium.

Problems with the transverse sinus

To differentiate the space from the left atrium or left atrial appendage (roof lies in transverse sinus) use colour flow Doppler. There will be no flow in the sinus. Beware, because of the position of the sinus it can be mistaken for abscess or cyst or—if containing fat—an atrial mass.

Oblique sinus lies between the pulmonary veins on back of left atrium.
- Use 4-chamber 0° view.
- Fluid or haematoma in sinus appears as a space between left atrium and the probe tip in the oesophagus.

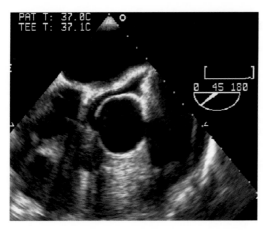

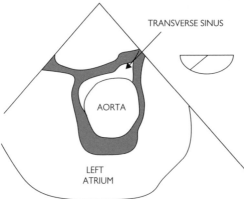

Fig. 7.18 Mid-oesophageal, ~50° view just above aortic valve. Fluid in transverse sinus is seen as echolucent area between aorta and left atrium.

Pericardial effusion

Assessment
Global effusions
- Use all views. Seen well in 4-chamber 0° view or transgastric short axis 90° view (Fig. 7.19).
- Report depth in several different sites and report where the measurements were made.
- Gauge global effusion on same parameters as transthoracic imaging (<0.5cm; 0.5–1cm: mild; 1–2cm: moderate; >2cm: large).
- Comment on appearance (fibrin strands, masses, haematoma).

Differentiate between pleural and pericardial fluid by using descending aorta and left atrium (as for transthoracic imaging). In 4-chamber view rotate probe to focus on the left ventricle and descending aorta. Pericardial fluid will pass between aorta and left atrium (sometimes widening the gap) whereas pleural fluid will extend to the lateral side of the aorta.

Localized effusions
- Common sites are in *oblique sinus* behind left atrium or a *posterolateral collection* against right atrium or right ventricle.
- Both can be seen in the 4-chamber 0° view.
- Space between probe and left atrium is the *oblique sinus* collection.
- Rotate probe to focus on right heart. Look at right ventricle and atrium for evidence of localized compression or collapse from a *posterolateral* effusion.
- Use long axis 135° view to check *transverse sinus*.

Cardiac tamponade

Features of cardiac tamponade can usually be assessed with transthoracic imaging. If assessment is required during transoesophageal imaging use the 2D and Doppler parameters as for transthoracic studies (□ p.300). Remember that tamponade is a clinical diagnosis (hypotension, tachycardia etc.) and echocardiography will only provide supportive evidence.

Problems in ventilated post-surgery/ITU patients

- There will not be the normal respiratory variation in Doppler indices of mitral and tricuspid inflow and these should not be used. Rely on 2D features.
- Look for right or left ventricular or atrial collapse.
- Look for localized collection compressing left or right ventricle or atria reducing chamber function.
- With *oblique sinus* collection look at pulmonary vein flow. Local compression will reduce flow velocity in vein.

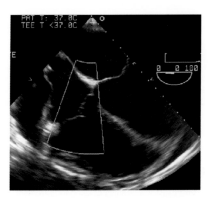

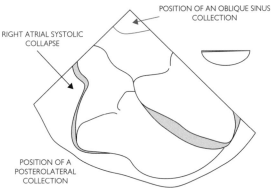

POSITION OF AN OBLIQUE SINUS COLLECTION

RIGHT ATRIAL SYSTOLIC COLLAPSE

POSITION OF A POSTEROLATERAL COLLECTION

Fig. 7.19 Mid-oesophageal 4-chamber 0° view showing global pericardial effusion with exaggerated right atrial collapse during atrial systole. Annotation demonstrates where an oblique sinus and posterolateral collection would be seen in this view.

Aorta

The close proximity of the oesophagous to the aorta makes transoesophageal imaging ideal for assessment of the ascending and descending thoracic aorta. Parts of the aortic arch including the origin of the brachiocephalic vessels can also be visualized. The views allow diagnosis and assessment of aortic dissection and severity of aortic atheroma. The portability of transoesophageal imaging also permits assessment of traumatic aortic trans-section.

Normal findings

Views

The key aortic views are the 50° short axis aortic valve view both at aortic valve level and withdrawn slightly, the 135° long axis view, and dedicated descending aorta and aortic arch views (Fig. 7.20). Deep transgastric and 110° long axis transgastric views can be used for alignment of Doppler in the ascending aorta.

Proximal ascending aorta

- Proximal ascending aorta is best seen in the 50° short axis view with slight withdrawal of the probe to scan up the aorta. The 135° long axis view also allows measures of aortic root size. Transgastric views sometimes allow Doppler alignment through the proximal ascending aorta.

Aortic arch

- Seen as the last views as the probe is withdrawn in the aortic views and can be seen in long and short axis.

Descending thoracic aorta

- The descending thoracic aorta can be seen in short (0°) and long axis (90°) with the dedicated posteriorly-directed aortic views. Advancing and withdrawing the probe allows scanning of the entire length of the aorta. This view can help demonstrate descending aortic aneurysm and atheroma,. Rotation will differentiate artefact from true abnormality, particularly when dissection suspected.
- Aortic views can also demonstrate the aortic isthmus, and the ostium, and proximal part, of the left subclavian artery. This landmark is used to describe extent of dissection or help assess placement of intra-aortic balloon pumps.

Emergency evaluation of the aorta

In an emergency where aortic dissection is a major indication proceed immediately to the 135° long axis view. This view shows the aortic annulus, aortic valve, and proximal ascending aorta with sinuses of Valsalva and right and non-coronary leaflets of the aortic valve. A proximal aortic dissection flap or excessive dilatation of the sinus of Valsalva is therefore readily diagnosed. Pericardial fluid and aortic regurgitation can also be detected.

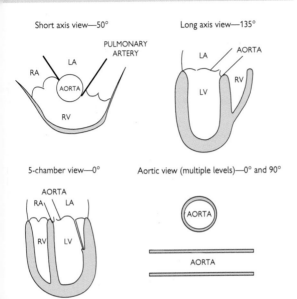

Fig. 7.20 Key views to assess the aorta.

Aortic size

Proximal aorta

- Make measurements in 2D imaging from mid-oesophageal 135° long axis view in systole (with valve leaflet tips open to their maximum). Standard measures are annulus, sinus of Valsalva at aortic leaflet tip level, sinotubular junction, proximal ascending aorta (Figs. 7.21 and 7.22)

3D TOE to measure aortic annulus

Measurement of the aortic annulus and proximal aorta is of particular importance in determining suitability of patients for transcutaneous aortic valve implantation (TAVI) and selecting appropriate prosthesis size. Use of 3D imaging and the X-plane modality helps ensure true cross-sectional diameter being measured.

- Either obtain short-axis 50° view of aortic valve and then position X-plane cursor though centre of valve to obtain true long-axis cut, or preferably, obtain a full volume 3D dataset of the aortic valve and post process to get a precise cross section at the different levels. The key level is at the level of the aortic annulus and measurements should be taken from hinge point to hinge point. Measurements in 2 axes should also be performed as the annulus is often not circular.
- It is likely that measurement of true orifice (aortic annulus) from 3D images will become viewed as the standard. 3D measures are often slightly larger than 2D measures.

Arch and descending aorta

- In aortic short axis 0° view measure aortic diameter at different levels. Record the distance from incisors (40cm, 35 cm, 30cm) for each measure. When withdrawn to the aortic arch rotate to 90° to get a cross-section and measure diameter.

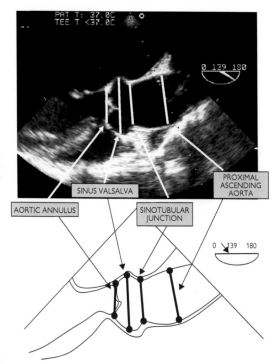

Fig. 7.21 Standard measures of aortic root and proximal aorta in long axis 135° view.

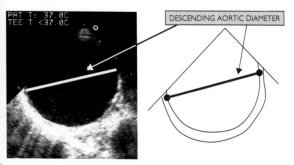

Fig. 7.22 Standard measures of descending aorta diameter from short axis aortic view.

Aortic atherosclerosis

Aortic atherosclerosis is easily seen with TOE. Assessment is importan
when hunting for embolic source or before surgery for impression of like
coronary atherosclerotic disease. Risk of embolic events increases incr
mentally with extent of atheroma and is dramatically higher once plaqu
extends beyond 4mm. Severity is strongly associated with risk factors fo
atheroma and, incidence and severity of carotid and coronary diseas
Site of atherosclerosis is not always correlated with stroke localizatio
and presence of atherosclerosis may simply be a marker of generalize
atherosclerosis.

Assessment

Atherosclerosis is seen as wall thickening, irregular plaque, or as ulcerate
thrombotic, mobile plaque. Significant atherosclerosis increases the ris
for dissection and aneurysm formation.

- In aortic views scan up the descending aorta and aortic arch. Also
  assess proximal ascending aorta.
- Measure wall thickness at several sites and in particular at any positio
  where there are irregularities. Aortic thickness is *intima–media
  thickness*. The wall is seen as 2 white lines separated by a black space.
  Intima–media thickness is the thickness of the inner white and black
  bands added together (Fig. 7.23).
- Grade atherosclerosis within the different sections of the aorta as *mil*
  moderate, or *severe* (Fig. 7.24).
  - Normal wall thickness <2mm.
  - Mild atherosclerosis wall thickness 2–4mm moderate
    atherosclerosis wall thickness >4mm.
  - Severe atherosclerosis irregular protruding plaque (Fig. 7.25).
- Comment on specific lesions, such as thrombus or ulcerated plaques,
  and comment on location and depth.

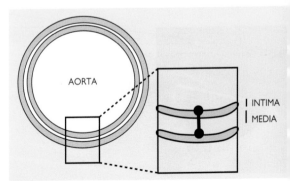

Fig. 7.23 Measurement of aortic intima media thickness.

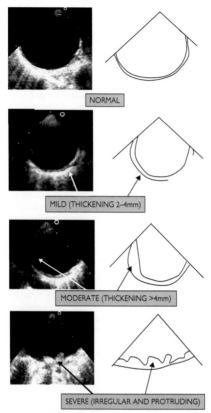

NORMAL

MILD (THICKENING 2–4mm)

MODERATE (THICKENING >4mm)

SEVERE (IRREGULAR AND PROTRUDING)

Fig. 7.24 Grades of atheroma within the aorta. See 🎞 Video 7.12.

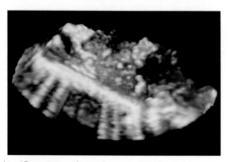

Fig. 7.25 Live 3D acquisition of aorta demonstrating atheroma.

Aortic dissection

TOE allows diagnosis and serial monitoring of aortic dissection. Diagnostic utility with experienced operator is good and comparable to other modalities (sensitivity and specificity >97%).

Diagnosis

- TTE should routinely be performed first as this may be diagnostic and negate need for TOE.
- For transoesophageal imaging adequate sedation and good technique are essential. Excessive retching can cause acute blood pressure rise, which could extend dissection and cause acute haemodynamic deterioration. Therefore, if concerns particularly if haemodynamic instability consider performing study in theatre with cardiac surgeon available.
- Use all aortic views to scan all of aorta in short and long axes (Fig. 7.26). In short axis, look for an enlarged aorta with a line across lumen dividing *true* and *false* lumens. True lumen is usually smaller. Colour flow mapping can be used to demonstrate high velocity flow in the true lumen and no, or slow flow, in false lumen. In long axis views *dissection flap* may be seen as a linear mobile structure with motion independent of the aortic wall. See Table 7.4.

Limitations—false negative and false positive findings

- The distal ascending aorta cannot be assessed by TOE due to interposition of trachea and left bronchus. Thus pathology in about 5cm in length may be missed. However, isolated dissection in this location is rare. False negative studies can occur due to localized root dissection with pericardial haematoma but no false lumen.
- Linear artefacts have to be distinguished from real intimal flaps. Reverberation is the most frequent source of these artefacts. Strong backscatter from various tissue-fluid interfaces such as the anterior aortic valve or Swan–Ganz catheters in the pulmonary artery can cause linear echoes in the aortic lumen. They are typically found at double the distance from the transducer compared to the source of the reverberation. Also mirror artefacts showing a reduplication of the aortic lumen are possible. A real intimal flap should be visible in at least 2 planes. See Table 7.5.
- 3D echocardiography is particularly useful in differentiating dissection flap from artefact: a true flap can be visualized as a sheet, rather than a linear structure if artefactual.

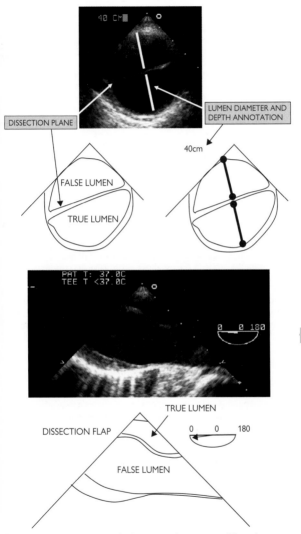

Fig. 7.26 Short axis (top) view of a dissection with measures or false and true lumen. Long axis view (bottom) of aorta demonstrating dissection flap. See 📹 Video 7.13 and 📹 Video 7.14.

Assessment

If an aortic dissection is diagnosed (Fig. 7.27) or the study is for serial monitoring of a known dissection the objectives of the investigation should be to:

- Perform all standard aortic measures and measure diameter of true and false lumens at different levels.
- Try and identify start and end of dissection and record positions. This allows serial monitoring of size and length of dissection. In the ascending aorta dissections tend be along the greater curvature and in the descending aorta may spiral around the true lumen.
- Multiple tears may be present and sometimes it is not possible to locate the entry site with transoesophageal imaging. As you scan up the aorta use colour flow to identify connections between true and false lumens (will be seen as colour flow jets). If seen, measure positions and direction of flow.
- Comment on and quantify aortic regurgitation. Aortic valve insufficiency can occur due to dilatation of the aortic root, impaired cusp movement by ring haematoma, impaired cusp support and cusp prolapse, or prolapse of the dissecting flap into outflow tract.
- Comment on pericardial fluid and evidence of tamponade.
- Assess global and regional left ventricle function in case of coronary artery involvement. 10% of dissections involve the coronary ostia.
- Use 3D assessment to confirm nature and extent of dissection flap. Orientate the probe in 2D just above aortic valve in cross section initially. Look for coronary ostia to confirm or exclude involvement: this may be better visualized and appreciated in 3D. Perform 3D colour flow study to look for additional tears, the number and extent of which may be under-appreciated on 2D imaging.
- When monitoring dissection, review last study and repeat all measures. Highlight any changes in appearances or size.

Surgery for aortic dissection

Preoperative

If performing echocardiography before Type A dissection surgery:

- Check diagnosis and differentiate between acute dissection, leaking aneurysm or intramural haematoma. Type and timing of surgery will vary significantly.
- Look at aortic valve cusps and aortic root. If normal cusps, and aortic annulus and sinotubular junction normal size, then even if regurgitation is seen, inter-position ascending aortic graft replacement, rather than total aortic root replacement, can be considered.

Postoperative

Ensure successful repair and no residual evidence of dissection. If native valve was preserved, ensure normal valve function.

Table 7.4 Differentiating true from false lumen

	True lumen	False lumen
Diameter	True < false	False > true
Pulsation	Systolic expansion	Systolic compression
Blood flow	Systolic, antegrade	Reduced
Spontaneous contrast	Rare	Frequent
Thrombus	Rare	Frequent, depending on flow communication
Localization	Inner, anterior contour	Outer, posterior contour

Table 7.5 Differentiating intimal flap from artefact

	Intimal flap	Artefact
Borders	Definite	Indistinct
Movement	Rapid, oscillatory	Parallel to strong reflector proximal to artefact
Extension	Within aorta	Beyond aortic wall
Colour Doppler	Homogenous colour on both sides	Different colour communicating jets
3D	Sheet like appearance	Linear

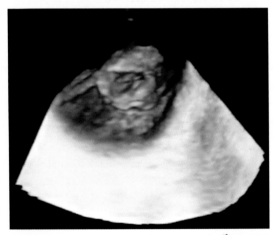

Fig. 7.27 3D TOE demonstrating dissection flap in the aorta. See 📼Video 7.15.

Intramural haematoma

There is debate as to whether aortic intramural haematoma is a discrete pathological entity or precursor of aortic dissection. Haematoma tends to occur in older patients with hypertension.

Diagnosis and assessment

- Intramural haematoma is seen as a generalized thickening of the media without obvious disruption of the intima and no flow communication.
- Wall thickness >7mm suggests haematoma (normal <4mm).
- Can affect any area of aorta. Intramural haematoma in ascending aorta is usually managed similar to type A dissection.

Differential diagnosis of haematoma is atherosclerotic disease with a penetrating aortic ulcer. Penetrating ulcer is always: associated with heavy atheroma; predominantly affects descending aorta; intima is irregular with thickening above the intima. Atherosclerosis is also suggested by inward displacement of any intimal calcification with homogenous mottled thickening of wall either side of the displacement.

Aortic transection or traumatic aortic disruption

Usually occurs at aortic isthmus following acceleration/deceleration injury (e.g. restrained passenger or driver in road traffic accident). Usually other traumatic injuries.

To differentiate from dissection:
- Transection is disruption of media rather than intima, resulting in relatively thick flap, usually very mobile, and perpendicular to aortic wall (aortic dissection is intimal, with thin flap parallel to wall).
- There is usually no thrombus in the false lumen but there may be a mediastinal haematoma.
- Usually asymmetric aortic shape. >4mm difference in anteroposterior and longitudinal aortic dimensions (dimensions similar with dissection).
- Colour flow mapping reveals similar velocities on both sides of any flap, with turbulence around the point of disruption (turbulence unusual in dissection and usually slower velocities in false lumen).

Aortic coarctation

Usually diagnosed from transthoracic assessment of Doppler flow suprasternal view. Accurate transoesophageal imaging can be difficult b images are best obtained by examining the descending aorta at 0° in m tiple sections to identify the isthmus. At level of isthmus, rotate to a 9 longitudinal view to identify the origin of the left subclavian artery. Lo for irregularity of aortic lumen. Morphology of aortic coarctation is ofte complex and further imaging is usually necessary.

Assessment

- Measure size of aorta proximal, distal, and at the coarctation. For follow-up, post-repair, compare with previous studies to look for repair dilatation or persistent gradient.
- PW Doppler in long axis aortic views can be used to look for flow acceleration across a coarctation.
- 3D volume set acquired at level of maximal narrowing can help appreciate complexity of coarctation.

Sinus of Valsalva aneurysm

A rare, congenital abnormality (<1:1000 patients). Acquired aneurysm are even rarer and are predominantly due to endocarditis, trauma, syphil or tuberculosis. Often an incidental finding. When symptomatic, ruptur causes chest pain and breathlessness or, with smaller ruptures, more insidio onset congestive cardiac failure.

Assessment

- Use the 135° long axis view (>95% originate from either right or non-coronary cusps, both visualized). Aneurysm usually has a wind-sock appearance blowing in either right atrium or right ventricle.
- 3D imaging from this view can clarify relationship to cardiac chambers and aid with planning of interventional approach.
- Colour flow mapping will show an aortic to cardiac chamber shunt. CW Doppler assessment confirms continuous flow.
- Use a 50° aortic short axis view with slight probe withdrawal to level of coronary sinus to identify coronary arteries and exclude coronary artery fistula as an important differential diagnosis.
- Haemodynamic effect of a ruptured coronary sinus is best assessed fror size of atria and left ventricle, reflecting extent of volume overload.

Thoracic aortic aneurysm

Thoracic aortic aneurysm is usually suspected on chest X-ray or TTE Confirmation can be by CT, magnetic resonance imaging, or TO (Fig. 7.28). CT and magnetic resonance imaging have the advantage c showing the true extent of the aneurysm and clear identification of th origin of the head and neck vessels, while TOE more accurately delineate flow patterns within the aneurysm, the presence of thrombus, and th presence of atherosclerotic debris.

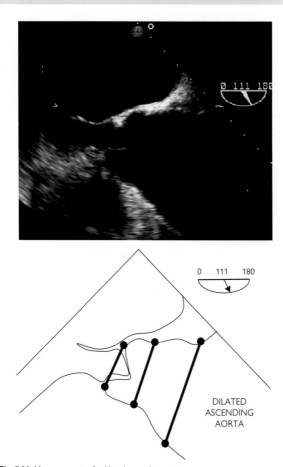

Fig. 7.28 Measurements of a dilated ascending aorta.

Masses

Masses are usually much clearer on TOE than TTE and therefore TOE is indicated for definition of masses (Fig. 7.29). Abnormal masses are vegetations or very rarely thrombi or tumours (see 📖 p.326).

Report position, size, and functional effects. Comment on any suspicions as to the nature of the mass but remember that echocardiography is unlikely to give the definitive diagnosis.

Differential diagnosis of masses

Like TTE, transoesophageal imaging does not provide a specific tissue pattern of the tumour (the exception being lipomas). Therefore it is not possible to differentiate masses (tumours, thrombi, and vegetations) according to their structure on echocardiography. However there are associated features, which help to make a diagnosis.

Myxomas

Myxomas are the most frequent cardiac tumours and usually originate from the fossa ovalis of the interatrial septum. They also may be found in other chambers.

Fibroelastoma

Fibroelastoma are mobile tumours on the upstream side of the aortic valve (rarely mitral valve). In comparison to vegetations there are usually no other valvular lesions.

Lipomatous interatrial hypertrophy, lipoma in the tricuspid ring

These lipomatous changes have a characteristic high density appearance but do not result in acoustic shadowing like calcification.

Thrombi

Thrombi are usually associated with reduction in blood flow (atrial fibrillation, dilated heart chambers, altered or artificial valves or atheroma)

Exceptions to this principle are thrombi associated with coagulopathy and left ventricular non compaction or on aortic atherosclerosis.

Vegetations

Vegetations are associated with other clinical signs of endocarditis (e.g. raised inflammatory markers, positive blood cultures).

If the study is for benign or malignant tumours, and there is suspicion of an extracardiac tumour, consider whether there might be oesophageal involvement. If this is possible then consider an endoscopy or other imaging before performing transoesophageal imaging.

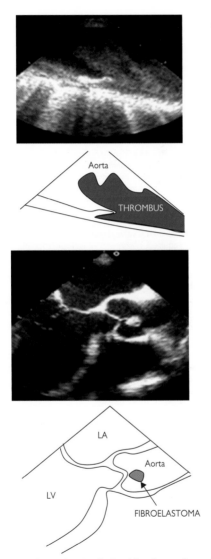

Fig. 7.29 Examples of aortic thrombus (top) and fibroelastoma (bottom). See ▣ Video 7.16 for an example of myxoma.

Cardiopulmonary bypass and coronary artery surgery

If cardiopulmonary bypass is used for coronary artery surgery in a patient with normal left ventricular function and no significant valve disease, it remains a matter of debate whether intraoperative TOE is used routinely. However, a comprehensive study performed before establishing cardiopulmonary bypass, provides a comparison for postoperative studies in particular in patients with suboptimal target vessels and challenging grafting.

Indications

- TOE is strongly indicated in coronary artery surgery complicated by: severe cardiac dysfunction; significant ischaemic mitral regurgitation; large left ventricular aneurysm; mural thrombus; left ventricular remodelling (Dor procedure); recent myocardial infarction; ischaemic ventricular septal defect; requirement for left ventricular assist device support post surgery.
- TOE should be used when a patient preoperatively has mild to moderate aortic or mitral valve disease to determine whether valve surgery is also required. Postoperative echocardiography is required to assess cardiac function and valve performance whether the valve was operated on or not.

Coming off bypass

Start monitoring with transoesophageal imaging soon after the aortic cross clamp is removed. Monitor de-airing of the left heart and aorta and then watch to ensure restoration of cardiac function. After the patient is weaned off bypass, ensure stable systemic haemodynamics (i.e. systolic blood pressure >90–100mmHg, adequate left ventricular filling) then assess effectiveness of surgery. For all surgery, determine global and regional cardiac function using standard techniques. If global cardiac dysfunction develops consider:

- Was there satisfactory myocardial preservation, in particular with concomitant coronary artery disease?
- Was there a large amount of air emboli into a coronary (particularly the right as this is uppermost in the supine patient)? Usually causes severe right, and some left, ventricular failure with significant tricuspid and mitral regurgitation. Further cardiopulmonary bypass may be required to wash out air emboli. Monitor recovery with echocardiography.
- Is there insufficient flow in the bypass grafts (kinking, sutures, etc.) causing regional wall motion abnormality?

Failure to wean off bypass

A possible urgent call for TOE is to evaluate a patient who has failed to come off bypass following surgery. Ensure you are familiar with what surgery is being performed and what the preoperative investigations and transoesophageal findings were i.e. valve disease, left ventricular function, and degree of coronary disease. Although there could be many causes look for:

• Massive mitral or aortic regurgitation due to prosthesis failure
• Acute right ventricular failure due to air emboli (the right coronary artery is particularly prone to air emboli because of its proximal position and therefore 'upper' position in the supine patient).

Left ventricular failure due to intraoperative myocardial infarction. This could be due to concomitant coronary disease without sufficient coronary protection or surgical injury (to a coronary ostia in aortic surgery or the circumflex coronary artery in mitral surgery). Check regional wall motion abnormalities as a guide to which artery may be affected. Look at coronary ostia lumen size and flow in short axis views.

Off-pump coronary artery bypass

Transoesophageal monitoring can be useful in off-pump coronary artery bypass graft surgery to monitor cardiac function and potential mitral regurgitation. Beware of the following aspects of off pump surgery:

- Imaging of left ventricular wall motion is limited by the stabilizer apparatus, which tethers the adjacent myocardium.
- During right coronary artery and circumflex grafting major displacement of the heart does not allow reliable imaging.
- Distortion of the heart can also cause transient mitral regurgitation or increase in right atrial pressure and a shunt via a patent foramen ovale.
- It is best to restart imaging after completion of anastomoses and release of the stabilizer.
- For a short period after the anastomosis regional wall motion abnormalities are seen, representing stunned myocardium. If wall motion abnormalities are persistent, graft patency should be checked.

Ischaemic mitral regurgitation

Ischaemic mitral regurgitation is regurgitation due to incompetent mitral valve systolic coaptation with normal valve leaflet structure, in the presence of ischaemic heart disease. Commonly due to tethered mitral leaflets after basal posterior myocardial infarction, combined with mild to moderate mitral annulus dilatation. Less frequently due to papillary muscle dysfunction or detachment.

- It is usually present before surgery. In this case imaging has to assess the severity to decide on the need for mitral valve repair or replacement. To plan surgery (approach, mitral valve ring size etc.) measure leaflet tethering distance (distance between posterior papillary muscle and mitral valve posterior annulus) and mitral valve annulus diameter.
- Ischaemic regurgitation may also evolve during coronary bypass surgery due to insufficient grafting to the right coronary artery or diffuse myocardial ischaemia. Ischaemic mitral regurgitation is dynamic so tends to be less severe during surgery because of the reduced left ventricular afterload and the general anaesthetic. Moderate to severe regurgitation on intraoperative echocardiography requires surgical intervention.

Aneurysm repair

Before and during ventricular aneurysm resection or apex remodelling (Dor procedure) echocardiography should focus on:

- Presence, mobility, and distribution of mural thrombus.
- Involvement of mitral valve apparatus and papillary muscle.
- Mitral regurgitation caused by surgery.
- Amount and function of residual myocardium.

Haemodynamic instability

On the Intensive Care Unit and during intraoperative monitoring TOE provides a quick and reliable way to investigate the cause of haemodynamic instability. *Haemodynamic instability* usually means *unexplained hypotension* in some cases associated with *unexplained hypoxaemia*. TOE provides information on both intrinsic cardiac causes (e.g. ventricular function, valve function) and extracardiac factors (e.g. left ventricular preload and afterload). Assessment should take into account the clinical history and follow a standard routine to try and exclude common cause (Table 7.6). Chapter 11 provides information on how to use TTE in this setting.

Hypotension due to hypovolaemia

Hypovolaemia causes reduced left ventricle preload/filling. A simple measure of preload/filling is the *left ventricular end-diastolic area* in the short-axis transgastric view. This view can be used for monitoring during surgery. It is useful if a baseline area is known (e.g. preoperative or at start of surgery) in order to judge change from normal filling.

• Hypovolaemia causes a reduced end-diastolic left ventricular volume and, with preserved left ventricular function, an even greater reduction in end-systolic volume. This results in a very high fractional area change.
• If hypovolaemia is diagnosed, the response to fluid therapy should be monitored. Optimal filling of the left ventricle is achieved when further volume supplements do not result in further increases in end-diastolic left ventricular area. Further volume then merely causes increase in left ventricular end-diastolic pressure.

Hypotension due to reduced peripheral resistance

Reduced peripheral resistance (e.g. due to sepsis) results in much higher stroke volumes. End-diastolic volume therefore remains normal but the end-systolic volume is reduced. This again leads to an increased fractional area change.

Hypotension due to ischaemia

If there is clinical suspicion of myocardial ischaemia it is useful to compare any new findings to the preoperative assessment of cardiac function. Look for:

• Left ventricular systolic global and regional function.
• Right ventricular systolic dysfunction. Right ventricular dysfunction is often associated with right ventricular dilatation, tricuspid regurgitation, paradoxical septal movement and a decrease in left ventricular chamber size can sometimes occur.
• True or pseudo-aneurysm and/or right ventricular rupture in those known to have had an infarct.
• Ischaemic ventricular septal defect or papillary muscle rupture.
• Pericardial effusion or tamponade.

Table 7.6 Conditions causing hypotension. Severe aortic stenosis can also be associated with hypotension and is identified from changes to the aortic valve and transvalvular gradient. Aortic dissection can cause hypotension due to associated pericardial effusions and tamponade, hypovolaemia or aortic regurgitation

Condition Associated findings	End-diastolic volume*	End-systolic volume*	Ejection fraction**	Cardiac output
Decreased preload Hypovolaemia	↓	↓↓	↑	↓
Decreased afterload Vasodilation/sepsis	↔	↓↓	↑↑	↑
LV dysfunction Global/regional wall motion, rupture	↑	↑↑	↓↓	↓
RV dysfunction Dilated right heart thrombus in pulmonary artery	↓	↓	(↓)	↓
Tamponade Effusion	↓	↓	↓	↓

*Left ventricle end-diastolic and end-systolic areas in the short axis transgastric views may be used as markers of left ventricle volume.

**Fractional area change can be substituted for ejection fraction.

Unexplained hypoxaemia

Hypoxaemia suggests inadequate lung perfusion. In ventilated patients this may be a greater than normal need for respiratory support. Cardiac causes can include right ventricle dysfunction, pulmonary embolism, or right-to-left shunts. Investigations should also look for primary lung pathology (e.g. pneumonia with associated sepsis).

Pulmonary embolism

Pulmonary embolism is not easy to diagnose (and can not be excluded) because large emboli are needed to induce haemodynamic changes or to be visualized. Helpful features to suggest pulmonary embolism include:

Indirect signs

- Dilated right atrium. Dilated and diffusely hypokinetic right ventricle. Dilated pulmonary artery. (An increased right ventricle wall thickness suggests a more chronic problem, e.g. pulmonary hypertension.)
- An increase in tricuspid regurgitation because of raised pulmonary artery pressure. Judge pressure from the tricuspid regurgitation. (However, cardiac shock can lead to a normal gradient.)

Direct signs

- Thrombus in the inferior or superior vena cavae, or pulmonary artery.
- There are 2 types of thrombi. Type A are highly mobile and vermiform. They derive from deep veins and can become trapped in a Chiari network, tricuspid valve chordae or right ventricle trabeculae. Type B originate from chamber walls, leads, or prostheses.
- To see the pulmonary artery withdraw the probe slightly from an aortic 50° view and angulate the probe forward. The right pulmonary artery can be seen wrapping around the aorta. The left pulmonary artery is obscured by the bronchus.

Patent foramen ovale

In suspected pulmonary embolism always assess the inter-atrial septum. High right atrial pressure opens the foramen and can cause significant right-to-left shunting. With successful treatment of the embolism the shunt reduces and then disappears. Paradoxical embolism is possible and sometimes thrombi can be trapped in the septum.

Right-to-left shunt

Right-to-left shunts can be intracardiac or intrapulmonary. Base initial survey on colour flow mapping of the atrial and ventricular septa. If no shunt is displayed by colour flow mapping use agitated saline contrast, injected through a central line.

- If an *intracardiac shunt*, contrast will pass from right to left atrium, or from right to left ventricle immediately after arrival in the right atrium.
- If an *intrapulmonary shunt*, contrast will appear in the left atrium via the pulmonary veins at least 3 beats after the right atrium.
- If there is a known pre-existing left-to-right shunt this may be turned into a right-to-left shunt by the type of surgery, ventilation, or a super-added pulmonary embolism. Positive end-expiratory pressure ventilation may open a patent foramen ovale in the presence of severe pulmonary embolism.

Mechanical cardiac support

Intra-aortic balloon pump

TOE can be used to identify contraindications to a balloon pump and ensure the balloon is correctly placed in the thoracic descending aorta, distal to the subclavian artery (Fig. 7.30).

Complicating factors

Possible contraindications include: descending aortic aneurysm, moderate to severe aortic regurgitation, severe atheroma.

Placement

To localize the balloon tip start with an aortic arch view. Try and locate the left subclavian artery origin then advance the probe until the tip of the balloon pump comes into view. It should be several centimetres below the left subclavian artery. The tip appears as a bright mark in the centre of the aorta, with associated artefacts. If the probe is advanced further the balloon may be seen deflating and inflating in the aorta.

Left ventricular assist devices

Left ventricular assist devices take blood from a cannula placed in the left atrium or left ventricle, pass it through an extracorporeal pump, and then pump the blood back into the circulation via a tube inserted into the ascending aorta. TOE can help in placement, assessment of device function, and device weaning.

Complicating factors

Before placement, imaging should be used to identify possible contraindications and complications.

- Aortic regurgitation may deteriorate after device placement because of increased backflow into a relatively decompressed left ventricle. In moderate aortic regurgitation valvular surgery has to be considered prior to device placement.
- Thrombi within the ventricular cavities may be mobilized by assist device tubes and should be excluded.
- Aortic atheroma may be dislodged during cannula insertion.
- Right ventricular dysfunction should be assessed in case right ventricular assistance is required.
- Patent foramen ovale should be identified. Significant right-to-left shunting can be found after left ventricular assist device placement. The device significantly offloads the left heart and drops left atrial pressure, whereas the right atrium remains at a relatively high pressure.

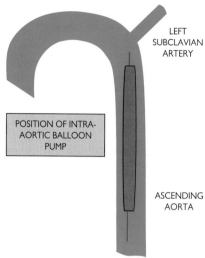

Fig. 7.30 Position of intra-aortic balloon pump in aorta. The top of the balloon can be imaged in aortic views.

Placement

During placement of a left ventricular assist device use TOE to report to the surgeon:

Cannulae

- Position of the atrial cannula (should be in centre of atrium). It should not lie against a wall and be away from the subvalvular apparatus.
- Flow in the cannulae (can be displayed using colour flow mapping).
- Flow pattern in the descending aorta.
- De-airing of the system by observing clearing of bubbles through the ascending or descending aorta.

Changes to valves and septum

- Patent foramen ovale, which may have been missed pre-placement.
- Presence of tricuspid regurgitation.
- Competence of the aortic valve.

Changes to chamber function

- Whether adequate left ventricle offload is achieved.
- Left atrium filling status and size.
- Right ventricle volume status and contraction.

During use

After placement, TOE should monitor for bleeding and pericardial effusion. This is common during the first 24 hours of support and can cause cardiac tamponade.

Weaning

On removal, TOE should be used to judge weaning of left ventricle assist support. The emphasis should be on watching the effect of reducing support on left ventricular function. The left ventricle should gradually improve and take over haemodynamic function.

- Monitor response of the left ventricle to resumed volume loading at both regional and global levels.
- Look at mitral valve competence and systemic haemodynamics.
- Check that improvement in left ventricle function is sustained with minimal support rather than just a shorted-lived improvement of left ventricle contraction.

Pleural space and lungs

As the probe is rotated during the study the lungs and pleura may come into view. It is difficult to give accurate information about lung pathology because they are full of air which does not allow good ultrasound views. Pleural effusions are easily recognized as crescent or 'tiger claw' shaped areas of fluid. The principle to determine whether it is a right or left effusion is to look at the way the 'tiger claw' points. If it points to the right it is a right-sided effusion and if to the left, a left-sided effusion (Fig. 7.31).

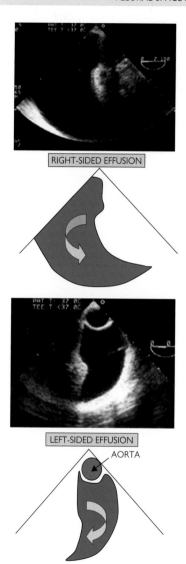

Fig. 7.31 Pleural effusions.

Pacing wires and other implants

As well as prosthetic valves a series of other artificial devices will be seen during transoesophageal studies. Right-sided implants include pacing and defibrillator wires in the right atrium and ventricle and central lines in the superior vena cava and right atrium (Fig. 7.32).

Increasingly, percutaneous closure devices are being implanted. Most commonly these are seen across the atrial septum but can also be positioned in the ventricular septum or beside prosthetic valves to close para-prosthetic leaks. Left atrial appendage occluder devices are also implanted in some centres. Make sure you check the notes before and during the procedure if there is an unusual feature identified.

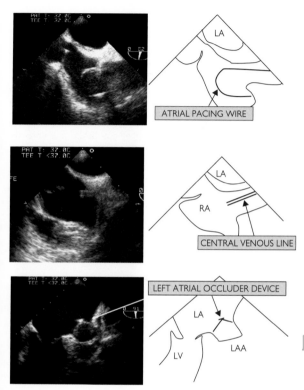

Fig. 7.32 Examples of pacing wires, central lines, and an atrial occluder.
See 🎬 Video 7.17, 🎬 Video 7.18, 🎬 Video 7.19, 🎬 Video 7.20.

Intracardiac echocardiography

Background

- Since its initial use over 30 years ago, intracardiac echocardiography (ICE) has become increasingly available and important as an alternative to TOE primarily to guide percutaneous interventions and support electrophysiological procedures.
- The limitations of the earliest ICE catheters used (poor tissue penetration and difficult manipulation) have been overcome with catheters that use lower frequencies (enabling tissue penetration of up to 12cm) and have better manoeuvrability (Table 8.1).
- ICE provides high-resolution images of cardiac structures which can be displayed as M- and B-modes, with Doppler (CW, PW, or colour flow imaging) or reconstructed into 3D (mainly used in research only at the moment but clinical 3D ICE is not far off now).
- Advantages of ICE over TOE during percutaneous interventions include clearer imaging, shorter procedure times and the use of local (rather than general) anaesthesia.
- ICE catheters are for single-use only and the additional cost that this incurs is the principal disadvantage although this may be offset by the shorter procedure times, improved patient turnaround, and reduced personnel costs.
- ICE is ideal for imaging PFO closures as these procedures can now be performed as a day case under local anaesthetic with total procedure times of around 30min.
- As visualization of the septum is so accurate, ICE has also been shown to reduce the need for fluoroscopy when compared to TOE-guided procedures with a reduction in radiation doses used, shorter procedure times, and shorter hospital stays.
- ICE catheters are not inserted 'over a wire' and are relatively stiff so careful intravascular and intracardiac manipulation is required to avoid perforation.

Indications

- Percutaneous ASD/PFO closure.
- Percutaneous closure of perimembranous ventricular septal defects.
- Balloon mitral commissurotomy.
- Left ventricular or atrial septal pacing.
- Septal ablation for hypertrophic cardiomyopathy.
- Guiding the biopsy of cardiac masses.
- Pulmonary valvuloplasty.
- Guiding transseptal access during electrophysiological procedures.
- Catheter ablation of arrhythmias for defining anatomy.
- Paravalvular leak closure.
- Left atrial appendage occlusion.
- Transcatheter aortic valve implantation.

Table 8.1 Commercially available ICE catheters

ICE catheter Name	Company	Features
AcuNav®	Biosense Webster	8F or 10F 5.5–10MHz 64-element phased-array. PW Doppler, colour Doppler 4-way head articulation for multiple steering
ViewFlex®	St Jude Medical	9F 4.5–8.5MHz 64-element linear phased-array Pulsed wave Doppler, tissue Doppler Bidirectional curved tip
Ultra ICE™	Boston Scientific	9F Mechanical catheter Greyscale imaging
SoundStar™3D	Biosense Webster	10F 5.5–10MHz 64-element linear phased-array Embedded position sensor allows location and beam orientation of catheter

Equipment

Mechanical catheters
- Mechanical transducers have a rotating element (9MHz) which creates a 360° imaging plane perpendicular to the long axis of the catheter.
- The transducers provide a tissue penetration of around 4cm.
- The main limitations of mechanical catheters are the limited imaging plane (horizontal only), reduced catheter manoeuvrability (versus more recent phased-array catheters), and the inability to perform Doppler studies.

Phased-array catheters
- Phased-array 64-element transducers are able to scan in a longitudinal plane, creating a 90° sector image.
- Lower range frequencies (5–10MHz) allow better tissue penetration (up to 12cm).
- Improved manoeuvrability is achieved as the head of the catheter has a multidirection articulation tip and steering locks can maintain catheter angulation (Fig. 8.1).

Procedure

Patient preparation
Patient preparation relates to the interventional procedure that is to be undertaken. Normally this will involve:
- Pre-procedural fasting for 4 hours. An important aspect for ICE is that the patient should not be dehydrated so give IV fluids if necessary.
- Insertion of a peripheral cannula to allow delivery of sedation if needed. Both inguinal areas should be prepared and draped.

Catheter preparation
- A connector is used to link the ICE catheter to the ultrasound machine. The connector is covered in a sterile sleeve then connected to the ICE catheter. Check the catheter steering mechanism before use.

Vascular access
- Venous access is usually obtained via the right femoral vein using a Seldinger technique although the right jugular vein has also been used.
- The catheter is manipulated into the right atrium. Special caution is needed when manipulating the catheter through the pelvic veins and fluoroscopy screening is recommended to avoid the catheter catching on venous branches (Fig. 8.2).
- Sometimes gentle AV steering is needed tortuous vessels.
- Placement of a guidewire through an adjacent sheath can help guide the catheter into the right heart, or insertion of a longer sheath (e.g. 12Fr Mullins sheath) to the IVC or right atrium in particularly difficult cases.

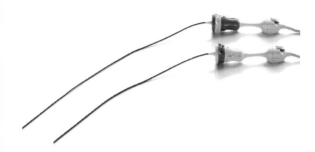

Fig. 8.1 AcuNav intracardiac echocardiography catheters. Image courtesy of Biosense Webster, Inc.

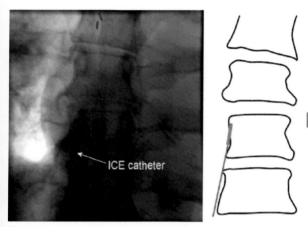

Fig. 8.2 Fluroscopy of the ICE catheter in the right atrium.

Imaging planes

With the use of a phased array catheter, all cardiac anatomical landmarks can be imaged with the probe positioned either in the right atrium or right ventricle. A structured system of steering and manipulation of the catheter is recommended to allow a detailed thorough examination, improving operator orientation and recognition of landmarks.

Standard view

The 'standard view' (Fig. 8.3) is achieved with the ICE probe sited in the mid-right atrium and with the scan plane facing anteriorly.
* This provides excellent views of the right atrium, right ventricle, and tricuspid valve.
* Withdrawing the catheter to the inferior right atrium brings the Eustachian ridge and the tricuspid valve isthmus into view.

What do you see?
* Right atrium.
* Right ventricle.
* Tricuspid valve.

Atrial septum

Slowly advancing the catheter whilst gently retro-flexing and rotating the catheter tip manipulates the probe towards the intra-atrial septum, highlighting the fossa ovalis (Fig. 8.4).
* In order to avoid foreshortening some left-to-right manipulation may be needed.
* Detailed interrogation of the atrial septum and fossa ovalis can be obtained and, if needed, agitated saline bubble contrast studies (📖 p.506) can be performed to assess for the presence of a patent foramen ovale.
* This position of the catheter for assessment of the atrial septum is employed for percutaneous septal procedures as it sits in a neutral position, without interfering with interventional catheters.

What do you see?
* Right atrium.
* Atrial septum.
* Left atrium.

Aortic valve and root

To view the aortic valve in the short axis the catheter tip is retroflexed and then rotated clockwise towards the aorta (Fig. 8.5).

What do you see?
* Aortic valve.
* Ascending aorta.
* Left ventricle.

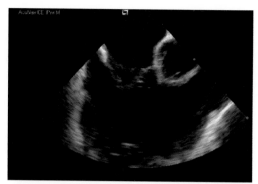

Fig. 8.3 Standard view showing the right atrium (RA), right ventricle (RV), tricuspid valve (TV), and part of the aortic valve (AV). See ▣ Video 8.1.

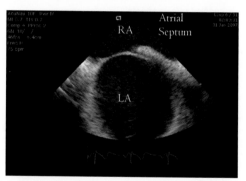

Fig. 8.4 Atrial septum view showing the right atrium (RA), atrial septum, and left atrium (LA). See ▣ Video 8.2.

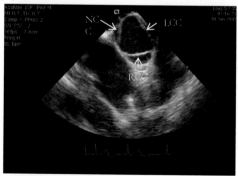

Fig. 8.5 Aortic valve view. See ▣ Video 8.3. NCC = non-coronary cusp, LCC = left coronary cusp, RCC = right coronary cusp.

Pulmonary veins

The left superior and inferior pulmonary veins can be viewed by increasing the depth from the atrial septum view (Fig. 8.6). For finer adjustment inferior angulation may be needed. The right pulmonary veins can be seen by gentle clockwise rotation and superior advancement of the catheter.

What do you see?
- Left and right pulmonary veins.
- If needed, Doppler studies can be performed to analyse the venous flow.

Left atrial appendage

Advancing the catheter towards the atrial septum and rotating clockwise brings the left atrial appendage into view.

What do you see?
- Left atrial appendage.
- Left ventricle.
- Mitral valve.

Mitral valve and left ventricle

Advancing the catheter towards the atrial septum and rotating clockwise brings the left atrial appendage and mitral valve into view (Fig. 8.7).

What do you see?
- Left atrium.
- Mitral valve.
- Left ventricle.

Right ventricle

From the initial standard view the catheter can be flexed and gently advanced towards the tricuspid valve. With further careful manipulation under fluoroscopic control the catheter can be placed in the right ventricle (Fig. 8.8). Typically the catheter lies against the septum and rotated to scan either the right ventricular free wall or the left ventricle.

What do you see?
- Ventricular septum.
- Right ventricular free wall.
- Left ventricular lateral wall.

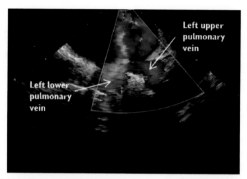

Fig. 8.6 Identifying the pulmonary veins.

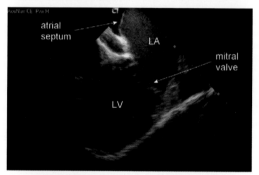

Fig. 8.7 Mitral valve and left ventricle (LV) view. The atrial septum and left atrium (LA) are also seen. See 📹 Video 8.4.

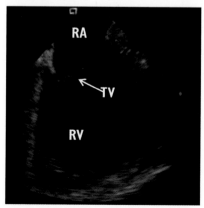

Fig. 8.8 Right ventricle (RV) view. RA = right atrium; TV = tricuspid valve. See 📹 Video 8.5.

Atrial septal interventions

Visualization of the interatrial septum and fossa ovalis with ICE allows a detailed assessment of the size and length of the PFO 'tunnel' and additional information gained on the mobility of the atrial septum (Figs. 8.9 and 8.10). The ICE catheter is usually quite stable for guiding the percutaneous closure of PFO and atrial septal defects (ASDs).

Key views

The following steps in sequence allow full assessment of the atrial septum during atrial septal interventions:

- After advancing the ICE catheter from the inferior vena cava into the mid-right atrium rotate the probe clockwise. The aorta and LVOT will initially be seen. Further clockwise rotation will allow visualization of the lower atrial septum.
- Posterior deflection with continued clockwise (posterior) rotation will obtain a long axis view of the atrial septum.
- Moving the catheter cranially and caudally shows the entire atrial septum.
- If appropriate a bubble contrast study can be performed from this position to document the presence of a PFO.
- From here, the left upper and lower pulmonary veins can be visualized with the aid of Doppler colour flow.
- Clockwise rotation of the catheter allows visualization of the right upper and lower pulmonary veins.
- Gentle anterior flexion and clockwise rotation shows the superior vena cava.
- With anterior and lateral movement of the catheter tip a short axis view of the atrial septum is obtained.

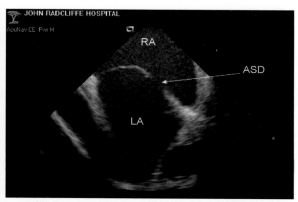

Fig. 8.9 Atrial septal defect (ASD). LA = left atrium; RA = right atrium.
See 📹 Video 8.6.

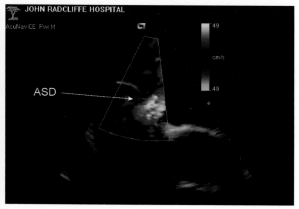

Fig. 8.10 Colour flow Doppler showing flow across atrial septal defect (ASD).
See 📹 Video 8.7 and 📹 Video 8.8.

Balloon sizing
- The long axis view of the atrial septum usually provides the best imaging plane for balloon sizing (Fig. 8.11).
- Colour flow imaging is used whilst obtaining multiple views of the inflated balloon to demonstrate complete coverage of the defect.
- The balloon size can be obtained from anterior and lateral fluoroscopy images.

Device deployment
- Following sizing, a sheath is positioned over a stiff wire into the left upper pulmonary vein through which the device is delivered.
- After device insertion, prior to and following deployment the adjacent structures should be interrogated to ensure that there was no encroachment of the device on the atrioventricular valves, the right pulmonary vein or the inferior or superior vena cava (Fig. 8.12).

Evaluation of the defect during atrial septal intervention

During atrial septal intervention the key views will allow ASD size estimation by measurement of the distance between the defect to the:
- Aortic valve (superior-anterior rim).
- Coronary sinus (posterior rim).
- Mitral valve (inferior-anterior rim).
- Inferior vena cava (inferior-posterior rim).

Special care should be taken to also evaluate the relationship of the defect to:
- Pulmonary veins.
- Atrioventricular valve.
- Aortic root.

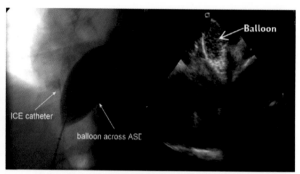

Fig. 8.11 Fluoroscopy showing balloon crossing atrial septal defect (ASD) (left). Balloon sizing of ASD (right). See 📹 Video 8.9.

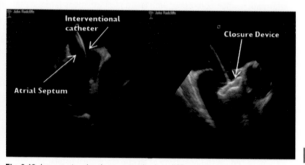

Fig. 8.12 Interventional catheter passed across ASD—device starting to deploy in image shown (left). ICE imaging during percutaneous ASD closure. See 📹 Video 8.10, 📹 Video 8.11, 📹 Video 8.12, 📹 Video 8.13, 📹 Video 8.14.

Electrophysiological interventions

The advantage of accurate visualization of anatomical structures means that ICE can be used to guide interventional physiology. Clinical applications of ICE during electrophysiology include:

Transseptal puncture guidance

- During electrophysiology transseptal puncture is very important to obtain access into the left atrium for ablation procedures.
- Historically fluoroscopy has been used to guide the transseptal puncture. Here, the anatomical structures are not displayed directly and the needle puncture is guided by the movement during pullback from the superior vena cava and position in the cardiac shadow relative to a catheter in the aortic root.
- ICE offers the opportunity to guide the transseptal puncture by directly visualizing the needle tip within the fossa ovalis region. By detailing the relevant anatomy, ICE can offer the operator further information when confronted with anatomical variations (atrial septal aneurysm or lipomatous hypertrophy of the atrial septum, etc).
- Colour flow Doppler can also be helpful to identify the puncture site should the interventional catheter fall back into the right atrium.

Catheter ablation of arrhythmias

The detailed anatomical orientation provided by ICE has the following advantages during ablation procedures:

- A detailed understanding of the anatomy of the pulmonary veins.
- ICE provides the ability to confirm stable, complete catheter-tissue contact which ensures more complete ablation and reduces the incidence of clot formation on the catheter.
- To identify the presence of thrombus within the left atrial appendage.
- To confirm the anatomy of the oesophagus in relation to the left atrium, to reduce the possibility of atrio-oesophageal fistula.
- Assists accurate placement of both mapping and ablation catheters.
- Operators are able to prevent tissue overheating (and resultant scar formation, thrombosis, or stenosis) by delivering ablation therapy until the onset of microbubble formation, ensuring maximal safety.
- Images acquired using ICE have recently been combined with 3D electrophysiological mapping catheters to provide additional anatomical information during ablation.

Additional uses

ICE has also been used to guide catheter occlusion of the left atrial appendage by deploying the ICE catheter in the pulmonary artery via a long sheath, and to guide transcatheter aortic valve implantation (see 📖 p.464), utilizing both transvenous and transarterial placement.

Radiological interventions such as fenestration of aortic dissection flaps can also be guided with the use of 8Fr intra-arterial ICE.

Contrast
echocardiography

Introduction

Contrast imaging relies on the use of an injected agent that is very echogenic in order to increase the brightness of the ultrasound image. Broad types of contrast used are those that are normally only held in the venous circulation and then absorbed in the lungs (right-heart contrast agents) and those that are present in both the venous and systemic circulation (left-heart contrast agents).

Both right and left contrast agents essentially consist of gas bubbles of varying size. On the right this is air contained in saline and on the left a gas in a lipid or albumin shell (Figs. 9.1–9.3).

Right-heart contrast agents

- Right-heart contrast agents such as agitated saline consist of air microbubbles (of a relatively large size when compared to left-heart contrast agents). These are short lived and normally diffuse into the lungs when crossing the pulmonary circulation. The presence of agitated saline microbubbles in the left heart indicates either the presence of a right-to-left intracardiac shunt or an arteriovenous shunt elsewhere in the body, typically in the pulmonary circulation.
- The stability of these bubbles can be improved if the agitation is performed with blood (<0.5ml in 10ml saline).
- Other agents used because they contain bubbles include Gelofusine® (gelatine) but have the risk of allergic reaction.

Uses

- To identify the presence of a right-to-left intracardiac shunt due to an atrial septal abnormality.
- To identify the presence of a right-to-left intrapulmonary shunt.
- To enhance the delineation of Doppler signals, e.g. the use of agitated saline contrast can provide a better Doppler signal assessment of the tricuspid valve.

Left-heart contrast agents

- Left-heart contrast agents must be durable and small enough to be able to cross the pulmonary circulation and pass into the left atrium following an intravenous injection.
- Left-heart contrast agents comprise a microbubble gas centre with an outer shell. This makes it durable but also small enough for safe passage across the pulmonary circulation.

Uses

- To improve LV endocardial border definition in order to:
  - improve image quality and the percentage of wall segments visualized
  - improve the confidence of interpretation of wall motion abnormalities during stress imaging.
  - improve accuracy of ventricular volumes and EF measures.
- To improve LV cavity opacification to detect pathology e.g. thrombus, apical HCM, LV non-compaction.
- To enhance the delineation of Doppler signals.
- To assess myocardial perfusion.

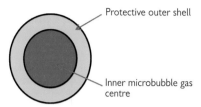

Protective outer shell

Inner microbubble gas centre

Fig. 9.1 Representation of a left-heart contrast molecule.

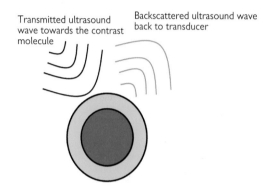

Transmitted ultrasound wave towards the contrast molecule

Backscattered ultrasound wave back to transducer

Fig. 9.2 The bubble causes backscatter from the transmitted ultrasound wave which is picked up by the ultrasound transducer.

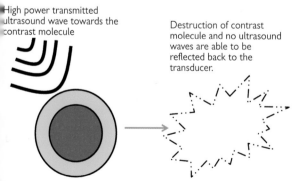

High power transmitted ultrasound wave towards the contrast molecule

Destruction of contrast molecule and no ultrasound waves are able to be reflected back to the transducer.

Fig. 9.3 Higher power ultrasound waves will cause the destruction of left-heart contrast agents by causing them to resonate.

Specific contrast agent preparation

Left-heart contrast agents

SonoVue® (Bracco International BV)

- *Structure*: a phospholipid shell filled with sulphur hexafluoride (SF_6).
- *Preparation and storage*: it is reconstituted with sodium chloride (Fig. 9.4). The authors recommend that the contrast is constituted within a few minutes of injection and to agitate the vial before each injection is withdrawn. If given as an infusion it needs to be agitated in a special agitating pump during delivery.
- *Bolus*: recommended dose is 2.0mL. However, the dose derives from studies using fundamental imaging, which should be avoided. For harmonic imaging bolus injections of 0.2–0.4mL are adequate. The bolus should be followed by a 3–5mL bolus of 0.9% sodium chloride or 5% glucose. Total dose should not exceed 1.6mL.
- *Infusion*: for SonoVue® a special agitation pump is used (Fig. 9.5). For stress studies 2 vials should be drawn up into the syringe. The rate of infusion should be initiated at 0.8mL/minute, but titrated as necessary to achieve optimal image enhancement (the range is 0.6–1.2mL/min).

Optison® (Amersham)

- *Structure*: Optison® (Amersham) an albumin shell containing perflutren gas.
- *Preparation and storage*: it comes in a vial that requires reconstitution and manual agitation. It is then drawn up into a 2mL or 1mL syringe. A second needle is used to vent the vial (this can be removed if repetitive doses are withdrawn). The authors recommend that the agent is reconstituted directly before injection and the vial agitated before each dose is withdrawn. It should be stored in a refrigerator between 2–8°C.
- *Dose and administration*: the recommended dose is 0.5–3.0mL per patient injected into a peripheral vein. However, that dosage derives from studies using fundamental imaging, which should be avoided. For contrast-specific imaging modalities bolus injections of 0.2–0.4mL are adequate. Total dose should not exceed 8.7mL. The bolus should be followed by a 3–5mL bolus of 0.9% sodium chloride or 5% glucose.

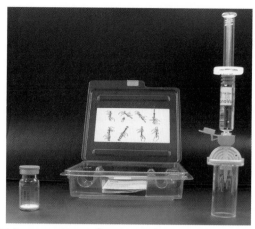

Fig. 9.4 Preparation of SonoVue®. The agent is packaged as dry powder and reconstituted using saline. Image courtesy of Bracco International BV.

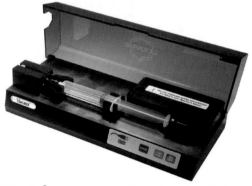

Fig. 9.5 SonoVue® pump Image courtesy of Bracco International BV. The pump provides continuous rotation of the syringe in order to prevent accumulation of the microbubbles in the upper parts of the syringe.

Luminity® (Bristol Myers Squib)
- *Structure*: Luminity® is composed of lipid-encapsulated perflutren microspheres. The spheres are between 1–10 micrometres in diameter.
- *Preparation and storage*: it should be stored in a refrigerator at 2–8°C until activated. It needs to be activated by a mechanical shaking device (Vialmix) and then can be used for up to 12 hours (although if left standing for more than 5min it requires 10sec of shaking by hand before further use). It can be reactivated once more within 48 hours.
- *Dose and administration*: recommended bolus dose is of 0.1–0.4mL followed by a bolus of 3–5mL of 0.9% sodium chloride or 5% glucose. Diluting 0.3mL in 10mL saline (0.9% sodium chloride) and injecting 1–2cc is an alternative and provided good contrast in IE33 scanners. Total dose should not exceed 1.6mL. The recommended intravenous infusion is of 1.3mL Luminity® added to 30ml of 0.9% sodium chloride. The rate of infusion should start at 1mL/min and be titrated to achieve optimal image enhancement (not to exceed 10mL/min).

Right-heart contrast agents
- Agitated saline contrast can be used to demonstrate the presence of right-to-left shunts across the atrial septum, or to improve the Doppler envelope when examining the tricuspid valve (Fig. 9.6).
- Insert a cannula ideally into the right antecubital fossa.
- Attach a 3-way tap to the cannula.
- Obtain 2 10mL Luer lock syringe. In one syringe draw up 9mL of saline and 1mL of air. 0.5mL of the patient's blood can also be drawn up.
- Ensure both Luer lock syringes are firmly attached to the cannula and force the mixture back and forth between the syringes until frothy.

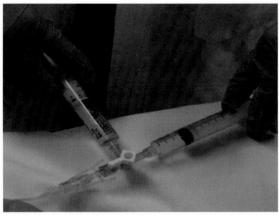

Fig. 9.6 A three-way tap with Luer lock syringes should be used for agitated saline injections.

Administration of contrast agents

Left-heart contrast agents

- Patient preparation requires insertion of an intravenous cannula usually into an antecubital vein and its connection to a 3-way-tap or small-bore Y connector. Ultrasound contrast agents can be injected through this line by bolus injection or an infusion.
- The use of smaller diameter cannula should be avoided as the bubbles from the contrast will be subjected to a large pressure drop as the fluid exits the tip of the lumen. The faster the injection and the smaller the diameter of the lumen, the larger the pressure drop and there is increased chance of damage to the contrast bubbles.

Bolus injection

- Slow bolus injections (0.2mL) of all agents (SonoVue®, Luminity®, and Optison®) can be used followed by a slow 5mL saline flush over 20s. However, these are not as controllable or reproducible as infusions.
- Agitate the contrast immediately before injection slowly and withdraw the contrast agent from the syringe avoiding high negative pressure.
- If giving a bolus injection for left-heart contrast studies, a saline flush (5mL) may be considered to push the agent into the central blood stream if there is delayed contrast appearance. Lifting the arm is often sufficient.

Contrast infusion

- Because of microspheres behaviour, continuous agitation of the contrast is necessary for optimum contrast.
- Agitation can be performed manually by slowly rocking the pump to and fro. A special infusion pump has been developed for SonoVue®. A constant infusion of SonoVue® 0.8mL/min from the start is usually satisfactory and need not be changed in the majority of patients.
- The pump is particularly useful in stress echocardiography; the infusion can be stopped at any time and resumed when needed. Between infusion periods, the contrast agent is gently agitated.

Right-heart contrast agents

- Patient preparation also requires insertion of an intravenous cannula, usually into an antecubital vein.
- Need to be given as a bolus injection through a relatively large bore cannula in a relatively proximal location.
- Need to be given as a rapid bolus to ensure complete opacification of the right atrium. Blood from both the superior and inferior vena cavae streams into the right atrium and it is possible with slow boluses for the bubbles not to mix into the flow from the inferior vena cava and therefore not reach the interatrial septum.
- Another way some people use if they are having difficulties with opacification of the atrium near the interatrial septum is to give an injection into the femoral vein so that the bubbles travel up the inferior vena cava.

Advantages of bolus injections

- Easy to perform.
- Wash-in period and wash-out is visible.
- Agent is quickly used with little stability problems.
- Allows the highest peak enhancement.

Disadvantages of bolus injections

- Contrast is short-lived.
- The contrast effect changes during study.
- Timing of injection of bolus can be difficult.
- Comparative contrast studies difficult.

Advantages of contrast infusion

- Prolongs the period of contrast enhancement.
- Provides a steady (constant) effect.
- Allows the dose of the agent to be optimized and used efficiently.

Disadvantages of contrast infusion

- More complex than bolus injections to perform.
- Titration of contrast takes time.

Contrast safety

Left-heart contrast agents

The safety of ultrasound contrast agents has been assessed in cohorts of several thousand patients. Side effects have been noted but they are usually mild and transient. Most frequent side effects of SonoVue® in clinical trials were: headache (2.1%), nausea (1.3%), chest pain (1.3%), taste perversion (0.9%), hyperglycaemia (0.6%), injection site reaction 0.6%), paraesthesia (0.6%), vasodilation (0.6%), injection site pain (0.5%). Serious adverse events in particular allergic reactions are very rare (0.01%) and less frequent than for X-ray contrast agents.

- Allergic reactions: They may happen as acute sensitivity reactions (IgE mediated type I), but Complement Activation Related Pseudo Allergy (CARPA) seems to be more typical for the contrast agents with a phospholipid membrane (SonoVue® and Luminity®). In comparison to IgE mediated reactions, CARPA reactions need no prior exposure to the agent, the reaction is milder or absent upon repeated exposures and spontaneous resolution is possible. Although serious adverse events are very rare, appropriate allergy and emergency equipment as well as a physician with knowledge in emergency medicine should be present or close by.
- Acute coronary disease: Only Optison® and Luminity® may be used in acute coronary syndromes, since their contraindication on the use in these conditions has been recently withdrawn by FDA, based on the evidence of their favourable risk:benefit profile and safety. SonoVue® may be used 7 days after acute coronary syndrome.
- Special considerations and precautions with use: mechanical ventilation, clinically significant pulmonary disease (including diffuse interstitial pulmonary fibrosis and severe chronic obstructive pulmonary disease), adult respiratory distress syndrome, severe heart failure (NYHA IV), endocarditis, acute myocardial infarction with ongoing angina or unstable angina, hearts with prosthetic valves, acute states of systemic inflammation or sepsis, known states of hyperactive coagulation system, recurrent thromboembolism.

Right-heart contrast agents

Reports of serious side effects from the use of agitated saline injection are rare. There have been a few case reports of agitated saline contrast causing ischaemic complications such as stroke or transient ischaemic attacks. Available data is not sufficient to estimate the incidence of these events, although such complications appear to be extremely rare.

Management of allergic reactions[1]

- Recognize signs and symptoms of an allergic reaction: itching, erythema, urticaria, wheeze, laryngeal obstruction, tachycardia, hypotension.
- Ensure airway is secure and give 100% O_2.
- If any signs of airway obstruction seek anaesthetic help to maintain airway patency.
- If suspected anaphylaxis give IM adrenaline 0.5mg (i.e. 0.5mL of 1:1000). Repeat every 5min if needed as guided by blood pressure, pulse, and respiratory function until better.
- Secure IV access
- Chlorpheniramine 10mg and hydrocortisone 200mg IV.
- IV normal saline titrated against blood pressure.

Ensure appropriate monitoring on ward: cardiac monitor, regular blood pressure review.

Left-heart contrast agents in pregnant or lactating women

- No left-heart ultrasound contrast is approved for use in pregnant or lactating women.
- In women of childbearing age the physician has to ask for confirmed or possible pregnancy.
- Ultrasound contrast injections should be avoided unless there is no alternative imaging method to answer the clinical question and the clinical need for information is felt to be greater than any potential risks.

Reference

1 Longmore M et al. (eds) (2010). *Oxford Handbook of Clinical Medicine*, 8th edn. Oxford: Oxford University Press.

Right-heart contrast study applications

Contrast study for atrial shunts and patent foramen ovale

Microbubble contrast studies can be used to identify atrial shunts and confirm the presence of a patent foramen ovale (Fig. 9.7). There are 3 elements to a good contrast study for an atrial shunt:

A stable image

- Use apical 4-chamber view (or subcostal view) optimized so that all 4 chambers are seen. Try the view with the patient doing a Valsalva to ensure you can keep all chambers in view.

Agitated saline injection

- Inject rapidly through a Venflon® inserted into an antecubital vein. It must completely and rapidly opacify the right atrium.

A good Valsalva

- Shunting may be evident at rest so the first contrast injection should be without Valsalva.
- If no bubbles appear in the left heart repeat the injection with a Valsalva manoeuvre.
- The critical time of a Valsalva is when the patient relaxes. It is then that right-sided pressures transiently elevate relative to the left and contrast shunts.
- Get the patient to take a breath and bear down hard. Inject the contrast and when it has filled the right atrium tell them to relax. If there is a shunt a few bubbles will appear in the left atrium and left ventricle within 5 beats of the patient relaxing. If bubbles appear later this is more consistent with a pulmonary arteriovenous malformation.
- Set the system to capture 10–20 beats and start acquisition on contrast injection. Look back through the loop for bubbles. Repeat the study with more contrast until all three elements of the study are perfect.
- The appearance of bubbles in the left heart within 5 cardiac cycles following right chamber opacification and release of Valsalva suggests an intracardiac shunt.

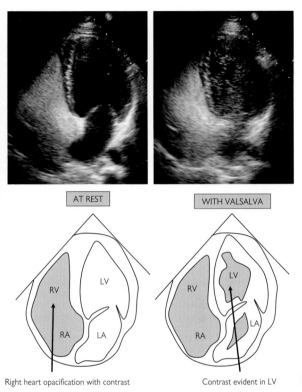

Right heart opacification with contrast   Contrast evident in LV

Fig. 9.7 Contrast injection: left-sided bubbles with Valsalva (on right) demonstrating a patent foramen ovale. Also note septal aneurysm. See 📖 Video 9.1.

Contrast study for pulmonary shunts

Intrapulmonary shunts are often the result of pulmonary arteriovenous malformations. Intravenous agitated saline contrast can be used to aid the diagnosis of intrapulmonary shunts.

- A stable image position and adequate agitated saline injection should be used as described on 📖 p.572.
- The appearance of bubbles in the left heart only after 5 cardiac cycles suggests an intrapulmonary shunt.

Contrast study for Doppler enhancement

Intravenous injection of agitated saline and other contrast agents can be used to enhance the tricuspid regurgitation signal (Fig. 9.8). The contrast enhancement of a weak TR velocity jet signal allows more accurate estimation of right heart haemodynamics. Right-heart contrast agents may also enhance the appearance of hepatic vein flow reversal.

- Acquire the TR jet CW signal by placing the CW cursor across the TR jet as in the normal examination (see 📖 p.162).
- Inject the agitated saline or left-heart contrast.
- The contrast is likely to generate a lot of noise on the spectral trace so reduce the gain until the enhanced Doppler envelope is evident.

Diagnosis of persistent left superior vena cava

The diagnosis of a persistent left SVC is usually made incidentally following identification of a dilated coronary sinus or because there are difficulties with pacemaker lead insertion from the left side. This is because a persistent left-sided SVC most frequently drains directly into the coronary sinus.

A good view of the coronary sinus and its insertion into the right atrium is required. This can often be best done on TOE or with TTE using a modified apical 4-chamber view tilted down to cut through the coronary sinus.

- Following injection of agitated saline into the left arm the contrast is seen to appear in the coronary sinus before the right atrium.
- In the majority of patients a right (normal) SVC is then also present. Therefore when agitated saline is injected into the right arm it is seen to enter the right atrium before any appearing in the coronary sinus. However, if the right SVC is absent then this injection will also appear in the coronary sinus first.

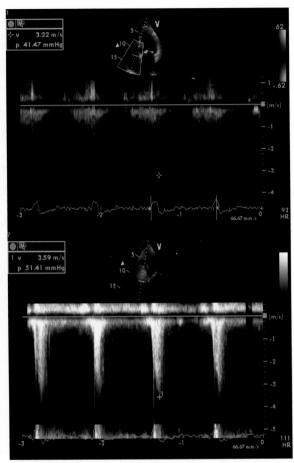

Fig. 9.8 Above: TR velocity jet continuous wave Doppler without the use of contrast. Below: TR velocity jet continuous wave Doppler augmented by contrast.

Imaging techniques for left ventricular opacification

The durability of the contrast agent within the left ventricle is highly dependent upon both the bubble composition and also the ultrasound settings. Optimizing the ultrasound settings is vital to ensure good opacification of the LV (Table 9.1).

Imaging presets and analysis

- When ultrasound contrast agents are used, contrast-specific imaging modalities should be employed (Fig. 9.9) based on the use of harmonic frequencies and low transmit power from the transducer.
- There are a range of manufacturer specific presets. The standard is a real-time, low power mode. The low-power contrast-specific imaging technology provides excellent ventricular opacification and often simultaneous myocardial opacification.
- In systems without contrast-specific imaging modality use harmonic imaging but with a mechanical index of <0.6.

Contrast specific imaging

- When exposed to ultrasound waves, the contrast bubbles resonate and emit harmonic frequencies in addition to the frequency that comes from the transducer, the fundamental frequency. The harmonic frequencies are two times greater than the fundamental (second harmonic), three times (third harmonic), and so on. With increasing frequency the amplitude of the ultrasound waves decreases.
- Myocardial tissue shows the same response to ultrasound but only with high transmit power (MI>1). Microbubbles will resonate at low powers (MI=2).
- Thus, if the transducer is set to low power imaging the harmonic signals from the contrast in the blood will be significantly stronger than any signals from the myocardium and therefore excellent blood to myocardial contrast is obtained.

Image settings to prevent microbubble destruction

The transmitted ultrasound frequency from the ultrasound machine can destroy the microbubbles. Bubble destruction can be done purposefully in some forms of imaging such as myocardial flash perfusion imaging but usually stable micro-bubbles are needed to optimize image quality. To increase the length of time microbubbles persist in the circulation there are two imaging aspects that can be varied:

- Low mechanical index: The higher the mechanical index, the greater the transmitted acoustic power and the higher the chance of microbubble destruction. Using lower mechanical indexes will therefore also reduce the destruction of micro-bubbles. However, this needs to be balanced against the need for penetration to achieve adequate depth of imaging, for which higher mechanical indexes can be used.
- Intermittent imaging: Continuous imaging with the transducer on the chest wall will cause a gradual depletion of microbubbles. Therefore intermittent imaging is recommended to increase microbubble durability.

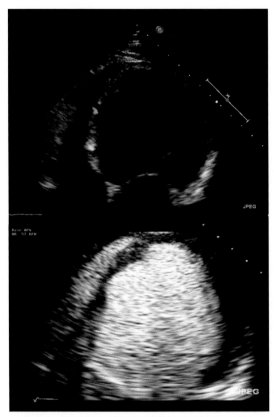

Fig. 9.9 Example of contrast-specific imaging. Without contrast agent there are only faint signals from myocardial tissue. After contrast injection there is bright opacification of the blood within the left ventricle cavity and excellent delineation of the endocardium. Opacification of the myocardium is not as intense as the cavity but provides a good display of left ventricle wall thickness. See 📹 Video 9.2.

Left-heart contrast study applications

Contrast study for left ventricular opacification

European Association of Echocardiography indications for resting left ventricular opacification contrast are as follows:

In patients with suboptimal images:

- To enable improved endocardial visualization and assessment of LV structure and function when 2 or more contiguous segments are *not* seen on non-contrast images.
- To have accurate and repeatable measurements of LV volumes, and ejection fraction by 2D/3D echo (e.g. before CRT, follow-up echocardiograms for assessment of cardiac toxicity) (Fig. 9.10).
- To increase the confidence of the interpreting physician in the LV function, structure, and volume assessments.
- To confirm or exclude the echocardiographic diagnosis of the following LV structural abnormalities, when non-enhanced images are suboptimal for definitive diagnosis:
  - Apical hypertrophic cardiomyopathy, LV non-compaction.
  - Ventricular non-compaction.
  - Apical thrombus (Fig. 9.11).
  - Ventricular pseudoaneurysm.

Contrast study for Doppler enhancement

- Intravenous injection of left-heart contrast agents can be used to enhance Doppler signals. The technique is as for right-heart agents (see 📖 p.574).
- As left-heart contrast agents pass from the right to the left heart, they can be used to augment Doppler traces from the right heart (e.g. tricuspid valve) and also the left heart.
- In the left heart, contrast can be used to enhance mitral Doppler traces or pulmonary vein Doppler traces for the assessment of diastolic dysfunction.
- Since only small amounts of contrast are needed for this indication, Doppler enhancement can be achieved in the wash-out phase after LV opacification. Usually the Doppler and/or power gain needs to be reduced to achieve normal intensity spectra.

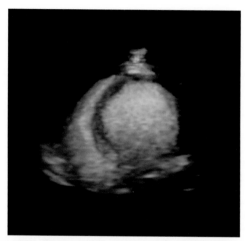

Fig. 9.10 3D LV contrast opacification. See 📹 Video 9.3 and 📹 Video 9.4.

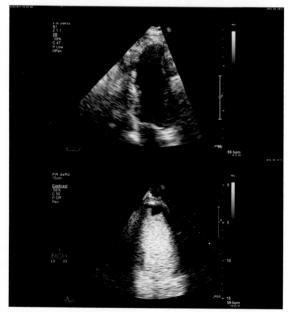

Fig. 9.11 The use of LV opacification to demonstrate the presence of LV apical thrombus. The LV apical thrombus is not clearly seen without contrast (upper image) and its presence confirmed following LV contrast opacification (lower image). See 📹 Video 9.5.

Contrast study in dobutamine stress echocardiography

Since image quality is crucial for reliable stress echocardiography, review all baseline images prior to beginning the stress procedure. If endocardial borders are not visible (or barely visible) in 2 or more myocardial segments consider using an ultrasound contrast agent (Fig. 9.12).

Indications for use of contrast in stress echocardiography

- When 2 or more endocardial border contiguous segments of LV are not well visualized.
- To obtain diagnostic assessment of segmental wall motion and thickening at rest and stress.
- To increase the proportion of diagnostic studies.
- To increase reader confidence in interpretation.

Contraindications

- Known or suspected significant intracardiac shunts.
- Known hypersensitivity to the agent.

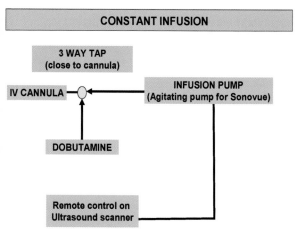

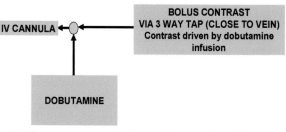

Fig. 9.12 Most contrast agents can be given as a bolus or an infusion. When given with a dobutamine infusion it can be given via the same cannula using a 3-way tap. The contrast agent is driven by the dobutamine infusion. No boluses of saline are necessary. There is no risk of dobutamine boluses since the amount of contrast is very low.

Contrast study for myocardial perfusion

The use of left-heart ultrasound contrast agents for the assessment of myocardial perfusion has the potential to significantly improve myocardial assessment during stress echocardiography. Myocardial contrast echocardiography is quick, easy to perform, and potentially a bedside technique (as long as facilities for an infusion of contrast are available). Contrast echocardiography supplements wall motion information with perfusion judged from the appearance of contrast within the myocardium.

Principle

- Myocardial contrast echocardiography (perfusion imaging) describes echocardiography with intravascular ultrasound contrast agents.
- This results in opacification of the cavities and the intramyocardial blood vessels.
- The amount of myocardial opacification depends on the settings of the ultrasound scanner, the density of the myocardial micro vessels (where most of the myocardial blood is located), and the myocardial blood flow.
- Differences in the intensity of myocardial opacification and in the speed of filling the myocardium with contrast can be used to identify areas of non-viability and/or ischaemia.

Indications

- At present most guidelines for echocardiographic assessment of ischaemia and viability are based on assessment of LV wall motion alone.
- Ultrasound contrast agents are approved for LV opacification and endocardial definition. At present, assessment of myocardial perfusion is not an approved indication for ultrasound contrast agents.
- However, using state-of-the-art equipment myocardial opacification often is inevitable when performing contrast echo for LV opacification (Table 9.1).
- It is worth including these findings when assessing the patient for myocardial viability and ischaemia as the perfusion data can confirm sometimes questionable findings on LV wall motion.
- Protocols that exclusively make the diagnosis from perfusion images may be an option in the future.

Table 9.1 Common pitfalls seen in myocardial contrast echocardiography and their solutions

Pitfall of myocardial contrast echocardiography	Solution
Insufficient contrast dosage and/or setting causing inhomogeneous opacification and swirling	Increase contrast dose and/or correct setting
Nearfield destruction artefacts in the apical parts of the left ventricle setting causing inhomogeneous opacification and swirling	Stepwise reduce transmit power (MI) in 0.1 step and/or change focus to farfield
Very strong signals in the nearfield and poor LV contrast in the farfield particularly in the basal part of the LV segments	Increase transmit power or just wait several beats, for subsequent injections use a small dosage or a slower bolus
Rib shadows can be found in all segments: look for the typical band of low echogenicity	Try modified view

How to set imaging parameters

A balance between having sufficient power of the ultrasound and an adequate signal-to-noise ratio without significant microbubble destruction is important to achieving adequate perfusion imaging. Both high power and low power (MI <0.2) have been used.

- High power: High power provides good signal-to-noise ratio although there is destruction of microbubbles and so assessment of myocardial perfusion cannot be performed in real time nor can it be performed simultaneously with assessment of wall motion.
- Low power: Low power imaging reduces microbubble destruction allowing simultaneous assessment of perfusion and wall motion although has a lower sensitivity for the detection of microbubbles.

How to assess myocardial perfusion

The myocardial contrast distribution can be visually assessed to give the operator an impression of overall myocardial perfusion (Fig. 9.13). Continuous infusion of contrast is used and the microbubbles are destroyed by a high burst of ultrasound at a high mechanical index causing a 'flash'. Following this the replenishment of the contrast agent within the myocardium and its distribution can be visually assessed (Fig. 9.13).

- The presence of an intact coronary microvasculature and normal myocardial blood flow allows an even replenishment of contrast within the myocardium.
- If there is diminished epicardial flow (e.g. following myocardial infarction) the speed and amount of contrast replenishment will be reduced in this territory.

Training and accreditation

Basic and stress echocardiography training including BLS/ALS is needed. As long as there are no approved procedures for accreditation in contrast echocardiography the following approach appears to be reasonable:

- Introduction by a physician with experience in contrast echocardiography (>50 studies/year).
- Participation in a course on contrast echocardiography in order to learn the performance, interpretation, pitfalls, and adverse effects in contrast echocardiography.
- Perform at least 20 contrast echoes under guidance or supervision.
- Experience with contrast agent for left ventricular opacification in at least 50 cases is a prerequisite for moving on to assess perfusion and function with contrast agents.

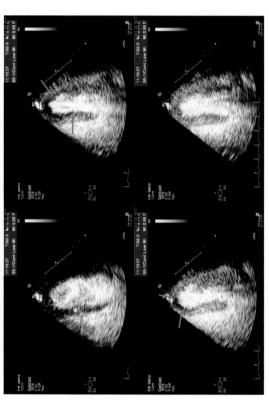

Fig. 9.13 4-Chamber view showing delayed filling in the apicoseptal myocardium after injection of contrast. Top left: LV opacification; top right and bottom left: early opacification of the myocardium; bottom right: late filling. Note the perfusion defect (arrows) indicating ischaemia in the LAD territory.

Chapter 10

Stress echocardiography

Introduction

Stress echocardiography has become a valuable method for cardiovascular stress testing. It plays a crucial role in the initial detection of coronary artery disease, in determining prognosis, and in therapeutic decision-making. The major use of stress echocardiography is to assess myocardial ischaemia or viability in patients with coronary artery disease. Stress echocardiography can also be applied to evaluation of valvular disease and cardiomyopathies.

Stress echocardiography or other non-invasive imaging tests?

Non-invasive imaging techniques have greatly improved the evaluation of patients with known or suspected coronary artery disease. Stress echocardiography and myocardial scintigraphy are widely available and provide similar diagnostic accuracy along with an incremental value over clinical risk factors for detection of coronary artery disease. Cardiovascular magnetic resonance (CMR) is the most recent addition to the functional cardiac imaging armamentarium. It offers a comprehensive assessment of myocardial ischaemia which may include wall-motion analysis at rest and during dobutamine stress, or rest and stress first-pass myocardial perfusion during vasodilatory stress. Myocardial viability is evaluated with either the late gadolinium enhancement technique (infarct imaging) or the low-dose dobutamine test. Positron emission tomography has high diagnostic performance to detect ischaemia and viability, but continues to have limited clinical use because it is not widely available. Cardiac computed tomography allows coronary calcium scanning along with non-invasive anatomic assessment of the coronary tree, but no functional information on ischaemia/hibernation. Therefore, it should be combined with a functional test (ideally stress echocardiography or CMR, and not myocardial scintigraphy which also involves radiation), to provide a complete assessment of the physiological significance of stenotic lesions in coronary arteries.

There are clinical situations where myocardial scintigraphy is relatively contraindicated (left bundle branch block, bifascicular block, and ventricular paced rhythms). In these situations dynamic exercise leads to perfusion abnormalities of the septum and adjacent walls in the absence of obstructive coronary disease. If there is local expertise, stress echocardiography is an option. On the other hand, in patients with known extensive coronary artery disease and regional wall abnormalities at rest, the diagnostic accuracy of stress echocardiography is somewhat reduced. If available, CMR with adenosine first-pass perfusion and late gadolinium enhancement is an attractive option for those patients. No single imaging modality has been proven to be superior overall. Available tests all have advantages and drawbacks, and none can be considered suitable for all patients. The choice of the imaging method should be based on the clinical history and also on local expertise and availability.

Pre-test probability

In patients referred for stress echocardiography the likelihood of having coronary artery disease can usually be estimated from their symptoms and history. This *pre-test probability* is useful because the gain by performing a stress test depends on the pre-test probability (Table 10.1). Based on the accuracy of stress echocardiography to detect coronary artery disease it is also possible to calculate the probability of coronary artery disease with a negative or positive result of stress echocardiography (*post-test probability*).

If there is a *high* pre-test probability (e.g. typical angina and risk factors) the risk of a cardiac event remains high even if there is a negative test. In patients with a *low* pre-test probability (e.g. young patients with atypical chest pain) a positive test does not predict poor prognosis. Therefore, when used for diagnosis, stress echocardiography (like nuclear perfusion imaging) is ideal for patients with *intermediate* pre-test probability (e.g. women with atypical chest pain and some risk factors). In this group of patients a negative test predicts a low risk of further cardiac events, whereas a positive test indicates a high risk and warrants further invasive diagnostics.

Although stress echocardiography in patients with high pre-test probability is of limited *diagnostic value*, it is still of *clinical value*. In patients with known coronary artery disease stress echocardiography can help to define the location and extent of ischaemia.

Table 10.1 Combined Diamond–Forrester and CASS data of pre-test likelihood of coronary artery disease in symptomatic patients. (Modified from Committee on the Management of Patients with chronic stable angina. ACC/AHA 2002 guideline update for the management of patients with chronic stable angina. *J Am Coll Cardiol* 2003; **41**(1):159–68.)

Age	Atypical angina		Typical angina	
	Men	Women	Men	Women
30–39	34	12	76	26
40–49	51	22	87	55
50–59	65	31	93	73
60–69	72	51	94	86

Values represents % with coronary artery disease on angiography

■ >70%   ■ 30–70%   ■ <30%

Indications

The main indication for stress echocardiography is the assessment of coronary artery disease patients (Fig. 10.1). ECG stress testing is the most frequently used initial stress test to evaluate patients with suspected coronary artery disease. Stress echocardiography is used in addition to stress ECG or as the initial diagnostic tool. However, stress echocardiography has been applied to several other pathologies. The key indications are to aid management of patients with:

Suspected coronary artery disease

- As part of an investigational strategy for the diagnosis of patients in whom stress ECG was inconclusive.
- For people for whom treadmill exercise is difficult or impossible because of poor mobility or inability to perform dynamic exercise.
- For people for whom stress ECG poses particular problems of poor sensitivity or difficulties in interpretation, including women, patients with cardiac conduction defects (for instance, left bundle branch block and resting ST segment abnormalities), and diabetes
- For people with a lower likelihood of coronary artery disease and future cardiac events. Likelihood of coronary artery disease depends on clinical assessment of risk factors including age, gender, ethnic group, family history, associated comorbidities, clinical presentation, physical examination, and results from other investigations (e.g. blood cholesterol levels or resting ECG).

Known coronary artery disease

- To determine the likelihood of future coronary events, for instance after myocardial infarction or risk assessment for proposed non-cardiac surgery.
- To assess myocardial viability and hibernation, particularly with reference to planned myocardial revascularization.
- To guide strategies of myocardial revascularization by determining the haemodynamic significance of known coronary lesions.
- To assess the adequacy of percutaneous and surgical revascularization.

Valvular heart disease

- Aortic stenosis with a low gradient and poor left ventricular systolic function (see Chapter 3).
- Aortic stenosis with a high gradient in asymptomatic patients.
- Mitral stenosis with discrepancy between haemodynamic and clinical findings (e.g. dyspnoea despite low gradient at rest, asymptomatic patient with high-grade stenosis).
- Mitral regurgitation (organic, severe) in asymptomatic patients.
- To establish evidence of inducible ischaemic mitral regurgitation.
- To evaluate aortic regurgitation (severe) in asymptomatic patients.

Hypertrophic cardiomyopathy or subaortic muscular obstruction

- Assessment for dynamic gradient.

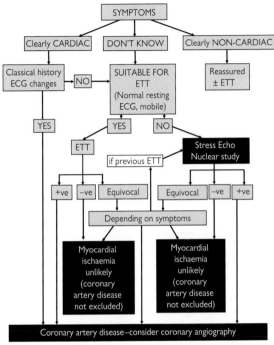

Fig. 10.1 An approach to investigate a patient with suspected coronary artery disease.

Contraindications

Absolute contraindications for all stress modalities

- Non-ST-segment elevation acute coronary syndrome. Once stabilized, exercise stress can be considered 24–72 hours after chest pain, in low- or intermediate-risk patients. High-dose dobutamine should not be performed within the first week after a myocardial infarction.
- ST-segment elevation myocardial infarction within the previous 4 days.
- Left ventricular failure with symptoms at rest.
- Recent history of life-threatening arrhythmias.
- Severe dynamic or fixed LVOT obstruction (aortic stenosis and obstructive hypertrophic cardiomyopathy).
- Severe systemic hypertension (systolic blood pressure >220mmHg and/or diastolic blood pressure >120mmHg).
- Recent pulmonary embolism or infarction.
- Thrombophlebitis or active deep vein thrombosis.
- Known hypokalaemia (particularly for dobutamine stress).
- Active endocarditis, myocarditis, or pericarditis.
- Left main coronary artery stenosis that is likely to be haemodynamically significant.

Absolute contraindications for vasodilator stress

- Suspected or known severe bronchospasm.
- 2nd- and 3rd-degree atrioventricular block in the absence of a functioning pacemaker.
- Sick sinus syndrome in the absence of a functioning pacemaker.
- Hypotension (systolic blood pressure <90mmHg).
- Caffeine intake, xanthines, or dipyridamole use in the last 24 hours.

Relative contraindications to vasodilator stress

- Bradycardia of <40bpm. Initial dynamic exercise normally increases the rate sufficiently to start the infusion.
- Recent cerebral ischaemia or infarction.

Contraindications to contrast imaging

- Known allergy to any of the constituents of contrast agents.

Detection of ischaemia

Principle

The rationale for the diagnosis of myocardial ischaemia with stress echocardiography is a relative reduction in myocardial blood flow on stress sufficient to cause a decrease in myocardial contraction. The ischaemic changes in left ventricle wall motion appear earlier than ECG changes and angina (the *ischaemic cascade*, Fig. 10.2). During stress, in a normal subject, coronary and myocardial blood flow increases 3–4-fold to comply with the increased oxygen demand of the myocardium. This can occur because myocardial arteriolar resistance reduces. If there is a significant stenosis of an epicardial coronary artery the resistance of the arteriolar vessels is already reduced at rest. This is known as *auto-regulation* and allows preservation of coronary blood flow at rest, and at low levels of stress, in the territory supplied by the stenosed artery. Therefore, at rest severe occlusions do not result in wall motion abnormalities. However, with stress and increased oxygen demand the blood flow cannot be further increased and the corresponding myocardial segment cannot contract as well as myocardial segments supplied by patent arteries. The more severe the epicardial stenosis the smaller the possible increase in coronary blood flow and the earlier wall motion abnormalities occur.

Limitations

- Usually stenosis >50% results in wall motion abnormalities on stress. However, less severe stenosis in particular with long segments or vascular remodelling can also cause ab-normalities.
- There has to be a significant increase in oxygen demand to disclose regional wall motion abnormalities—in particular for moderate stenoses. This is only possible by reaching or exceeding target heart rates as in exercise ECG stress testing.
- Even severe stenosis may be missed if there is a well-developed collateral circulation.
- Worsening of wall motion or an inappropriate loss of contractility in comparison to other myocardial segments is the hallmark of stress echocardiography. However, this may be difficult to visualize if resting function is already reduced.
- Abnormal microvascular function, e.g. in arterial hypertension or diabetes, may reduce the auto-regulation and cause abnormal responses to stress. However, the changes are usually diffuse and not segmental as observed in coronary artery disease.

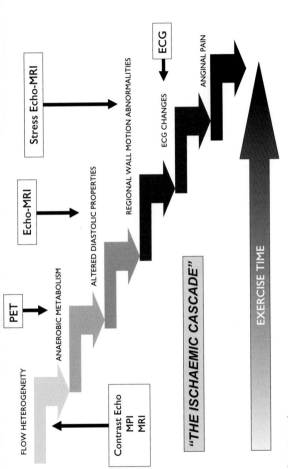

Fig. 10.2 The ischaemic cascade.

Viability assessment

- Viability studies based on left ventricular wall motion are performed when akinetic (or severely hypokinetic) segments are found and there is a question as to whether the patient will benefit from revascularization. If segments are reported as *viable* this implies the myocardial function is still preserved even though their blood supply is limited (Fig. 10.3).
- The rationale for the diagnosis of *myocardial viability* with stress echocardiography is to demonstrate that the akinetic (or severely hypokinetic) segments improve contractility when exposed to low doses of dobutamine. This ability to increase contractility is referred to as a *contractile reserve*.
- If there is a haemodynamically significant stenosis or an occlusion of the supplying artery, higher dosages of dobutamine may then result in ischaemia and the contractility decreases. This improvement and then deterioration is referred to as a *biphasic response*.

Limitations

- Dobutamine increases oxygen demand and at higher doses induces ischaemia in hibernating myocardium (biphasic response). This usually requires doses exceeding 20microgram/kg/min. However, very severe stenoses may cause ischaemia at the lowest doses of dobutamine and no improvement of contractility may be seen.
- Contractility depends on preservation of the inner layers of the myocardium. Therefore the lack of contractile reserve does not mean there is no viable myocardium in the outer layers. Although major recovery of function after revascularization appears to depend on preserved contractility, segments with irreversibly damaged inner layers but preserved outer myocardial layers still may benefit from improved blood flow and remodelling.
- It may be difficult to differentiate *passive* movement (*tethering*, i.e. being pulled with a normally moving segment) of a myocardial segment from *active* movement due to contraction. Image processing analysis tools, such as strain imaging and tissue tracking, may be useful to differentiate but there is limited experience.
- Viability assessment using stress echocardiography relies on good image quality. Contrast echocardiography is usually needed to improve border delineation.

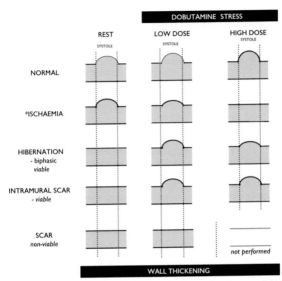

Fig. 10.3 Changes in wall thickening with dobutamine stress. *Decline in wall thickening with ischaemia can be variable in degree and timing.

Causes of akinetic left ventricle segments

Scar (non-viable)
- Irreversible loss of myocardium.
- Often reduced diastolic wall thickness <0.6cm.

Stunning (viable)
- Transiently reduced contractility after ischaemia.
- Usually spontaneous recovery (e.g. transient coronary occlusion in infarction with early recanalization, or post stress in severe stenosis).
- Stunning usually diagnosed by follow-up studies that demonstrate recovery in function.
- If complete occlusion during infarction this can take 4–6 weeks.

Hibernation (viable)
- Permanently reduced contractility.
- Permanent coronary occlusion or high-grade stenosis with insufficient collateral blood flow 'too little to live, too much to die'.
- Transient recovery with low-dose dobutamine.
- Worsening with high dose 'biphasic response'.

Intramural scar (viable)
- Scar in wall but with no significant stenosis in supplying artery and remaining viable myocardium in wall.

Perfusion assessment

Principle

- Normal viable and non-ischaemic myocardium can be recognized by observing the pattern of myocardial contrast enhancement (see Chapter 9 and Fig. 10.4).
- Usually with normal perfusion the microvessels fill with contrast and there is homogeneous opacification and prompt refill of contrast following microbubble destruction.
- After myocardial infarction, scar tissue replaces the myocytes and the density of intramyocardial vessels decreases. Similarly, in acute myocardial infarction without reperfusion, myocardial blood flow is absent in the necrotic area. Therefore the myocardial opacification decreases and 'dark' or 'black' areas are seen within the myocardium, usually in the subendocardial region.
- Typically infarct and scar tissue do not opacify because the amount of contrast within the few vessels remaining is not enough to cause an ultrasound signal. Therefore for viability assessment with contrast only a resting study is necessary. Nevertheless the echocardiographic method of choice for viability assessment is still low-dose dobutamine stress and perfusion imaging is only considered when contrast has been used for LV opacification or when dobutamine is contraindicated.
- If an area of myocardium starts to become ischaemic during a stress study, again the perfusion with microbubbles decreases and the refill of contrast reduces. Therefore the area becomes dark.
- Myocardial ischaemia is present when 2 or more myocardial segments show normal opacification at rest and a perfusion defect during stress.
- Assessment for inducible ischaemia can be performed with all approved stress protocols, but appear to be most suitable for vasodilator protocols.
- In the ischaemic cascade, stress-induced myocardial perfusion defects tend to precede wall motion abnormalities and as a result subtle wall motion abnormalities can often be identified when a perfusion defect has also become evident.
- It is important to remember that myocardial perfusion defects may be transient and are often better seen during the replenishment after the flash.

Limitations of perfusion assessment

- Scar tissue sometimes can cause a very echogenic tissue signal. This makes it very difficult to assess changes in myocardial opacification after contrast injection.
- A perfusion defect at rest is found in an akinetic segment, if not consider an artefact.

Perfusion defect criteria

- A relative decrease in contrast enhancement in segment/region in comparison to another region with comparable image quality/attenuation.
- First appearance in the subendocardial layers rather than transmurally.
- In areas of normal wall motion or reversible wall motion abnormalities.

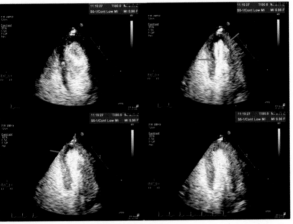

Fig. 10.4 4-chamber view showing delayed filling in the apicoseptal myocardium after injection of contrast. Top left: LV opacification; top right and bot-tom left: early opacification of the myocardium; bottom right: late filling. Note the perfusion defect (arrows) indicating ischaemia in the LAD territory. See 📹 Video 10.10 and 📹 Video 10.12.

Preoperative assessment for non-cardiac surgery

- In patients undergoing major vascular surgery a dobutamine stress echocardiogram allows determination of the perioperative risk for cardiovascular complications. This is particularly useful if patients have 3 or more of the characteristics: age >70 years; current angina; prior myocardial infarction; congestive heart failure; prior cerebrovascular event; diabetes mellitus; or renal failure.
- The main method to protect patients with known coronary artery disease perioperatively is to prescribe effective beta-blockade. The risk of perioperative cardiac complications has been assessed in clinical trials and is related to the number of wall segments that become ischaemic on dobutamine stress echocardiography.
- Patients without new wall motion abnormalities have a low risk (<5%). Patients with 1–4 segments showing new wall motion abnormalities have a slightly higher perioperative risk but can be protected with beta-blockers.
- If >4 segments exhibit new wall motion abnormalities during stress, there is a high risk (>30%) of cardiac complications perioperatively. This risk cannot be reduced by beta-blockers and there is therefore a potential theoretical benefit from revascularization (although currently unproven to reduce risk).
- The most recent guidelines (Fig. 10.5) were published in 2009[1]. These take into account the urgency of the surgery, the cardiac risk of the surgery, the patient's functional capacity, as well as cardiac risk factors.
- In patients with ≥3 cardiac risk factors then non-invasive testing can be considered. If this shows ≤moderate stress-induced ischaemia and the patient is stable then the planned surgery can go ahead. If non-invasive stress testing shows extensive ischaemia then each case should be considered individually considering the potential benefit of the proposed surgical procedure with the predicted outcome and the effect of medical therapy and/or coronary revascularization.

Reference

1 Task Force for Preoperative Cardiac Risk Assessment and Perioperative Cardiac Management in Non-cardiac Surgery; *et al*. Guidelines for pre-operative cardiac risk assessment and perioperative cardiac management in non-cardiac surgery. *Eur Heart J* 2009; **30**:2769–812.

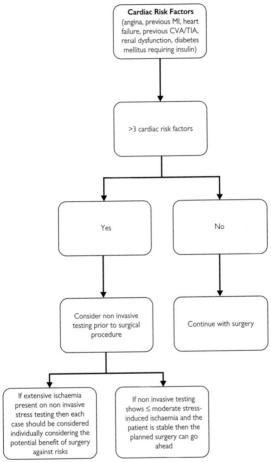

Fig. 10.5 Flow chart showing preoperative assessment for non-cardiac surgery.

Task Force for Preoperative Cardiac Risk Assessment and Perioperative Cardiac Management in Non-cardiac Surgery; *et al.* Guidelines for pre-operative cardiac risk assessment and perioperative cardiac management in non-cardiac surgery. *Eur Heart J* 2009; **30**:2769–812.

Equipment and personnel

Equipment

Because analysis of wall motion abnormalities is difficult and not reliable in the presence of poor quality images, every effort has to be made to optimize visualization of the endocardial border and the myocardium.

- The scanner should provide tissue harmonic imaging and a contrast-specific imaging modality in order to be applicable in the majority of patients.
- Use of digital frame grabbers and split or 'quad-screen' displays allow side-by-side comparison of rest and stress images using the same echocardiographic views and is the current standard for performing stress echocardiograms.
- Tissue Doppler imaging is optional but may add clinical information (e.g. detection of post-systolic shortening).
- 3D imaging, which is becoming increasingly available, offers the ability to eliminate apical foreshortening and shorten the time needed for acquisition of stress images.

Personnel and experience

- Two people are required to record and monitor stress echocardiography—one of them should have substantial experience in the evaluation of patients with ischaemic heart disease and in analysis of wall motion/thickening abnormalities.
- Recordings should be performed by a skilled echocardiographer (technician or physician).
- If a physician is not participating in the study, one should be available in the immediate locality in case of acute problems. One of the personnel present should be qualified in advanced life support.
- Recording and interpretation of stress echocardiograms requires extensive experience in echocardiography and should be performed only by technicians and physicians with specific training in the technique. Most recommendations suggest physicians have performed and interpreted a minimum of 100 studies under supervision before they can perform stress echocardiography independently. Supervised over-reading of at least 100 stress echocardiograms is required to attain the minimum level of competence for independent interpretation.

Drugs

- Depending on the stress protocol chosen the appropriate drugs (dobutamine, adenosine, dipyridamole, atropine) and agents to reverse their effects should be prepared (aminophylline if dipyridamole used, beta-blockers).
- Standard resuscitation drugs and equipment will need to be available in the room.

Patient preparation

Patients should be provided with information or have a detailed verbal explanation. Informed consent is usually considered appropriate especially for pharmacological stress or with the use of contrast agents.

Safety

A large international study of stress echocardiography reported on 85,997 patients undergoing stress echocardiography.[1] The incidence of life-threatening adverse events in those undergoing stress with exercise was 1:6574, dobutamine 1:557, and dipyridamole 1:1294. There were 6 deaths (1:14333) related to the procedure (5 with dobutamine, and 1 with dipyridamole). These were mainly due to ventricular arrhythmias. It was pointed out that the subgroup of patients receiving dobutamine may have been at higher risk because of viability studies in those with established coronary disease.

Reference

1 Varga A et al. Safety of Stress Echocardiography (from the International Stress Echo Complication Registry). Am J Cardiol 2006; **98**:541–3.

Example information sheet

You have been asked to attend for stress echocardiography. A stress echocardiogram is an ultrasound scan of your heart, which is performed after increasing your heart rate. A stress echocardiogram provides information about the performance of your heart at stress and helps your doctors to identify symptoms you may have on exertion.

Before the procedure?

Please continue to take all your medications as usual except for your beta-blocker which should not be taken on the morning of the test. You will be seen by the doctor who will take a medical history and after explaining the procedure will ask you to sign a consent form. If you have any concerns, please do not hesitate to ask, as we would like you to be as relaxed as possible and are happy to answer questions.

What happens during the procedure?

The doctor will insert a small tube into your arm (cannula) to infuse the drug (dobutamine), which increases the heart rate. A blood pressure cuff will be placed on your arm. You will be asked to lie on your left side and the ultrasound scan will be performed. Dobutamine will be given via the cannula, which will gradually increase the heart rate. In addition ultrasound contrast agents may be given to improve image quality. There will be a doctor present and also a technician. The procedure takes 20–30min to examine all areas carefully. When the examination is finished the dobutamine is stopped and the heart rate will come down quickly.

Benefits?

The benefits from stress echocardiography are that it can: Define the nature of cardiac symptoms; Point out the status of the cardiovascular system; Decide which further therapeutic and diagnostic procedures you have to undergo following the information derived from this examination.

Risks?

Usually the investigation is tolerated well, some patients could have some mild symptoms during the test (mostly palpitations, tremor, light headed sensation). Serious risks are very rare less than 0.3% (1 in every 330 patients) and include heart rhythm problems, myocardial infarction and low blood pressure. Your doctor would not recommend that you have a stress echocardiogram unless she/he felt that the benefits of the procedure outweighed these small risks.

After the procedure?

After the procedure you will be asked to stay for another 30min. This is the time needed to completely clear the infused drugs. You will be offered refreshments. The doctor will return and discuss the results of your procedure. Any relevant advice and literature will then be given. Your cannula will be removed and you may go home with your relative/ friend. A letter with the results of your procedure will be sent to your GP and any referring doctor.

Performing the study

General

The image acquisition is structured to make it easy to identify changes from baseline in wall motion and thickening of the left ventricle. The fundamental requirement is high-quality 2D echocardiographic recordings with good endocardial border definition in all segments. These basic images need to be acquired confidently and quickly during stress. Additional data can include tissue Doppler profiles (global and regional parameters of function) and direct assessment of myocardial perfusion by myocardial contrast enhancement (depending on local licences).

Views

Multiple views are required to ensure all left ventricular segments are monitored and all 3 major coronary distributions are assessed. The key 4 views are: apical 4- and 2-chamber, parasternal short and long axis (or apical long axis) (Fig. 10.6). Subcostal or additional short-axis views can be substituted when necessary or when more appropriate for visualization of specific anatomy.

Set-up

- Spend time ensuring good patient position (they will be in this position throughout the stress). A clear, stable ECG recording is required.
- Study all 4 views and spend time optimizing the images.
  - *Machine settings*: select harmonic imaging and adjust focus zone. Ideally, frame rate should be >25 frames/s (if heart rate >140 then frame rates >30 frames/s may be better).
  - *Probe position*: be very careful not to foreshorten apical views (Fig. 10.7). The patient may need to do held inspiration or expiration for clear, stable, unforeshortened images.
  - *Contrast*: decide whether there is good endocardial border definition in each view and whether images can be acquired confidently and smoothly during the stress in each window. If 2 or more segments are not seen or the images are difficult use contrast.

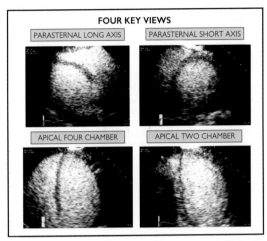

Fig. 10.6 There are 4 key views. The parasternal long axis and apical 3-chamber provide very similar information. See 📹 Video 10.1, 📹 Video 10.2, 📹 Video 10.3, 📹 Video 10.4, 📹 Video 10.5, 📹 Video 10.6, 📹 Video 10.7, 📹 Video 10.8.

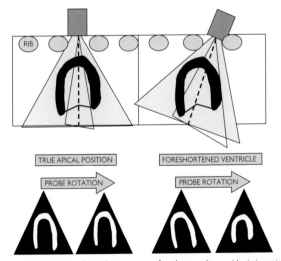

Fig. 10.7 It is vital that all apical views are not foreshortened to avoid missing apical wall motion abnormalities. If the probe is not on the true apex then even though the apex may be included in the initial plane probe rotation for the next view will create a foreshortened image.

Image acquisition

- Record a set of baseline images (use a stress protocol preset if available). Use a standard acquisition order, e.g. parasternal long axis, parasternal short axis, apical 4-chamber and apical 2-chamber (alternatively the apical views can be recorded first).
- Start the stress (e.g. pharmacological/physical).
- At the preset time-points (depending on stress and clinical response) record a complete set of images. Some machines have a 'compare' mode to ensure your images are in exactly the same position.
- Look for changes in wall motion and thickening during image acquisition so that you interpret the test as you go along.
- Once all the images are acquired, review them off-line, ideally with a second experienced reviewer, to create the final report.

3D stress applications

3D stress echocardiography

- Real-time 3D stress echocardiography allows the acquisition of a full volume image of the left ventricle. This has several advantages: all segments are imaged quickly and during the same time interval and accurate comparisons can be made.
- The cropping of 3D volumes allows planes to be chosen which are 'on axis' which is sometimes difficult to achieve exactly with 2D stress echocardiography.
- The reduced temporal resolution of stress echocardiography means that LV contrast agents are invariably used.
- The presence of stitching artefacts can also hinder image analysis, particularly if there is quick variability in the heart rate.
- However, acquisition of 3D datasets allows for other potential assement of ischaemia such as changes in strain (Fig. 10.8).
- Whilst the advantages of 3D stress echocardiography are clear, the reduced image quality and problems with stitching has limited its uptake by cardiology departments.

iRotate

- This mode, offered by Phillips allows the 2D image to be rotated to a different plane whilst maintaining the probe in the same position.
- This mode can be of use during stress echocardiography where for instance following acquisition of the apical 4-chamber view the ultrasound waves are transmitted in a different direction to obtain a 2-chamber apical view and then a 3-chamber apical view without moving the ultrasound probe.

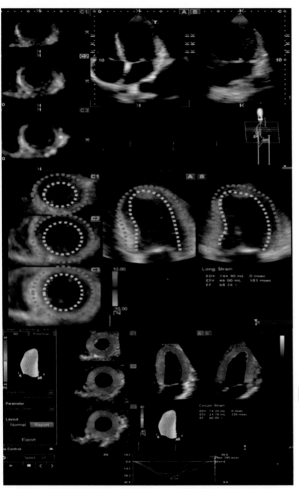

Fig. 10.8 3D strain acquisition and postprocessing on Toshiba Artida system. Top: from the apical LV window, the LV is displayed in two apical views and three short axis views. Middle: contouring of the epicardial and endocardial border. Bottom: normal LV 3D circumferential strain analysis.

Monitoring and termination criteria

Monitoring

As with other forms of stress testing, standard ECG and blood pressure monitoring should be performed. This may provide diagnostic and prognostic information during exercise studies. With pharmacological stress ECG monitoring has limited diagnostic value but is needed to trigger loop recording and monitor for arrhythmias. However, if a 12-lead ECG is not performed during pharmacological stress, a 12-lead ECG recorder should be readily available in case of problems.

Termination criteria

Treadmill exercise echocardiography should be terminated at traditional endpoints:
- Attainment of target heart rates.
- Cardiovascular symptoms.
- Significant ECG changes or arrhythmias.

Bicycle exercise and pharmacological stress provide additional echocardiographic endpoints because they allow online, continuous visualization of wall motion and thickening. Stress echocardiography with online monitoring should be terminated at:
- Traditional endpoints (previously listed).
- The development of wall motion abnormalities corresponding to 2 or more coronary territories.
- Wall motion abnormalities associated with ventricular dilation and/or global reduction of systolic function.

Target heart rates for stress

Maximum age predicted heart rate = 220 − Age of patient

Target heart rate = 85% × Maximum age predicted

e.g. Age = 67

Maximum age predicted = 220 − 67 = 153bpm

Target heart rate = 0.85 × 153 = 130

Target heart rate according to age

Age	100%	85%
85	135	115
80	140	119
75	145	123
70	150	128
65	155	132
60	160	136
55	165	140
50	170	145
45	175	149
40	180	153
35	185	157
30	190	162
25	195	166
20	200	170

Exercise stress protocols

Exercise is the most physiological stressor for assessment of myocardial ischaemia in patients able to exercise.

Stress protocol

- The protocols are the same as for exercise stress ECG testing.
- A Bruce treadmill protocol with 3-min stages of graded increases in speed and gradient, or an ergometer with 3-min stages of graded cycling resistance at a fixed cycling rate (Fig. 10.9).
- Treadmill exercise should be terminated at traditional endpoints such as attainment of target heart rates, cardiovascular symptoms, and/or significant ECG changes suggestive of ischaemia.
- Supine and upright bicycle exercise appear to have equivalent degrees of accuracy. Supine bicycle ergometry on a special bed, which can be rotated, provides additional echocardiographic endpoints because it allows continuous visualization of wall motion at incremental levels of stress, including peak exercise. Bicycle exercise should be terminated at traditional endpoints and, if a supine bicycle is used, when wall motion abnormalities develop that correspond with 2 or more coronary territories, or wall motion abnormalities associated with ventricular dilation and/or global reduction of systolic function.

Image acquisition

Imaging should be performed at:
- Baseline.
- Post treadmill exercise (because ischaemia-induced wall motion abnormalities may resolve quickly, post-exercise imaging should be accomplished within 60–90sec of termination of exercise). If the patient is asymptomatic and there are no ECG changes then extending the exercise up to 100% of target heart rate provides more time post-exercise to acquire images.
- If supine bicycle ergometry is used imaging should also be performed during exercise and an intermediate stage can be recorded.

Exercise or dobutamine?

For the diagnosis of myocardial ischaemia, there appears to be no difference in the accuracy and prognostic information obtained with dobutamine compared to exercise stress. It is possible that for milder forms of coronary artery disease, treadmill may be advantageous. Exercise stress echocardiography presents a challenge to obtain good quality images. For patients unable to exercise, dobutamine is indicated. An advantage of dobutamine is that it has a rapid onset and cessation of action, and its effects can be reversed by beta-blocker administration. If there is a contraindication to dobutamine then dipyridamole, adenosine or pacing may be used. For risk assessment prior to non-cardiac surgery the accuracy of dobutamine stress echocardiography is proven. For assessment of myocardial viability use of low- and high-dose dobutamine seems to be the best stress method for echocardiography.

BRUCE EXERCISE PROTOCOL

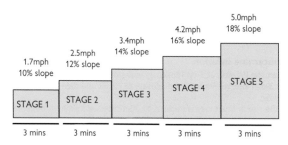

Modified Bruce has 2 extra 3 minute stages at start
(1.7mph/0% slope and 1.7mph/5% slope)
then continues as above

ERGOMETER PROTOCOL

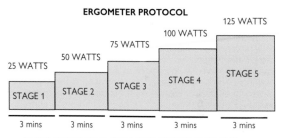

AT CONSTANT PEDAL RATE OF 50 CYCLES PER MINUTE

Fig. 10.9 Standard protocols for exercise testing.

Dobutamine stress for ischaemia

Myocardial ischaemia is assessed by graded dobutamine infusion. This increases myocardial oxygen demand in a fashion analogous to staged exercise. Contractility, heart rate, and systolic blood pressure are all increased.

Dobutamine infusion

- Start the infusion at 5 or 10microgram/kg/min dobutamine.
- At 3-min intervals increase the infusion to 20, 30, and then 40microgram/kg/min.
- If the rise in heart rate is minimal by 30microgram/kg/min dobutamine then consider using atropine (Fig. 10.10). Check for contraindications to atropine, in particular glaucoma, before administration.
- Atropine should be used at the minimum effective dose. Administer 0.3mg doses at 60sec intervals until the desired heart rate response is seen. Maximum dose should be 1.2mg. The effect on accuracy is not fully established but appears beneficial.

Dobutamine stress and beta-blockers

In patients with ongoing beta-blocker treatment a reduced sensitivity for reversible ischaemia has been found. This is seen even if target heart rate is reached with additional atropine injections due to the negative inotropic effect of beta-blockers. Therefore, it is recommended to stop beta-blockers ideally 48 hours prior to the test to increase sensitivity (avoid false negatives). However, if not possible, patients can still be accepted for exercise or dobutamine stress with atropine accepting that sensitivity is lower.

Image acquisition

See ♣ Video 10.9, ♣ Video 10.10, and ♣ Video 10.11 for examples of wall motion abnormalities. Images should be recorded at:

- Baseline.
- Intermediate stage (70% of the age-predicted heart rate).
- Peak stress (>85% of the age-predicted heart rate).
- Recovery.

The minimal images are baseline and peak. More than 4 stages can be recorded as felt clinically needed.

Termination of test

Diagnostic endpoints of stress echocardiographic testing are: maximum dose (for pharmacological) or maximum workload (for exercise testing): achievement of target heart rate; obvious echocardiographic positivity (with akinesis of ≥2LV segments); severe chest pain; or obvious ECG positivity (with >2mV ST-segment shift). Submaximal non-diagnostic endpoints of stress echo testing are non-tolerable symptoms or limiting asymptomatic side effects such as hypertension, with systolic blood pressure >220mmHg or diastolic blood pressure >120mmHg, symptomatic hypotension, with >40mmHg drop in blood pressure; supraventricular arrhythmias, such as supraventricular tachycardia or atrial fibrillation; and complex ventricular arrhythmias, such as ventricular tachycardia or frequent, polymorphic premature ventricular beats.

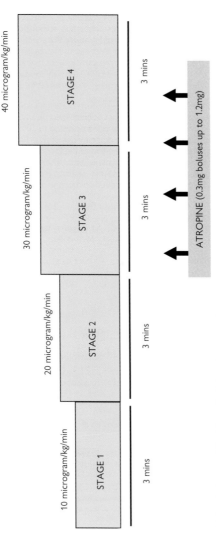
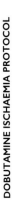

Fig. 10.10 Standard protocol for dobutamine ischaemia stress testing.

Dobutamine stress for viability

The basis for the diagnosis of myocardial viability is contraction of the myocardium either spontaneously or after inotropic stimulation by activating *contractile reserve*. The principle of low-dose dobutamine stress is to assess *contractile reserve*, i.e. look for evidence of improvement in wall motion abnormalities or clear inotropic response in areas that are thought to have coronary stenoses (Fig. 10.11). The need for viability assessment is usually to determine the value of performing revascularization.

Dobutamine infusion

- Start the infusion at 5microgram/kg/min dobutamine.
- Continue the infusion for up to 5min and then increase to 10microgram/kg/min. This can be increased to 20microgram/kg/min (Fig. 10.12).
- A 10% increase in heart rate marks the end of the low-dose protocol.
- After completing the low-dose protocol higher doses of dobutamine (30 and then 40microgram/kg/min for 5-min periods) may be given to look for a biphasic response (improved contraction at low dose followed by reduced contraction at peak).
- The presence of a biphasic response indicates inducible myocardial ischaemia and is perhaps the strongest predictor for recovery of myocardial dysfunction following revascularization. It will indicate a viable but jeopardized myocardial region.

Image acquisition

A full set of images should be recorded at:
- Baseline.
- Low stress (10% increase in heart rate).
- High stress (if performed).

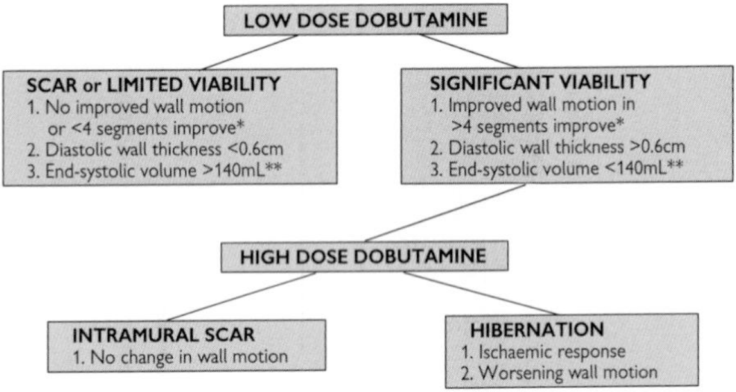

*Improvement in ≥4 segments is a good predictor for recovery of left ventricle function after coronary revascularization in patients with hibernating myocardium.
** End systolic volume >140mL indicates an advanced stage of remodelling. Revascularization may not result in reverse remodelling.

Fig. 10.11 Viable or non-viable?

DOBUTAMINE VIABILITY PROTOCOL

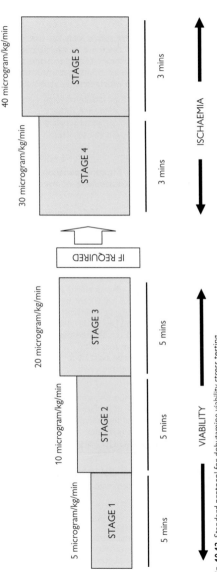

Fig. 10.12 Standard protocol for dobutamine viability stress testing.

Vasodilator stress

Vasodilator stress echocardiography should only be considered when physical stress is not possible and there are contraindications to dobutamine. It is less sensitive for identification of mild to moderate coronary artery disease. Vasodilator stress, however, may become more important as perfusion imaging becomes more widely clinically applicable.

Vasodilators are effective because they induce regional variation in coronary blood flow. Dipyridamole or adenosine cause a 2- or more fold increase in myocardial blood flow in segments supplied by normal coronary arteries whereas in segments supplied by stenotic arteries flow is unchanged or decreased. If oxygen demand increases with flow changes, regional abnormalities in wall motion and thickening appear.

Because vasodilator stress acts via change in perfusion, theoretically, it should be more suitable for direct assessment of myocardial perfusion using contrast echocardiography.

Dipyridamole protocol for myocardial ischaemia

The protocol for dipyridamole is based on continuous ECG and echocardiographic monitoring during a 2-stage infusion.

Infusion
- Check for contraindications to dipyridamole.
- Initially infuse 0.56mg/kg of dipyridamole over 4min.
- Monitor for 4min. If there are no adverse effects and no clinical or echocardiographic endpoints occur (significant anginal symptoms, wall motion abnormalities) infuse 0.28mg/kg over 2min.
- As with dobutamine (📖 p.614 and Fig. 10.13), atropine (doses of 0.25mg up to a maximum of 1mg) can be used after the second stage to increase heart rate and improve sensitivity.
- Aminophylline (240mg; IV) should be available for immediate use in case of an adverse dipyridamole-related event.

Imaging
Imaging should be performed continuously, and images captured at baseline, end of phase 1, end of phase 2 (if performed), and during recovery. The minimal images are baseline and hyperaemia. When ultrasound contrast is used during the stress test (indicated for improved endocardial definition) myocardial opacification can be assessed in addition to LV wall motion (see 📖 p.582).

Adenosine protocol for myocardial ischaemia

Adenosine works on a 6-min protocol with ECG and echocardiographic monitoring.

Infusion
- Check for contraindication to adenosine.
- Infuse at a maximum dose of 140microgram/kg/min over 6min.
- Stop the infusion if clinical or echocardiographic endpoints are reached (limiting symptoms or wall motion abnormalities).

Imaging

Image continuously and record at baseline, 3min, 6min, and during recovery. Adenosine is less sensitive than other stress modalities for detecting coronary disease by ischaemic wall motion abnormalities compared to other stress modalities.

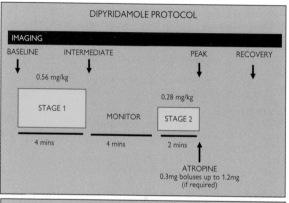

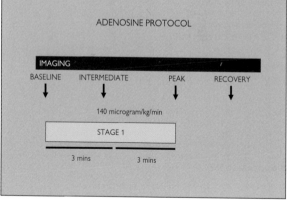

Fig. 10.13 Standard protocols for vasodilator stress testing.

Pacing stress

- This may be considered in patients with a permanent or temporary pacemaker.
- Pacing by temporary intravascular or oesophageal leads is usually not needed for clinically-indicated stress echocardiography.
- In most paced patients exercise, dobutamine, and vasodilator protocols are applicable.
- Pacing stress can be considered when an increase in heart rate cannot be achieved by exercise or dobutamine. Since pacing alone only produces chronotropic stress, it is usually considered to have lower sensitivity than the inotropic and chronotropic stress achieved by pharmacological stress.
- Dobutamine can be given at the same time as increasing the pacing rate to create both chronotropic and inotropic stress.

Pacing protocol

- Pacing stress should preferably be performed with atrial pacing to ensure natural ventricular contraction and to avoid pacing-induced wall motion abnormalities.
- In patients with permanent pacemakers, ensure the assistance of a pacemaker programmer and experienced operator.
- Record baseline images.
- Start pacing at 100bpm.
- Increase every 2min by 10bpm until the target heart rate (85% of age-predicted maximal heart rate) is achieved or until other standard endpoints are reached.
- After reaching target heart rate, reduce heart rate every minute by 20bpm till baseline heart rate is reached.

Image acquisition

- Record baseline images and then at every stage and in recovery.

Analysis

Echocardiographic recordings have to be evaluated during image acquisition in order to assess for echocardiographic endpoints. This should be followed by a comprehensive assessment after the stress test with side-by-side comparisons of recordings captured at baseline and stress.

Stress echocardiograms can be analysed on several planes of complexity, which range from a qualitative assessment of segmental wall motion in response to stress, to highly detailed schemes for quantitative analysis.

For image interpretation, multiple cine loop display allows up to 4 different stress levels for each imaging plane to be displayed simultaneously.

Standard review

- Start with assessment of image quality. Endocardial border definition can be used as an indicator of image quality. If endocardial border is not seen or is barely visible, wall motion and thickening cannot be reliably assessed in this segment. Grade image quality as *good*, *acceptable*, or *poor* and identify non-diagnostic segments.
- On resting images assess global function by LV ejection fraction using a visual estimate or from measuring end-diastolic or end-systolic volumes in 2 apical views.
- Compare rest and stress images for the development of global LV dysfunction (left ventricular enlargement and shape changes) and remeasure global function at stress if there appears to be a change.
- Then evaluate segmental wall motion at rest and at each level of stress using a 16- or 17-segment model. Use a 4-step visual score for each segment: 1—*normal*, 2—*hypokinetic*, 3—*akinetic*; 4—*dyskinetic*.
- Calculate a wall motion score at each stage, if required, to facilitate serial comparison. Divide the sum of the points by the number of segments analysed. Normal contraction has a wall motion score of 1; a higher score indicates wall motion abnormalities.
- For assessment of myocardial viability wall thickness is useful. Diastolic wall thickness <5mm at rest indicates non-viability and increases diagnostic confidence in combination with absent contractile response to dobutamine.
- If using contrast during stress echocardiography, it may be useful to assess the myocardial contrast enhancement. With current knowledge the results of perfusion imaging should be used in conjunction with the findings of visual left ventricular wall motion analysis.
- The adequacy of stress should be noted and records kept of the exercise time, symptoms, haemodynamic observations, and ECG changes.

Stress echo training

EAE recommends performing at least 100 exams under the supervision of an expert reader in a high-volume laboratory, and ideally with the possibility of angiographic verification, before starting stress echocardiography on a routine basis. Maintenance of competence requires at least 100 stress echo exams per year.

Audit and quality control

It is usually accepted that operators should interpret a minimum of 10 stress echocardiograms per month to maintain interpretational skills and sonographers should perform a minimum of 10 stress echocardiograms per month to maintain an appropriate level of skill.

Regular audits are useful to review the quality and accuracy of the stress echocardiograms. The audit should include the total number of stress echocardiograms performed per month for the time period audited: the number of procedures per sonographer and reads per physician; indications; imaging technology; use of contrast; stress protocols; quality of the studies; termination criteria; results (negative or positive for assessment of ischaemia, viable or non-viable for viability studies); and complications. For those patients undergoing coronary angiography, it would be ideal to have the results of coronary angiography for quality control with routine review of false positive and negative findings.

Future technologies

Echocardiography technology is progressing rapidly and has been developed to ensure assessment of left ventricular wall motion is more objective. Automatic wall tracking software, tissue Doppler imaging, and strain imaging are becoming clinically viable. The use of tissue Doppler velocity measurements during stress echocardiography allows the identification of post-systolic shortening—a known sign of regional ischaemia—which can be used in order to increase the sensitivity of the test. However, no data currently demonstrate the superiority of quantitative techniques over conventional wall motion analysis for the assessment of viable and ischaemic myocardium. 3D echocardiography has introduced a further exciting option for stress echocardiography with rapid acquisition of 3D volume datasets and reconstruction of 3D motion. The lower spatial and temporal resolutions of 3D imaging are limitations of the current 3D technique. However, 3D imaging eliminates apical foreshortening, which is common with 2D imaging, and may improve the detection of apical wall motion abnormalities. Moreover, 3D imaging generally shortens the time required for acquisition of stress images.

Sample report

Section 1. Demographic and other information

All the standard demographic details should be included. Stress echocardiography should also include:

- The clinical indication, including relevant clinical history and medications. This provides justification for the study and summarizes clinical information from a number of sources to focus the final conclusion.
- The stress protocol and imaging technique used with justification, including the name and dosage of contrast agents.
- Changes of blood pressure and heart rate should be described briefly. Reporting resting and peak stress blood pressure is usually sufficient.
- For exercise and dobutamine stress echocardiography the age, sex, and specific target heart rate should be included.
- Further measurements or details of ECG changes can be included if relevant.

Section 2. Description of observations and diagnostic statements

- Start with a statement about the completeness of the study and image quality, since diagnostic confidence heavily depends on high-quality recordings.
- Next report the baseline analysis. If global and/or regional left ventricular function is abnormal, the segments involved and the degree of abnormality (hypokinetic, akinetic, dyskinetic) should be demonstrated or listed. Schematics of the single views help to illustrate the distribution of wall motion abnormalities. Non-diagnostic segments can be marked (Fig. 10.14).
- Then report each of the stress recordings in the same way describing whether there was a normal response to stress or abnormal response with worsening wall motion. Segments that deteriorate should be listed or marked on the schematic and degree of abnormality noted.
- In viability studies it is important to evaluate whether the akinetic segments show improvement during stress.

Section 3. M-mode, 2D, and Doppler measurements

In stress echocardiography this section will include quantitative measures of LV function (e.g. ejection fraction) at baseline and on stress. There may also be information on left ventricular outflow velocities in patients with suspected stress-induced gradients or changes in mitral valve function. If tissue Doppler imaging or other analysis methods were used these can be documented.

Section 4. Conclusions

The conclusion should comment on any suboptimal aspect of the study (e.g. image quality, target heart rate reached, etc.) and any complications or adverse events. It should then address the clinical question and detail the main abnormalities that occurred during stress, or summarize the response as normal.

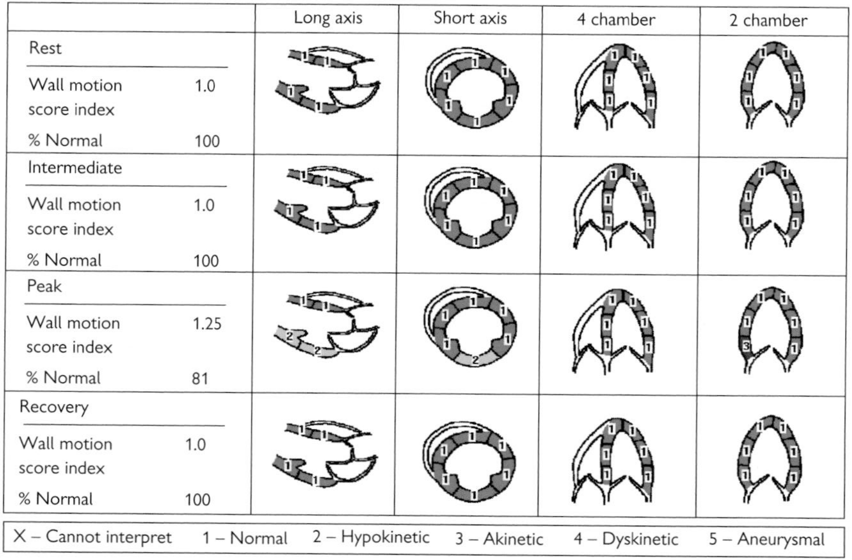

		Long axis	Short axis	4 chamber	2 chamber
Rest					
Wall motion score index	1.0				
% Normal	100				
Intermediate					
Wall motion score index	1.0				
% Normal	100				
Peak					
Wall motion score index	1.25				
% Normal	81				
Recovery					
Wall motion score index	1.0				
% Normal	100				

X – Cannot interpret 1 – Normal 2 – Hypokinetic 3 – Akinetic 4 – Dyskinetic 5 – Aneurysmal

Fig. 10.14 Example of an annotated report demonstrating segmental abnormalities.

Acute echocardiography

'Front door' echocardiography

Practice development

The last decade has seen the rapid development and refinement of portable echo technology. A simultaneous growth in interest in non-invasive diagnostic tools has driven a worldwide development of transthoracic echocardiography. As a result it has become a vital skill for those involved in acute patient care.

- 'Acute echocardiography' refers to the use of echocardiography at the bedside in the acute management of patients receiving urgent care in ward-based, high-dependency and critical care settings.
- The majority of this patient population do not have artificial airways and may have limited, established, invasive monitoring, particularly if they have become acutely unwell. Transthoracic echo therefore becomes an invaluable and powerful tool for rapid non-invasive haemodynamic assessment.
- This chapter focuses on the use of transthoracic echocardiography in the acute setting. This 'front door' echocardiography often operates in time critical situations and relies on more limited types of equipment with more focused data acquisition than might be expected in full echocardiographic studies. Local practice, and acceptability, may therefore vary and therefore local guidelines for use should be established.

A unique role for echocardiography

- The unique value of this tool comes from the fact it provides direct assessment of acute cardiac function combined with diagnostic echocardiographic information.
- Acute echocardiography is most powerful when viewed as part of a global patient assessment allowing full integration of clinical and echocardiographic findings.
- Acute echocardiography supports and augments:
  - Peri-arrest and resuscitation care.
  - Acute medical and trauma diagnostics.
  - Stabilization and management of the critically ill.

Safeguarding patient care

Practice safety framework

- Where a new practice is being established to provide acute echocardiography it is essential that the practitioners delivering the service have a level of echocardiographic expertise that allows them to make independent, and correct, clinical decisions based on their images.
- Therefore the service needs to develop approaches for appropriate operator training and accreditation.
- The individual arrangements for experience and training in an acute echocardiography service will vary between institutions, but, for many, this may be best achieved with a service that has some devolved autonomy from the parent cardiology echocardiography department.

Governance pathways

- As with any investigation that is routinely performed within a department effective clinical governance pathways must be established.
- This should include:
  - Systems for reporting and storing studies whilst maintaining patient confidentiality.
  - A forum for reviewing images with the parent cardiology department.
  - Established pathways to obtain urgent expert help.
  - Identification of a service lead to coordinate clinical governance.

Technology

- A primary requirement for the establishment of an acute echocardiography service will be acquisition of appropriate echo equipment.
- A good starting point is to align equipment with the parent cardiology department. This reduces operator errors and improves technological compatibility, for example, where sharing image storage systems.

Echocardiography training in the UK

Resuscitation echocardiography

There are a number of courses available in the UK; for example Focused Echocardiographic Evaluation in Life Support (FEEL) and Focus Assessed Transthoracic Echo (FATE). Prior to attending a course we recommend that a mentor is identified who will review and sign off the studies required to complete the log-book to the expected standard. Time investment from the mentor should be between 1–2 hours per 10 studies performed by the candidate. A time frame of 6 months is expected to complete the accreditation process. Certification entitles the operator to perform transthoracic studies in the arrest setting provided that they maintain reasonable competence. Practice must remain within the resuscitation framework.

Accreditation with the British Society of Echocardiography

Full transthoracic accreditation allows the operator to function as an independent practitioner and to perform comprehensive studies. Accreditation requires completion of a log-book of 250 specific cases, a written examination, and submission of 5 selected recorded studies illustrating specific pathologies. Completion of the accreditation process requires a significant time commitment from the operator over a 2-year period and provision of departmental supervision and training. Following achievement of accreditation, re-certification is required 5-yearly with demonstration of continued echo practice and learning.

Contemporary training issues

The qualifications described were not designed to address the specific practice requirements of clinicians working in acute care areas. At the time of writing in the UK the representative societies of Emergency Medicine, Acute medicine and Critical Care, in partnership with the British Society of Echocardiography, are individually considering certification processes to address clinicians' requirements and support the practice of acute echocardiography. It is likely that these certification processes will become available in the next 2 years. For more information please see the website of the relevant society:

- Acute Medicine: ℘ http://www.acutemedicine.org.uk
- Emergency Medicine: ℘ http://www.collemergencymed.ac.uk
- Critical Care Medicine: ℘ http://www.ics.ac.uk

Cardiopulmonary resuscitation

Introduction

- Although there are a number of courses providing training in peri-resuscitation echocardiography <u>F</u>ocused <u>E</u>chocardiographic <u>E</u>valuation in <u>L</u>ife Support has been developed as a consensus approach for the UK and is endorsed by both the British Society of Echocardiography and the Resuscitation Council.
- The FEEL algorithm guides the operator through rapid echocardiographic assessment during resuscitation using the Advanced Life Support protocol.
- The aim of the protocol is to identify reversible causes of cardiac arrest:
  - Cardiac tamponade.
  - Gross left ventricular overload and failure.
  - Gross hypovolaemia.
  - Massive pulmonary embolus.
- No measurements, colour imaging, or Doppler are used during the protocol; diagnosis relies solely on the operator's ability to observe pathology accurately.
- Echocardiographic assessment must be performed during the 10-s pulse check after 5 cycles of CPR and repeated only after completion of a further 5 cycles.
- Echocardiography must not delay the return of chest compressions.

The FEEL protocol

- The FEEL protocol is based on 4 views:
  - Parasternal long axis.
  - Parasternal short axis.
  - Apical 4-chamber.
  - Subcostal.
- It may be unnecessary to obtain all views: a single view may be adequate if diagnostic.
- The flow diagram in Fig. 11.1 can be used as a guide to asking pertinent clinical questions in a logical order during the resuscitation, the implications of key findings and urgent management.

Tips for success

- Clarity of *communication* is key to obtaining a useful echo study in this situation.
- Ensure the machine is set up and ready to go *before* approaching the patient.
- Negotiate the correct time to perform echocardiography with the *team leader*.
- Ask the *time-keeper* to count 10sec out loud while you perform the study.
- Communicate your *findings* to the team aloud.
- Do not compromise patient care: if you cannot locate adequate images obtain *senior help*.

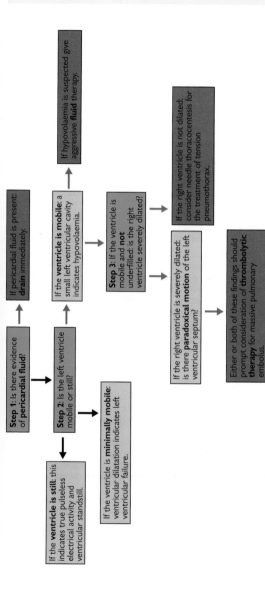

Fig. 11.1 Flowchart for FEEL algorithm.

Acute diagnostics

Diagnostic transthoracic echocardiography in the acute setting plays a particular role in the diagnosis and management of the patient presenting with:

- Acute shortness of breath.
- Suspected cardiac tamponade.
- Suspected sub-massive pulmonary embolus.
- Low cardiac output states.
- Clinical acute coronary syndromes.
- Blunt and penetrating thoracic trauma.

Transthoracic echocardiography is urgently indicated to assist in management decisions relating to:

- Thrombolysis in sub-massive pulmonary embolism.
- Urgent percutaneous coronary intervention in acute coronary syndromes.
- Drainage of pericardial fluid in cardiac tamponade.
- Management of acute cardiac failure.
- Transfer to cardiothoracic theatre for operative management of mechanical problems.

A full BSE minimum dataset should be the aim of all transthoracic studies in this setting. However, given the need for urgent management triggered by some echocardiographic findings, completion of a full study should not delay patient management. Fig. 11.2 outlines a practical guide to echocardiology in the acutely unwell patient.

It is good practice to repeat the echo study following patient stabilization to ensure a full dataset is achieved whenever possible and to record echocardiographic correlation with signs of improvement in the patient's clinical state.

Tips for success

- Optimize *patient comfort and safety* prior to attempting a study: for example, ensure they have adequate oxygen to maintain saturations and they are not in pain.
- Optimize *patient position* prior to commencing the study wherever possible: for example, left lateral position can be maintained with pillows, ask for help in turning the patient into a suitable position to optimize views, ask for assistance in maintaining the left arm in a suitable position.
- *Be prepared*: time available to perform a study may be limited. Think about what you need to look for and exclude in a systematic fashion using the protocol given in Fig. 11.2.
- *Minimize time wasted*: prepare the machine before optimizing patient position.
- Utilize all available *acoustic windows* to achieve answers to clinical questions: diagnostic acoustic windows can be achieved in 90–95% of acute cases.

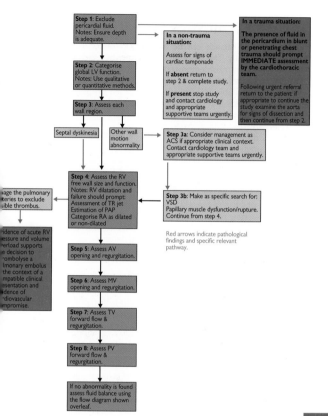

Step 1: Exclude pericardial fluid. Notes: Ensure depth is adequate.

In a non-trauma situation:

Assess for signs of cardiac tamponade

If **absent** return to step 2 & complete study.

If **present** stop study and contact cardiology and appropriate supportive teams urgently.

In a trauma situation:

The presence of fluid in the pericardium in blunt or penetrating chest trauma should prompt IMMEDIATE assessment by the cardiothoracic team.

Following urgent referral return to the patient; if appropriate to continue the study examine the aorta for signs of dissection and then continue from step 2.

Step 2: Categorise global LV function. Notes: Use qualitative or quantitative methods.

Step 3: Assess each wall region.

Septal dyskinesia

Other wall motion abnormality

Step 3a: Consider management as ACS if appropriate clinical context. Contact cardiology team and appropriate supportive teams urgently.

Manage the pulmonary arteries to exclude possible thrombus.

Step 4: Assess the RV free wall size and function. Notes: RV dilatation and failure should prompt: Assessment of TR jet Estimation of PAP Categorise RA as dilated or non-dilated

Step 3b: Make as specific search for: VSD Papillary muscle dysfunction/rupture. Continue from step 4.

Red arrows indicate pathological findings and specific relevant pathway.

Evidence of acute RV pressure and volume overload supports the decision to thrombolyse a pulmonary embolus in the context of a compatible clinical presentation and evidence of cardiovascular compromise.

Step 5: Assess AV opening and regurgitation.

Step 6: Assess MV opening and regurgitation.

Step 7: Assess TV forward flow & regurgitation.

Step 8: Assess PV forward flow & regurgitation.

If no abnormality is found assess fluid balance using the flow diagram shown overleaf.

Fig. 11.2 Transthoracic echocardiogarphy thought process in the acutely unwell patient.

Critically ill: volume status

Dynamic fluid balance can be effectively assessed using transthoracic echocardiography. The more profound the hypovolaemia or hypervolaemia the easier it is to demonstrate with echocardiography and the more parameters assessed the more accurate the evaluation.

- Fig. 11.3 and Table 11.2 provide details of the key parameters and imaging process that can help differentiate between hypovolaemia, normal volume status and volume overload. The key parameters to assess are:
  - IVC diameter and response, and right atrial size.
  - Parameters of left and right ventricular size.
- Change in measurements is of particular value. Therefore compare with previous images whenever possible and repeat assessments after therapy (diuresis or fluid) to determine whether fluid status is changing.
- Beware of:
  - Pre-existing regional wall motion abnormalities and chronic chamber dilatation: these will alter the measurements and reduce their value for assessment of volume status.
  - Body size: dimensions should be adjusted for body surface area (BSA) where possible:

$$BSA \ (m^2) = \sqrt{([Height(cm) \times Weight(kg)]/3600)}$$

Assessment of the inferior vena cava and right atrium

In spontaneously breathing patients the degree of collapse with inspiration correlates well with right atrial pressure. However, right atrial pressure itself only becomes an accurate assessment of volume status when significantly high or low (Table 11.1).

Measuring the IVC
- Use the subcostal view and get the vessel in its long axis (though a cross-section can be used).
- Measurement of IVC size should be taken 1–2cm below the entrance to the right atrium if possible, just above or below the hepatic vein.
- Accurate measurement in 2D requires the vessel to be followed throughout the respiratory cycle, keeping the junction of IVC and hepatic vein in view. If using 2D then you may need to capture 5 or more beats depending on the respiratory rate.
- M-mode gives better resolution and allows easy visualization of several cycles but keeping the vessel in view can be more difficult.

Measuring the right atrium
- Area measures are acquired from apical 4-chamber views.
- Beware of long-standing right atrial dilatation that will make correlations between size and right atrial pressure inaccurate.

Volume Status

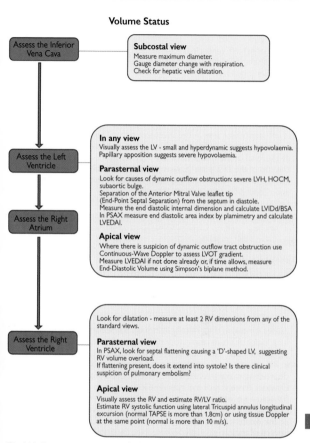

Fig. 11.3 Emergency assessment of inferior vena cava, left ventricle, right atrium, and right ventricle to guide volume status.

Table 11.1 Assessment of right atrial pressure

RAP (mmHg)	0–5	5–10	10–15	15–20	>20
IVC size (cm)	<1.5	1.5–2.5	1.5–2.5	>2.5	>2.5
Respiratory variation	Collapses	>50% collapse	<50%	<50%	No change

Assessment of the left ventricle

A very under-filled (small, cavity obliteration in systole) or severely dilated (large) left ventricle is easy to spot, but for more subtle states the measurement of dimensions and incorporation with other measures is imperative (Fig. 11.3).

A significant amount of information can be derived from measurements of left ventricular cavity size. The key measures that reflect cavity size are:
- Left ventricular internal diameter in diastole (LVIDd) (see 📖 p.196).
- Left ventricular end-diastolic area index (LVDAI) (See Table 11.)—this is left ventricular area in the short axis normalized for BSA.
- End-point septal separation—this is measured from the M-mode trace at the level of the mitral valve and represents the distance between the top of the first peak (E wave) of the mitral valve opening to the interventricular septum. It increases with both ventricular dilatation and reduced function (normal ≤6mm).
- Left ventricular end-systolic diameter (see 📖 p.196).

Hypovolaemia can convert lesser degrees of left ventricular hypertrophy into effective outflow obstruction because of the reduction in size of the end systolic left ventricular cavity.

Assessment of the right ventricle

Right ventricular dimensions can be measured in several different views so it is usually possible to get at least one accurate measurement. Standard measures should ideally be used (Table 4.6) or simplified 'rules of thumb' can be found in Table 11.3.
- Acute dilatation implies pressure or volume overload. The common causes for this in the critically ill include pulmonary embolus and acute lung injury or acute respiratory distress syndrome; less common are right ventricular infarction or acute tricuspid valve disease.
- In RV dilatation the right ventricular output is unlikely to be preload dependent, making detailed fluid balance decisions difficult.
- Diastolic flattening of the interventricular septum occurs with acute RV volume overload.
- Diastolic and systolic flattening suggests more severe volume overload or the existence of RV pressure overload. (see 📖 p.276).
- Severe dilatation is usually accompanied by systolic dysfunction and at least moderate TR.
- Beware of long-standing RV dilatation that makes inferences concerning size difficult in the acute setting.

Table 11.2 Parameters to help identify fluid status

	Suggests hypovolaemia	Normal range	Suggests volume overload
IVC diameter and response	<1cm and collapsing	1–2.5cm, collapsing 25–75%	>2.5cm, no response to respiration
LVIDd/BSA (cm/m²)	<2.4 women <2.2 men	2.4–3.2 2.2–3.1	>3.2 >3.1
LVEDAI (short axis)	<5.5	5.5–10	>10
End point septal separation	<0.5m	>0.5cm	–
LVESD	Papillary apposition	2.0–4.0cm	–
RV internal dimensions	–	See below	RVIDd >LVIDd
Interventricular septum	–	No flattening	Diastolic flattening
Right atrium	–	<20cm²	>30cm²

Table 11.3 Right ventricular dimensions

	Normal range (cm)
PLAX	AP dimension: 1.8–3.0
PSAX	RVOT: 2.0–3.2
A4C	TV annulus: 1.6–3.1 Mid RVIDd: 2.4–3.7 RV length (diastole): 6.9–8.9

Critically ill: fluid responsiveness

Any method of measuring change in stroke volume or cardiac output can be used to assess whether a patient responds to a given volume of fluid. Being able to *predict* whether a patient is likely to respond to that fluid ('fluid responsive') is even more useful as it can avoid the potential detrimental effect of excessive fluid administration.

• The term 'fluid responsive' implies that stroke volume will increase by 10–15% when a fluid load is delivered (usually 500mL, or 70–80mL/kg, of crystalloid or colloid given rapidly).
• Dynamic indicators of fluid responsiveness (such as parameters that change with respiration or patient position) are significantly more accurate than static (such as end-diastolic volumes).
• Mechanical ventilation allows more reliable assessment of the likelihood of fluid responsiveness.

IVC

Assessment of fluid responsiveness using the IVC is only reliable during mechanical ventilation. In this situation if the IVC collapses by >20% then the patient should respond to fluids (Fig. 11.4). In spontaneous ventilation complete collapse during inspiration is consistent with fluid responsiveness but may be confounded by respiratory effort and state of the right heart.

Left ventricle

A simple way to assess fluid responsiveness is to assess for variation in flow across the aortic valve or LVOT with different manoeuvres:

• Variation with respiration: variation with respiration in the vti across any valve or outflow tract can be used. However, the best validated method is flow variation across the aortic valve or LVOT. A change in left heart flow of >10% suggests the patient is likely to be 'fluid responsive'.
• Passive leg raising: Change in the vti (and therefore stroke volume) after passive leg raising is another method of fluid responsiveness assessment. This works because raising the legs effectively redistributes blood from the legs to the thorax which mimics a fluid challenge. To do a 'passive leg raise' raise both of the patient's legs to 45° for 1–2min. A change in SV of ~20% suggests fluid responsiveness.

Dysrhythmias reduce the utility of these measurements, but if present, then at least 3 or more representative waveforms should be recorded and the results then averaged.

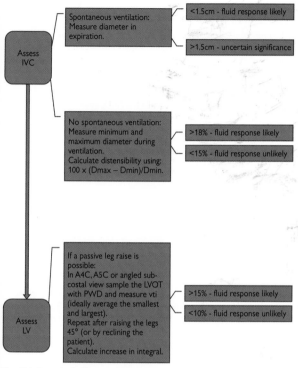

Fig. 11.4 Assessing fluid responsiveness.

Critically ill: advanced haemodynamics

A number of measurements may be of use in the critically ill both for diagnosis and to guide fluid, inotrope or vasopressor therapy (Fig. 11.5).

Serial focused assessments can eliminate the need for invasive monitoring in some instances.

Stroke volume (SV) and cardiac output (CO)

Stroke volume can be measured using PW Doppler of the LVOT (or the RVOT) combined with measurement of the outflow tract diameter (📖 p.230). Alternatively, it can be determined measuring change in area of the ventricle. CO is then derived from multiplying SV by heart rate. When assessing these parameters with echo beware:

- An accurate measurement of the outflow tract diameter is required as any error will be squared in the calculation.
- A clear Doppler trace, properly aligned through the aortic valve and LVOT is required, as a suboptimal trace may underestimate true velocities.
- Significant MR or TR will lead to inaccuracies in measurement of stroke volume based on PW Doppler in the outflow tract as it will not take account of the volume of blood that regurgitates into the atria.

Systemic vascular resistance (SVR)

SVR measurements can be used in diagnosis of underlying causes for haemodynamic problems, e.g. sepsis will lower systemic vascular resistance. Changes in systemic vascular resistance can be used as a guide to effectiveness of vasopressor therapy or changes in clinical status.

- To calculate SVR measure cardiac output, the mean arterial pressure, and the right atrial pressure. Then use the equation

$$SVR = 80 \times (MAP - RAP)/CO$$

(normal range is 770–1500 dynes/s/cm^{-5}).

Left atrial pressures (LAP)

Approximate LAP is most accurately confirmed by Doppler assessment of the MV inflow and annular tissue velocity, or by pulmonary vein flow pattern. The measure closely reflects LVEDP (see 📖 p.644). The two measures are therefore often discussed interchangeably but are presented in this chapter under both 'titles'. E/E' (septal) >15 suggests severely elevated LAP. A predominant and increased D wave in the pulmonary vein flow also suggests elevated pressures (a pre-dominant D wave is also seen in patients with severe mitral regurgitation although this is also, in part, due to a reduction in size of the S wave).

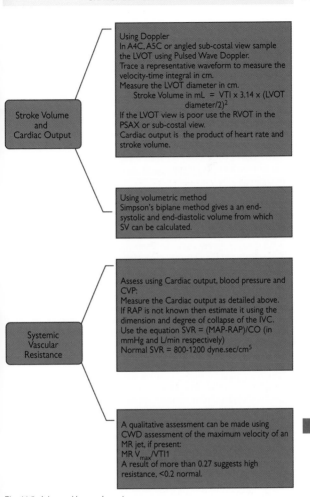

Stroke Volume and Cardiac Output

Using Doppler
In A4C, A5C or angled sub-costal view sample the LVOT using Pulsed Wave Doppler.
Trace a representative waveform to measure the velocity-time integral in cm.
Measure the LVOT diameter in cm.
   Stroke Volume in mL = VTI x 3.14 x (LVOT diameter/2)²
If the LVOT view is poor use the RVOT in the PSAX or sub-costal view.
Cardiac output is the product of heart rate and stroke volume.

Using volumetric method
Simpson's biplane method gives a an end-systolic and end-diastolic volume from which SV can be calculated.

Systemic Vascular Resistance

Assess using Cardiac output, blood pressure and CVP:
Measure the Cardiac output as detailed above.
If RAP is not known then estimate it using the dimension and degree of collapse of the IVC.
Use the equation SVR = (MAP-RAP)/CO (in mmHg and L/min respectively)
Normal SVR = 800-1200 dyne.sec/cm⁵

A qualitative assessment can be made using CWD assessment of the maximum velocity of an MR jet, if present:
MR V_max/VTI1
A result of more than 0.27 suggests high resistance, <0.2 normal.

Fig. 11.5 Advanced haemodynamics.

Estimated LV end-diastolic pressure (LVEDP)

LVEDP is useful in both the differentiation of pulmonary oedema from acute lung injury and estimating adequacy of preload. In pulmonary oedema LVEDP will increase whereas in acute lung injury it will decrease or not change. In estimation of preload, LVEDP will decrease as preload reduces. In the acute setting measures based on aortic or mitral regurgitation have been used. In the non-acute setting measures based on tissue Doppler imaging and pulmonary vein flow are routinely used to evaluate LVEDP to aid diagnosis of diastolic dysfunction and HFNEF (see Chapter 3). Estimated LV end-diastolic pressure also closely reflects left atrial pressure (see 📖 p.642).

- To measure LVEDP based on valvular regurgitation obtain a Doppler trace of the aortic regurgitation and measure the velocity at the end of the regurgitation trace. Get a measure of diastolic blood pressure at the same time as your measurement and then use the equation:

$$LVEDP = DBP - \text{end aortic regurgitation gradient}$$

- If the patient does not have aortic regurgitation but has some mitral regurgitation this can also be used to estimate LVEDP based on the initial slope of the regurgitation Doppler profile (see 📖 p.232).
- To measure LVEDP with tissue Doppler imaging, obtain a TDI trace based on movement of the mitral annulus in the 4-chamber view and get a Doppler spectral trace of mitral valve inflow. E/E' (septal) <8 suggests a normal LVEDP. E/E'>15 suggests LVEDP is elevated.

Corrected aortic flow time (FTc) and assessment of preload

Corrected aortic flow time can be used to assess preload. An increment caused by volume loading is a useful marker of fluid responsiveness (see 📖 p.642). It is however also affected by changes in inotropy and afterload, and also by the existence of bundle branch block. Normal FTc is 330–360ms. To measure corrected aortic flow time:

- Obtain an apical 5-chamber view (or suprasternal view) and align CW Doppler across the aortic valve and LVOT.
- On the Doppler tracing measure the duration (in ms) of forward flow across the aortic valve.
- Then correct this value for heart rate using the equation:

$$FTc = FT/\text{Square root of R–R interval } or$$

$$\text{(simplified) } FTc = FT + [1.29 \times (HR - 60)]$$

Pulmonary arterial occlusion pressure (PAOP)

PAOP is useful in the assessment of acute lung injury, respira-tory distress syndrome, and pulmonary oedema. PAOP can be assessed using a visual analysis of the interatrial septum, or by Doppler echocardiography. In any appropriate view:

- Watch the movement of the interatrial septum relative to the right atrium. If:
  - Septum persistently bows towards the right atrium PAOP = ~18mmHg.
  - Only bows in mid-systole but fully PAOP = ~13mmHg.
  - Only bows in mid-systole and only partially PAOP = ~10mmHg.

- Doppler indices suggesting PAOP <18mmHg are: E/A<1.4; E deceleration time >100ms; pulmonary vein S/D >0.65; pulmonary vein Doppler systolic fraction >44%; E/E'(lateral) <8. Also, E/Vp <1.7 (where V = propagation velocity, measured by calculating the velocity of the first aliasing time of the mitral inflow E wave using colour M-mode) predicts PAOP <18mmHg.

Critically ill: weaning from a ventilator

Difficulty in weaning a patient who has been critically ill from ventilatory support may occur whenever there is a mismatch between metabolic supply to the respiratory muscles and demand on those muscles.

The three most common factors affecting this balance are:
- Muscular weakness.
- Poor respiratory drive.
- Inadequate cardiac reserve.

The algorithm in Fig. 11.6 describes the thought processes and actions through which transthoracic echocardiography can assist in the management of the difficult to wean patient.

Tips for success

- *Image quality* should be maximized by taking time to optimize patient positioning.
- If previous echo images are available from the acute stages of the patient's illness it is important to comment on the *comparative* behaviour of the left ventricle in particular. The concept of the 'acute ventricle' is very relevant here. Systolic and diastolic dysfunction in acute illness from a range of causes including sepsis and polytrauma may take a variable time to resolve: optimization of the ventricle in the recovery phase of illness with interval monitoring thereafter is therefore optimal.
- Assessment of *diastolic dysfunction* should be based upon transmitral velocity assessment, tissue Doppler imaging of the mitral annulus, and PW Doppler assessment of the pulmonary venous inflow. Valsalva manoeuvre in this patient group will be either impossible or inadequate.
- This patient group is prone to the development of *pulmonary emboli*: clinician-echocardiographers should make a thorough assessment of pulmonary artery pressure and have a low threshold for further investigation of this potentially reversible cause of failure to wean.
- The pathway shown should be undertaken in conjunction with a full assessment of *fluid balance* as shown in the flow diagram on 📖 p.639. This assessment should be made alongside clinical enquiry into fluid balance over the total length of the patient's illness: acute assessment of echocardiographic indicators of fluid balance may not reflect the need for fluid off-loading to facilitate weaning.

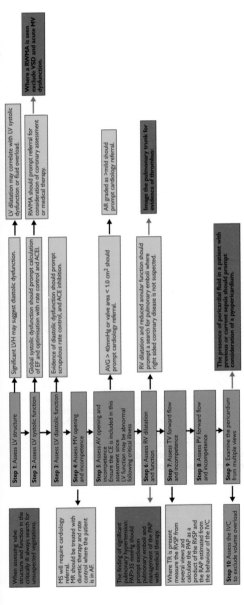

Step 1: Assess LV structure

When assessing valve structure and function in the critically ill always search for unsuspected vegetations.

Significant LVH may suggest diastolic dysfunction.

LV dilatation may correlate with LV systolic dysfunction or fluid overload.

Step 2: Assess LV systolic function

Global systolic dysfunction should prompt calculation of EF and optimisation with rate control and ACEI.

RWMA should prompt referral for consideration of coronary assessment or medical therapy.

Where a RWMA is seen exclude VSD and acute MV dysfunction.

Step 3: Assess LV diastolic function

Evidence of diastolic dysfunction should prompt scrupulous rate control, and ACE inhibition.

Step 4: Assess MV opening and incompetence

MS will require cardiology referral.
MR should be treated with diuretic therapy and rate control where the patient is in AF.

Step 5: Assess AV opening and incompetence
Ensure the CE is included in this assessment since LV function may be abnormal following critical illness.

AVG > 40mmHg or valve area < 1.0 cm² should prompt cardiology referral.

AR graded as >mild should prompt cardiology referral.

Step 6: Assess RV dilatation and function

The finding of significant pulmonary hypertension: PAP>35 mmHg should prompt exclusion of pulmonary embolism and management of the PAP with medical therapy.

RV dilatation and reduced annular function should prompt a search for pulmonary emboli where right sided coronary disease is not suspected.

Image the pulmonary trunk for evidence of thrombus:

Step 7: Assess TV forward flow and incompetence

Where TR is present measure the RVSP from several views and calculate the PAP as a product of the RVSP and the RAP estimated from the behaviour of the IVC

Step 8: Assess PV forward flow and incompetence

Step 9: Examine the pericardium from multiple views

The presence of pericardial fluid in a patient with previous or current sepsis should prompt consideration of a pyopericardium.

Step 10: Assess the IVC to exclude volume overload

Fig. 11.6 Thought processes and actions through which transthoracic echocardiography can assist in the management of the difficult to wean patient.

Chapter 12

Reporting and normal ranges

Reporting

A standard approach to reporting ensures complete studies, and improves comprehension for other readers during interpretation or follow-up. Here we describe a suggested structure for a report and anatomical structures are listed with examples of appropriate descriptions (📖 'Section 2', p.650). The calculations (📖 'Section 3', p.650) will have been collected as part of the minimal dataset (described in Chapter 2) and can be interpreted based on tables of expected values for different anatomy and pathology (these tables have been replicated in this chapter).

Section 1. Demographic and other information

- Patient's name, date of birth, gender, hospital number.
- Date on which study was performed.
- Location (inpatient, outpatient) and urgency.
- Indications for test.
- Referring physician.
- Sonographer/physician performing and interpreting the study.
- Height, weight, blood pressure (if available).
- Ultrasound machine and data storage.
- Image quality and any suboptimal views (if applicable).

Section 2. Description of observations and diagnostic statements

A brief description should be given of each anatomical feature. The description should summarize findings from all views (comments should be able to be supported from measurements later in report). It is unpractical to include all statements if everything is normal and usually it is sufficient just to call them normal in structure and function. However, there should be a protocol or check list to ensure all comments are based on facts (visual and quantitative assessment). For each anatomical detail, when appropriate, there should also be a diagnostic statement, such as, appearances suggestive of rheumatic mitral disease.

Section 3. M-mode, 2D, and Doppler measurements

This section is based on a minimal dataset that should be included in every report (📖 p.85), supplemented with additional measures as required to describe any pathology. Ideally the report should include normal values for particular measurements.

Section 4. Conclusions

This section is often read first by the referring physicians, who may not be cardiologists. It has to be easily understood and should summarize the whole study. Identify any abnormality, its cause (if identifiable) and any secondary effect. This may involve repeating some of the information from Sections 2 and 3. The questions of the referring physicians should be answered. If not possible, then the reasons should be included and alternative methods suggested (e.g. transoesophageal echocardiography or contrast echocardiography). Medical advice should be separated from the report of the study.

Sample report: normal

John Smith   DoB: 10:07:1935 Inpatient: Ward A
Height: 182 cm Weight: 74kg   BP: 120/70
Indication:?LV function
Referring Physician: Dr Smith Sonographer: John Brown
Interpreting Physician: Dr Jones
Machine: Ultrasound Machine A Images saved: Server
Image Quality: Good

Descriptions

1. Left ventricle: normal cavity size, normal wall thickness, normal systolic and diastolic funtion
2. Right ventricle: normal size, normal wall thickness, normal systolic function
3. Ventricular septum: normal
4. Left atrium: normal size
5. Right atrium: normal size
6. Atrial septum: normal
7. Inferior vena cava: normal diameter, normal response during respiration
8. Aortic valve: normal structure and function
9. Mitral valve: normal structure and function
10. Tricuspid valve: normal structure and function
11. Pulmonary valve: normal structure and function
12. Pulmonary artery: normal diameter
13. Pericardium: no thickening, no effusion
14. Aorta: normal diameter of root and ascending aorta

Measurements

1. Left ventricle	LVED-5.0cm, LVES-3.5cm, FS – 30% IVS–1.0cm, LVPW-0.9cm normal diastolic LV function, E' (Medial) 6.9 cm/s, E' (lateral) 10.9, E/E' 12.0
2. Right ventricle	RVED – 2.0cm
3. Left atrium	LA diameter – 3.2cm
4. Right atrium	—
5. Inferior vena cava	—
6. Aortic valve	peak velocity – 1.2m/s
7. Mitral valve	E: A ratio – 1.1
8. Tricuspid valve	TR maximum velocity – 1m/s
9. Pulmonary valve	PW peak velocity – 1m/s
10. Pulmonary artery	Root diameter – 2.6cm
11. Pericardium	—
12. Aorta	Root diameter – 2.7cm

Conclusions

Normal echocardiogram. Normal left ventricle size. Normal left ventricle systolic and diastolic function.
Dr. Jones

Left ventricle

Descriptive terms

Cavity size
- Normal, dilated (mild/moderate/severe), decreased.

Wall thickness
- Normal, hypertrophy (mild/moderate/severe).
- Pattern (concentric, eccentric, asymmetric + location)
- Decreased.

LV Mass
- Normal, mild, moderate, severe increase.

Shape
- Normal, aneurysm, pseudoaneurysm (+ location).

Global systolic function
- Normal, borderline, low normal.
- Decreased (mild, mild to moderate, moderate, moderate to severe, severe).
- Increased (hyperdynamic).
- Estimated ejection fraction.

Regional systolic function
- Normal, hypokinetic, akinetic, dyskinetic, scar.
- Asynchronous, not seen. Describe for each segment of the walls:
  - Anterior (basal, mid, apical).
  - Anteroseptal (basal, mid).
  - Inferoseptal (basal, mid, apical).
  - Inferior wall (basal, mid, apical).
  - Posterior (inferolateral) wall (basal, mid, apical).
  - Lateral wall (basal, mid, apical).

Diastolic filling
- Normal, abnormal (Impaired relaxation, pseudonormal, restrictive).
- Elevated left atrial pressure (E/E' >15, normal <18).

Left ventricle outflow tract
- No obstruction, obstruction (mild/moderate/severe).
- Septal hypertrophy, subaortic membrane.
- Associated with mitral valve systolic anterior motion.

Thrombus
- Absent, present (+ location and description).

Mass
- Absent, present (+ location and description).

Left ventricular size, mass, and function (Tables 12.1 and 12.2)

Table 12.1 Ranges for measurements of LV size and mass

	Women			
	Normal	Mild	Moderate	Severe
LV dimension				
LVED diameter, cm	3.9–5.3	5.4–5.7	5.8–6.1	>6.1
LVED diameter/BSA, cm/m²	2.4–3.2	3.3–3.4	3.5–3.7	>3.7
LV volume				
LVED vol, mL	56–104	105–117	118–130	>130
LVED vol/BSA, mL/m²	**35–75**	**76–86**	**87–96**	**>96**
LVES vol, mL	19–49	50–59	60–69	>69
LVES vol/BSA, mL/m²	**12–30**	**31–36**	**37–42**	**>42**
Linear method: fractional shortening				
Endocardial, %	27–45	22–26	17–21	<17
2D method				
Ejection fraction, %	**>54**	**45–54**	**30–44**	**<30**
Linear method: wall thickness				
Relative wall thickness, cm	0.22–0.42	0.43–0.47	0.48–0.52	>0.52
Septal thickness, cm	**0.6–0.9**	**1.0–1.2**	**1.3–1.5**	**>1.5**
Posterior wall thickness, cm	**0.6–0.9**	**1.0–1.2**	**1.3–1.5**	**>1.5**
2D method				
LV mass, g	66–150	151–171	172–182	>182
LV mass/BSA, g/m²	**44–88**	**89–100**	**101–112**	**>112**

BSA, body surface area; d, diastolic; s, systolic. Bold rows identify best validated measures.

3D LV volume and ejection fraction
Upper normal values (mean + 2 standard deviations [SD])
LV end-diastolic volume index (LVEDVI)   82mL/m²
LV end-systolic volume index (LVESVI)   38mL/m²
Lower limit (mean − 2 SD)
LVEF   49%

EF, ejection fraction; LVEDVI, LV end-diastolic volume index; LVESVI, LV end-systolic volume index.

Table 12.2 Ranges for measurements of LV size and mass

	Men			
	Normal	Mild	Moderate	Severe
LV dimension				
LVED diameter, cm	4.2–5.9	6.0–6.3	6.4–6.8	>6.8
LVED diameter/BSA, cm/m²	2.2–3.1	3.2–3.4	3.5–3.6	>3.6
LV volume				
LVED vol, mL	67–155	156–178	179–201	>201
LVED vol/BSA, mL/m²	**35–75**	**76–86**	**87–96**	**>96**
LVES vol, mL	22–58	59–70	71–82	>82
LVES vol/BSA, mL/m²	**12–30**	**31–36**	**37–42**	**>42**
Linear method: fractional shortening				
Endocardial, %	25–43	20–24	15–19	<15
2D method				
Ejection fraction, %	**>54**	**45–54**	**30–44**	**<30**
Linear method: wall thickness				
Relative wall thickness, cm	0.24–0.42	0.43–0.46	0.47–0.51	>0.51
Septal thickness, cm	**0.6–1.0**	**1.1–1.3**	**1.4–1.6**	**>1.6**
Posterior wall thickness, cm	**0.6–1.0**	**1.1–1.3**	**1.4–1.6**	**>1.6**
2D method				
LV mass, g	96–200	201–227	228–254	>254
LV mass/BSA, g/m²	**50–102**	**103–116**	**117–130**	**>130**

BSA, body surface area; d, diastolic; s, systolic. Bold rows identify best validated measures.

3D LV volume and ejection fraction

Upper normal values (mean + 2 standard deviations [SD])

LV end-diastolic volume index (LVEDVI)	82mL/m²
LV end-systolic volume index (LVESVI)	38mL/m²

Lower limit (mean − 2 SD)

LVEF	49%

EF, ejection fraction; LVEDVI, LV end-diastolic volume index; LVESVI, LV end-systolic volume index.

Right ventricle

Descriptive terms

Cavity size
- Normal.
- Dilated (mild/moderate/severe).
- Decreased.

Wall thickness
- Normal.
- Hypertrophy.
- Decreased.

Global systolic function
- Normal.
- Decreased (mild, moderate, severe).
- Increased (hyperdynamic).

Regional systolic function
- Normal.
- Hypokinetic.
- Akinetic.
- Not seen.
- Describe for free wall/apex/outflow tract.

Thrombus
- Absent, present (+ location and description).

Mass
- Absent, present (+ location and description).

Right ventricular size and function

(Tables 12.3 and 12.4)

Table 12.3 2D parameters to assess right ventricle size and function (ASE guidelines)

Measure	Abnormal
Chamber dimensions	
RV basal diameter (RVD1)	>4.2cm
RV subcostal wall thickness	>0.5cm
RVOT PSAX distal diameter (RVOT2)	>2.7cm
RVOT PSAX proximal diameter (RVOT1)	>3.3cm
Systolic function	
TAPSE	<1.6cm
Tissue Doppler peak velocity at the annulus	<10cm/s
Pulsed Doppler myocardial performance index	>0.40
Tissue Doppler myocardial performance index	>0.55
Fractional area change (%)	>35%

Table 12.4 3D RV volumes and ejection fraction

	LRV (95% CI)	Mean (95% CI)	URV (95% CI)
3D RV EF (%)	44 (39–49)	57 (53–61)	69 (65–74)
3D RV EDV indexed (mL/m^2)	40 (28–52)	65 (54–76)	89 (77–101)
3D RV ESV indexed (mL/m^2)	12 (1–23)	28 (18–38)	45 (34–56)

CI, confidence interval; EF, ejection fraction; EDV, endiastolic volume; ESV, endsystolic volume; LRV, lower reference value; URV, upper reference value.

Ventricular septum

Descriptive terms

Abnormal septal motion

- Abnormal (paradoxical) motion consistent with right ventricle volume overload.
- Abnormal (paradoxical) motion consistent with postoperative status.
- Abnormal (paradoxical) motion consistent with left bundle branch block.
- Abnormal (paradoxical) motion consistent with right ventricle pacemaker.
- Abnormal (paradoxical) motion due to pre-excitation.
- Flattened in diastole ('D'-shaped left ventricle) consistent with right ventricle volume overload.
- Flattened in systole consistent with right ventricle pressure overload.
- Flattened in systole and diastole consistent with right ventricle pressure and volume overload.
- Septal 'bounce' consistent with constrictive physiology.
- Excessive respiratory change consistent with tamponade, constriction, ventilation-related.
- Other (specify).

Ventricular septal defect

- Absent, present.
- Location (perimembranous, subpulmonary/doubly committed, inlet, muscular, multiple.
- Size (small/moderate/large).
- Shunt (left-to-right/right-to-left/bidirectional).

Atrial septum

Descriptive terms

Atrial septal defect
- Absent, present.
- Location (primum, secundum, sinus venosus).
- Size (dimensions in 2 planes and area from 3D study).
- Shunt (left-to-right, right-to-left, bidirectional).
- Qp/Qs.

Patent foramen ovale
- Absent, present.

Contrast study
- Normal, shunt present (small <5 bubbles/moderate 5–20 bubbles/large >20 bubbles).

Left atrium

Descriptive terms
Cavity size
- Normal, dilated (mild/moderate/severe), decreased.

Thrombus
- Absent, present (+ location and description).

Mass
- Absent, present (+ location and description).

Spontaneous contrast
- Absent, present.

Other
- Cor triatriatum, hypoplastic left atrium, consistent with cardiac transplantation.

Right atrium

Descriptive terms
Cavity size
- Normal, dilated (mild/moderate/severe), decreased.

Thrombus
- Absent, present (+ location and description).

Mass
- Absent, present (+ location and description).

Catheter/pacing wire
- Absent, present.

Right atrial pressure
- Septum bowed to left consistent with elevated right atrial pressure.
- Dilated coronary sinus consistent with elevated right atrial pressure or left superior vena cava.
- Persistent left superior vena cava.
- Normal inferior vena cava size/respiratory variation—right atrial pressure normal.
- Normal inferior vena cava size/reduced variation—right atrial pressure mildly increased (10mmHg).
- Dilated inferior vena cava size/reduced variation—right atrial pressure moderately increased (15mmHg).
- Dilated inferior vena cava/absent variation/dilated hepatic veins—right atrial pressure severely increased (20mmHg).

Other
- Prominent Eustachian valve, Chiari network.

Atrial size (Table 12.5)

Table 12.5 Parameters to assess left and right atria

	Women			
	Normal	**Mild**	**Moderate**	**Severe**
Atrial dimension				
LA diameter, cm	2.7–3.8	3.9–4.2	4.3–4.6	>4.6
LA diameter, BSA, cm/m²	1.5–2.3	2.4–2.6	2.7–2.9	>2.9
RA minor axis, cm	2.9–4.5	4.6–4.9	5.0–5.4	>5.4
RA minor axis/BSA, cm/m²	1.7–2.5	2.6–2.8	2.9–3.1	>3.1
Atrial area				
LA area, cm²	<20	20–30	31–40	>40
Atrial volume				
LA vol, mL	22–52	53–62	63–72	>72
***LA vol/BSA, mL/m²**	**<29**	**29–33**	**34–39**	**>39**
	Men			
	Normal	**Mild**	**Moderate**	**Severe**
Atrial dimension				
LA diameter, cm	3.0–4.8	4.1–4.6	4.7–5.2	>5.2
LA diameter, BSA, cm/m²	1.5–2.3	2.4–2.6	2.7–2.9	>2.9
RA minor axis, cm	2.9–4.5	4.6–4.9	5.0–5.4	>5.4
RA minor axis/BSA, cm/m²	1.7–2.5	2.6–2.8	2.9–3.1	>3.1
Atrial area				
LA area, cm²	<20	20–30	31–40	>40
Atrial volume				
LA vol, mL	18–58	59–68	69–78	>78
***LA vol/BSA, mL/m²**	**<29**	**29–33**	**34–39**	**>39**

BSA, Body surface area. *Bold rows identify best validated measures.

Aortic valve

Descriptive terms

Structure
- Normal, degenerative, rheumatic.
- Bicuspid, fused (RCC-LCC/RCC-NCC/NCC-LCC).
- Unicuspid, quadricuspid.

Leaflet thickness
- Focal thickening (RCC/LCC/NCC), diffuse thickening.
- Severity (mild/moderate/severe).

Calcification
- Present (mild/moderate/severe).
- Focal calcification (RCC/LCC/NCC).
- Diffuse calcification.

Leaflet mobility
- Normal, reduced (mild/moderate/severe), doming.

Other
- Leaflet perforation (RCC/LCC/NCC).
- Leaflet prolapse/flail (RCC/LCC/NCC).

Vegetation
- Location (RCC/LCC/NCC).
- Mobility (non-mobile/mobile), pedunculated.
- Size (small/moderate/large) + dimensions.

Abscess
- Location (RCC-annulus/LCC-annulus/NCC-annulus).
- Size (small/moderate/large) + dimensions.

Mass
- Location (RCC/LCC/NCC), description (see 📖 p.530).

Aortic stenosis (Table 12.6)

- None, present (mild/moderate/severe).
- Quantification:
  - Peak and mean transaortic velocity/gradient.
  - Aortic valve area.

Aortic regurgitation (Table 12.7)

- None, present (trace, mild, moderate, severe).

Table 12.6 Parameters to assess severity of aortic stenosis

	Mild	Moderate	Severe
Peak velocity (m/s)	2.5–2.9	3.0–4.0	>4.0
Peak gradient (mmHg)	<35	35–65	>65
Mean gradient (mmHg)	<20	20–40	>40
Valve area (cm^2)	>1.5	1.0–1.5	<1.0

Table 12.7 Parameters to determine severity of aortic regurgitation

	Specific signs of severity	
	Mild	Severe
Vena contracta	<0.3cm	>0.6cm
Jet (Nyquist 50–60cm/s)	Central, <25% of LVOT	Central, >65% of LVOT
Descending aorta	No or brief early diastolic flow reversal	
	Supportive signs of severity	
	Mild	Severe
Pressure half time	>500ms	<200ms
Descending aorta	–	Holodiastolic flow reversal
Left ventricle (only for chronic lesions)	Normal LV	Moderate or greater LV enlargement (no other cause)

Report as **moderate** if signs of regurgitation are greater than **mild** but there are no features of **severe** regurgitation.

Mitral valve

Descriptive terms

Structure
- Normal, rheumatic, myxomatous, degenerative.

Annulus
- Normal, dilated, calcified (mild/moderate/severe).

Leaflet thickness
- Normal, thickened (mild/moderate/severe).
- Leaflet tips, Leaflet body (aMVL/pMVL).

Commissures
- Antero-lateral fusion, posteromedial fusion.

Calcification
- Focal calcification (aMVL/pMVL), diffuse calcification.
- Commissural calcification (anterolateral/posteromedial).

Cleft
- Anterior leaflet, posterior leaflet.

Chordal disease
- Shortening, fusion/thickening, elongation.
- Rupture, calcification.

Papillary muscle
- Rupture, partial rupture (anterolateral/posteromedial).
- Calcification/fibrosis (anterolateral/posteromedial).

Leaflet mobility
- Normal, reduced (mild/moderate/severe).
- Doming, prolapse, bowing.
- Systolic anterior motion (mild/moderate/severe—based on outflow tract gradient).
- Chordal systolic anterior motion.

Prolapse
- Anterior, posterior leaflet (mild/mod/severe/flail).
- A1, A2, A3, P1, P2, P3 (mild/mod/severe/flail).

Vegetation
- Location (aMVL/pMVL).
- Mobility (non-mobile/mobile), pedunculated.
- Size (small/moderate/large), dimensions.

Abscess
- Location (aorto-mitral/pMVL/annulus).
- Size (small/moderate/large), dimensions.

Mass
Location (aMVL/pMVL), description (see 📖 p.530).

Mitral stenosis (Table 12.8)

- None, present (mild/moderate/severe).
- Quantitative measurements:
  - Peak and mean transmitral velocity/gradient.
  - Pressure half-time, mitral valve area.
- Suitable for commissurotomy.

Mitral regurgitation (Table 12.9)

- None, present (trace, mild, moderate, severe).
- Jet direction:
  - Anteriorly-, posteriorly-, centrally-directed.
  - Wall-impinging jet, directed down pulmonary veins.
- Diastolic mitral regurgitation (present/absent).
- Quantitative measurements:
  - MR: LA area ratio, regurgitant volume.
  - Vena contracta width, EROA.
- Pulmonary venous flow (normal, blunted systolic flow, systolic flow reversal).

Table 12.8 Parameters to determine severity of mitral stenosis

	Mild	Moderate	Severe
MV area (cm^2)	2.2–1.5	1.5–1.0	<1.0
MV pressure half-time (ms)	100–150	150–220	>220
Mean pressure gradient (mmHg)	<5	Variable	>10
TR velocity (m/s)	<2.7	Variable	>3
PA pressure (mmHg)	<30	Variable	>50

Table 12.9 Parameters to assess severity of mitral regurgitation

	Specific signs of severity	
	Mild	Severe
Jet (Nyquist 50–60cm/s)	<4cm^2 or <20% left atrium	>40% left atrium
	Small & central	Large & central or wall impinging and swirling
Vena contracta	<0.3cm	>0.7cm
PISA r (Nyquist 40cm/s)	None/minimal (<0.4cm)	Large (>1cm)
Pulmonary vein flow	–	Systolic reversal
Valve structure	–	Flail or rupture
	Supportive signs of severity	
	Mild	Severe
Pulmonary vein flow	Systolic dominant	
Mitral inflow	A-wave dominant	E-wave dominant (>1.2m/s)
CW trace	Soft & parabolic	Dense & triangular
LV and LA	Normal size LV if chronic MR	Enlarged LV & LA if no other cause

Report as **moderate** if signs of regurgitation are greater than **mild** but there are no features of **severe** regurgitation.

Tricuspid valve

Descriptive terms

Structure
- Normal, rheumatic, myxomatous (redundant).
- Ebstein.

Annulus
- Normal, dilated.
- Calcified.

Leaflet thickness
- Normal, increased.
- Leaflet tips, leaflet body (anterior/posterior/septal).

Calcification
- Focal calcification (anterior/posterior/septal).
- Diffuse calcification.

Papillary muscle
- Rupture.

Leaflet mobility
- Normal, reduced (mild/moderate/severe).
- Doming, prolapse, bowing.

Prolapse
- Anterior leaflet (mild/mod/severe/flail).
- Posterior leaflet (mild/mod/severe/flail).
- Septal leaflet (mild/mod/severe/flail).

Vegetation
- Location (anterior/posterior/septal).
- Mobility (non-mobile/mobile), pedunculated.
- Size (small/moderate/large) + dimensions.

Abscess
- Location (anterior-annulus/posterior-annulus/septal).
- Size (small/moderate/large) + dimensions.

Mass
- Location (anterior/posterior/septal).
- Description (see 🕮 p.530).

Tricuspid stenosis
- None, present.
- Quantitative measurements.
  - Peak and mean transtricuspid gradient.
  - Tricuspid valve area.

Tricuspid regurgitation
- None, present (trace, mild, moderate, severe).
- Jet direction: free wall-directed, septal-directed, centrally-directed.
- Hepatic vein flow:
  - Normal, blunted systolic flow.
  - Systolic flow reversal.

Tricuspid regurgitation (Table 12.10)

Table 12.10 Parameters to assess severity of tricuspid regurgitation

	Mild	Severe
Qualitative		
Valve structure	Normal	Abnormal
Jet (Nyquist 50–60cm/s)	<5cm^2	>10cm^2
CW trace	Soft & parabolic	Dense & triangular
Semi-quantitative		
Vena contracta	–	>0.7cm
PISA r (Nyquist 40cm/s) <0.5cm		>0.9cm
Tricuspid inflow	Normal	E wave dominant >1m/s
Hepatic vein flow	Normal	Systolic reversal
Quantitative		
EROA	Not defined	>/40mm^2
R vol	Not defined	>45mL
RV/RA/IVC	Normal size	Usually dilated

Report as **moderate** if signs of regurgitation are greater than **mild** but there are few features of **severe** regurgitation.

Right atrial pressure (Table 12.11)

Table 12.11 Assessment of right atrial pressure

RAP (mmHg)	0–5	5–10		10–15	15–20	>20
IVC size (cm)	<1.5	1.5–2.5		1.5–2.5	>2.5	>2.5
Respiratory variation	Collapses	>50% collapse		<50%	<50%	No change

Pulmonary valve

Descriptive terms

Structure
- Normal, dysplastic, bicuspid.

Mobility
- Normal, reduced.
- Doming.

Vegetation
- Location.
- Mobility (non-mobile/mobile), pedunculated.
- Size (small/moderate/large) + dimensions.

Mass
- Location, description (see 📖 p.530).

Stenosis
- None, present (mild/moderate/severe).
- Location (valvular, infundibular, valvular +infundibular supravalvular, branch).
- Left or right main pulmonary artery.
- Quantitative measurements: peak and mean transpulmonary gradient.

Regurgitation
- None, present (trace, mild, moderate, severe).

Pulmonary pressure
- Normal.
- Elevated systolic pressure (mild/moderate/severe).
- Elevated diastolic pressure (mild/moderate/severe).
- Estimated pulmonary artery.

Pulmonary artery

Descriptive terms

Appearance
- Normal, abnormal.

Dilatation
- Absent, present (mild/moderate/severe).

Thrombus
- Main/right/left pulmonary artery.

Pulmonary artery stenosis
- Main/right/left pulmonary artery (mild/moderate/severe).

Patent ductus arteriosus
- Absent, present.

Pulmonary regurgitation (Table 12.12)

Table 12.12 Parameters to assess pulmonary regurgitation

	Mild	Severe
Pulmonary valve anatomy	Normal	Abnormal
Jet size on colour flow	<10mm long	Large with wide origin
CW density and shape	Soft and slow	Dense and steep
PR index		<0.77
Jet width of RVOT		>65%
PA flow	Increased	Greatly increased compared to systemic
Right ventricle size	Normal	Dilated

If features suggest more than **mild** regurgitation but no features of **severe** grade as **moderate**.

Pulmonary stenosis (Table 12.13)

Table 12.13 Parameters to determine severity of pulmonary stenosis

	Mild	Moderate	Severe
Peak velocity (m/s)	<3	3–4	>4
Peak gradient (mmHg)	<36	36–64	>64
Valve area (cm^2)	>1.0	0.5–1.0	<0.5

Prosthetic valves

Descriptive terms

Type
- Mechanical (tilting disk/bileaflet/ball and cage/other).
- Bioprosthesis (stented xenograft/homograft/stentless.
- Autograft (Ross)/other).
- Manufacturer & size.
- Annuloplasty ring, valve repair.

Sewing ring
- Well seated, rocking, dehisced.

Occluder mechanism
- Normal, thickened leaflets (bioprosthesis).
- Normal mobility, restricted mobility, flail.

Abnormal masses
- Strand(s), micro-cavitations, pannus, thrombus.
- Vegetation (+description), abscess (+description).
- Fistula.

Stenosis
- Present, severity (as for native valve).

Regurgitation
- Physiologic, prosthetic, paraprosthetic.
- Severity (as for native valve).

Prosthetic valve velocities

Table 12.14 provides a guide to maximal expected velocities for different valve types. Refer to manufacturer guidelines for definitive measures and take into account clinical scenario. Velocities depend on left ventricle function, volume, and ionotropic status. Therefore minimal gradients are not presented. In individual cases the threshold may be exceeded with a functionally normal prosthesis—in particular if there is a hyperdynamic state.

Table 12.14 Maximum prosthetic velocities

Aortic prosthetic valves:						
Bileaflet valve (e.g. St Jude)						
Size (mm)	19	21	23	25	27	29
Vmax (m/s)	4.5	3.5	3.5	3.5	3.1	2.5
Tilting disc (e.g. Medtronic Hall, BS)						
Size (mm)	—	21	23	25	27	29
Vmax (m/s)	—	3.7	3.0	2.4	2.1	2.1
Ball and cage (e.g. Starr–Edwards)						
Vmax (m/s)	3.6					
Bioprostheses (e.g. Hancock, Carpentier Edwards)						
Size (mm)	19	21	23	25	27	29
Vmax (m/s)	3.5	3.0	3.0	2.9	2.9	2.5
Mitral prosthetic valves:						
Bileaflet valve (e.g. St Jude)						
Size (mm)	19	21	23	25	27	29
Vmax (m/s)	4.5	3.5	3.5	3.5	3.1	2.5
Tilting disc (e.g. Medtronic Hall, BS)						
Size (mm)	—	21	23	25	27	29
Vmax (m/s)	—	3.7	3.0	2.4	2.1	2.1
Ball and cage (e.g. Starr–Edwards)						
Vmax (m/s)	3.6					
Bioprostheses (e.g. Hancock, Carpentier Edwards)						
Size (mm)	19	21	23	25	27	29
Vmax (m/s)	3.5	3.0	3.0	2.9	2.9	2.5

Aorta

Descriptive terms

Appearance
- Normal, abnormal.

Dilatation
- Absent, present (mild/moderate/severe).
- Location and dimensions:
  - Dilated atrioventricular annulus.
  - Dilated aortic root/sinuses.
  - Dilated sinotubular ridge.
  - Dilated ascending aorta.
  - Dilated transverse aorta.
  - Dilated descending thoracic aorta.
  - Dilated abdominal aorta.

Aneurysm
- Absent, sinuses of Valsalva (left/right/non-coronary).
- Aortic root, ascending aorta, transverse aorta.
- Descending thoracic aorta, abdominal aorta.
- Dimensions, type (fusiform, saccular).
- Ruptured sinus of Valsalva (to right atrium, right ventricle, left atrium, left ventricle).

Atheroma/thrombus
- Absent, present.
- Location (aortic root, ascending aorta, transverse aorta, descending thoracic aorta, abdominal aorta).
- Appearance (layered/mural, protruding, ulcer).
- Severity (mild/moderate/severe).
- Mobility (immobile/mobile).
- Graft (prosthetic/homograft) + location.

Dissection
- Location, entry point, exit point(s).
- False lumen thrombus (absent/partial/present).
- Stanford type A or B.
- Intramural haematoma and location.
- Transection and location.

Coarctation
- Absent, repaired/residual, present.
- Severity (mild/moderate/severe).
- Measurements (minimum diameter, gradient).

Aortic size (Fig. 12.1)

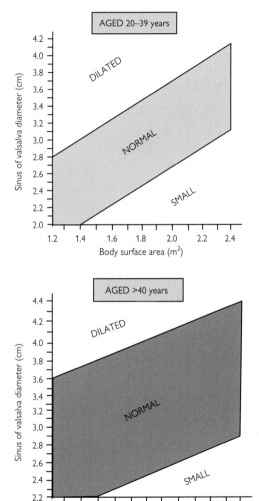

Fig. 12.1 Ranges of normal sinus of Valsalva size according to age.

Masses

Descriptive terms

Thrombus
- Absent, present.
- Size (small/moderate/large).
- Location.
- Description:
  • Shape (flat or mural/protruding/spherical/other).
  • Surface (regular/irregular).
  • Texture (layered/solid/part solid/calcified).
  • Mobility (mobile/fixed).
- Dimensions.

Tumour
- Absent, present.
- Size (small/moderate/large).
- Location.
- Description:
  • Shape (flat or mural/pedunculated/papillary/spherical/other).
  • Surface (regular/irregular/multilobular/other).
  • Texture (solid/layered/cystic/calcified/heterogeneous).
  • Mobility (mobile/fixed).
- Dimensions.
- Type (suggestive of myxoma/fibroelastoma/etc.).

Endocarditis

Descriptive terms

Vegetation
- Valvular/mural mass consistent with a vegetation.
- Location (atrial or ventricular side of valves, ventricular . . .).
- Mobility (non-mobile, mobile, pedunculated).
- Size (small, moderate, large).
- Dimensions.

Abscess
- Perivalvular or valvular cavity suggesting abscess.
- Location (annulus right coronary cusp etc.)
- Size (small, moderate, large).
- Dimensions.

Fistula
- From . . . to . . . .
- Size/haemodynamically relevant.

Severity of valvular lesion
- See native valves, Chapter 3.

Pericardial effusion
- See 📖 p.306.

Pericardium

Descriptive terms

Appearance
- Normal, abnormal.

Effusion
- Absent, present.
- Size (small/moderate/large).
- Location:
  - Circumferential.
  - Localized (near . . . left ventricle, right ventricle, left atrium, right atrium).
- Appearance/content (clear fluid, fibrinous, focal strands/masses, effusive-constrictive.

Thickening/calcification
- Absent, present.

Mass
- Absent, present.

Haemodynamic effects
- Septal bounce.
- Chamber collapse (absent/present + chamber).
- Increased respiratory variation (absent, present + location).
- Compatible with tamponade or constrictive.

Pericardial fluid (Table 12.15)

Table 12.15 Assessment of pericardial effusion based on thickness and volume

	Trace	Mild	Moderate	Severe
Thickness (cm)	<0.5	0.5–1	1–2	>2
Volume (mL)	50–100	100–250	250–500	>500

Index